中医经典译丛
Chinese-English Translation of Traditional Chinese Medicine Classics

汤液本草
Materia Medica for Decoctions
（汉英对照）

原　著　〔元〕王好古
主　译　范延妮
副主译　李　琳　张　洁
译　者　（按姓氏笔画排序）
　　　　王芳芳　李　琳　杨　凡
　　　　张　洁　张　爽　范延妮

本书为山东中医药大学"中医英译及中医文化对外传播研究"科研创新团队项目资助成果、山东中医药大学英语专业学科建设成果。

苏州大学出版社

图书在版编目(CIP)数据

汤液本草:汉英对照/(元)王好古原著;范延妮主译.—苏州:苏州大学出版社,2021.8
(中医经典译丛)
书名原文:Materia Medica for Decoctions
ISBN 978-7-5672-3323-2

Ⅰ.①汤… Ⅱ.①王… ②范… Ⅲ.①本草-中国-元代-汉、英 Ⅳ.①R281.3

中国版本图书馆 CIP 数据核字(2020)第 179520 号

书　　名:	汤液本草 TANG YE BEN CAO Materia Medica for Decoctions (汉英对照)
原　　著:	〔元〕王好古
主　　译:	范延妮
责任编辑:	汤定军
策划编辑:	汤定军
装帧设计:	刘　俊
出版发行:	苏州大学出版社(Soochow University Press)
社　　址:	苏州市十梓街1号　邮编:215006
印　　装:	广东虎彩云印刷有限公司
网　　址:	www.sudapress.com
邮　　箱:	sdcbs@suda.edu.cn
邮购热线:	0512-67480030
销售热线:	0512-67481020
开　　本:	700 mm×1 000 mm　1/16　印张:23　字数:377 千
版　　次:	2021 年 8 月第 1 版
印　　次:	2021 年 8 月第 1 次印刷
书　　号:	ISBN 978-7-5672-3323-2
定　　价:	88.00 元

凡购本社图书发现印装错误,请与本社联系调换。服务热线:0512-67481020

《汤液本草》序一

　　世皆知《素问》为医之祖，而不知轩岐之书实出于《神农本草》也。殷伊尹用本草为汤液，汉仲景广汤液为大法，此医家之正学，虽后世之明哲有作，皆不越此。予集是书，复以本草正条，各从三阴三阳十二经为例，仍以主病者为元首，臣、佐、使应次之。不必如编类者，先玉石，次草木，次虫鱼，以上中下三品为门也。如太阳经当用桂枝汤、麻黄汤，必以麻黄、桂枝为主，本方中余药后附之；如阳明经当用白虎汤，必以石膏为主，本方中余药后附之；如少阳经当用三禁汤，必以柴胡为主，本方中余药后附之。如太阴、少阴、厥阴之经，所用热药，皆仿诸此。至于《金匮》祖方，汤液外定为常制；凡可用者，皆杂附之。或以伤寒之剂改治杂病，或以权宜之料更疗常疾。以汤为散，以散为丸，变易百端。增一二味，别作他名；减一二味，另为殊法。《医垒元戎》《阴证略例》《癍论萃英》《钱氏补遗》等书，安乐之法，《汤液本草》统之，其源出于洁古老人《珍珠囊》也。其间议论，出新意于法度之中，注奇辞于理趣之外，见闻一得，久弊全更，不特药品之咸精，抑亦疾病之不误。夭横不至，寿域可期，其《汤液本草》欤。

时戊戌夏六月海藏王好古书

《汤液本草》序二

神农尝百草,立九候,以正阴阳之变化,以求性命之昏札,以为万世法,既简且要。殷之伊尹宗之,倍于神农,得立法之要,则不害为汤液;汉张仲景广之,又倍于伊尹,得立法之要,则不害为确论;金域洁古老人派之又倍于仲景,而亦得尽法之要,则不害为奇注。洁古倍于仲景,无以异仲景之倍于伊尹;仲景之倍于伊尹,无以异伊尹之倍于神农也。噫!宗之、广之、派之,虽多寡之不同,其所以立法之要,则一也。观洁古之说,则知仲景之言;观仲景之言,则知伊尹之意,皆不出于神农矣。所以先《本草》,次《汤液》,次《伤寒论》,次《保命书》,阙一不可矣。成无己《明理方例》云:自古诸方,历岁浸远,难可考凭。仲景方最为众方之祖。是仲景本伊尹之法,伊尹本神农之方。医帙之中,特为缜细,参合古法,不越毫末,实大圣之所作也。文潞公《药准》云:惟仲景为群方之祖也。晋唐宋以来,得医之名者,如王叔和、葛洪、孙思邈、范汪、胡洽、朱奉议、王朝奉、钱仲阳、成无己、陈无择辈,其议论方定增减变易,千状万态,无一有毫不出于仲景者。金域百有余载,有洁古老人张元素,遇至人传祖方不传之妙法,嗣是其子云岐子张璧,东垣先生李杲明之,皆祖长沙张仲景汤液,惜乎世莫能有知者。予受业于东垣老人,故敢以题。

丙午夏六月王好古书

《汤液本草》序三

刘禹锡云：《神农本经》以朱书，《名医别录》以墨书，传写既久，朱墨错乱，遂令后人以为非神农书，以此故也。至于《素问》本经，议者以为战国时书，加以"补亡"数篇，则显然非《太素》中语，宜其以为非轩岐书也。陈无择云：王叔和《脉诀》，即高阳生剽窃，是亦后人增益者杂之也。何以知其然？予观刘元宾注本，杂病生死歌后，比之他本即少八句，观此八句不甚滑溜，与上文书意重叠，后人安得不疑？与《本草经》朱书杂乱，《素问》之补亡混淆，何以异哉！宜乎，识者非之，继而纷纭不已也。吾不知他时谁为是正，如元宾与洁古详究而明称，其中凡有所疑而不古者，削去之；或不复注而直书本文，吾不知为意易晓不必云耶？为非圣贤之语辩之耶？二者必居一于此。又启玄子注《素问》，恐有未尽，以朱书，待明者改删增益，传录者皆以墨书，其中不无差误。如"刺热论"注五十九刺，首云王注，岂启玄子之自谓乎，此一篇又可疑也。兼与《灵枢》不同，以此经比之《素问》"八十九刺"，何者为的？以此观之，若是差别，劳而无益，学而安所适从哉！莫若以《金匮》考之，仲景所不言者，皆所不取，则正知真见定矣。卢若论血枯，举《太素》云：此得之年少时大脱血而成。又举子死腹中，秽物不消。又举犯月水入房，精与积血相射，入于任脉，留于胞中，古人谓之精积。元丰中，雄州陈邦济收一方，治积精及恶血淹留，胞冷绝娠，验者甚多，其意与《内经》相近。乌贼鱼骨本治漏下与经汁不断，茼茹去淹留恶血，古人用此，皆《本草》法。予观方注条云："古人用此，皆《本草》法"一句，何其知本哉！以是知轩岐之学，实出于神农也，又知伊尹《汤液》不出于轩岐，亦出于神农也。"皆"之一字，至甚深广也，岂独乌贼断汁之一法哉！故知张伯祖之学，皆出于《汤液》，仲景师而广之，迄今汤液不绝矣。晋唐宋以来，号名医者，皆出于此。至今大定间，洁古老人张元素及子云岐子张璧、东垣李杲明之三老者出，想千百载之下，无复有之也。何以知其然？盖当时学者虽多，莫若三老之实绝也。

时戊申仲夏晦日王好古书于家之草堂

汤液本草

MATERIA MEDICA for DECOCTIONS

翻译说明

1. 本次所译的《汤液本草》以明代王肯堂《古今医统正脉全书》吴勉学校刊本为底本,以四库本为主校本,并参考了多个通行本。

2. 为了更准确地展现和传递《汤液本草》的基本信息,本书采用中文原文、英文译文的顺序予以编排。

3. 本书中出现的中草药名称采取"四保险"的方法进行翻译,即每个本草名称均按拼音、汉字、英文和拉丁文的方式进行翻译,如:Fangfeng[防风,Divaricate Saposhnikovia Root, Radix Saposhnikoviae]。为便于编排,出现在表格中的中草药仅保留其拼音。

4. 本草名称如果是三个字及以下,其音译合并在一起;如果是四个字及以上,根据文意将其音译分开,便于阅读。

5. 古籍名称采用音译的方法翻译,括号中附以中文和英文翻译,书名中的每个字独立音译。例如,《汤液本草》译为 Tang Ye Ben Cao [《汤液本草》, Materia Medica for Decoctions]。书名为简称的,补充完整后进行翻译。例如,《珍》翻译为 Zhen [《珍珠囊》, Pouch of Pearls]。部分书名经考证仍无法确定为何种古籍的,采取拼音的方式呈现。例如,《本草》译为 Ben Cao,《经》译为 Jing。

6. 书中部分中草药名称经多方考证,至今仍无法确定为何种中药,在翻译成英文的时候,采取音译加 medicinal 的方法;翻译成拉丁文的时候,采取 materia medica 加音译的方法。

7. 本书中出现的人名为简称的,补充完整后音译。例如,"元宾"译为 Liu Yuanbin,"洁古"译为 Jie Gu(Zhang Yuansu),"仲景"译为 Zhang Zhongjing。

8. 书中出现的繁体字、异体字根据现行出版规范改为简体字、通行字。

9. 方剂名称的翻译根据现行标准,采取音译加直译方法。例如,"桂枝汤"

译为 Guizhi Decoction。

10. 书中涉及的剂量单位采用音译方法,基本形式和释义如下:

传统剂量单位	公制剂量单位	音译形式
尺	0.3333333 米	Chi
寸	0.0333333 米	Cun
丈	3.3333333 米	Zhang
升	200 毫升	Sheng
铢	1.303 克	Zhu
分	7.818 克	Fen
钱	3.125 克	Qian
两	31.272 克	Liang

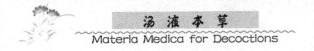

Preface One

Though *Su Wen* [《素问》, *Plain Conversation*] is commonly regarded as the origin of Chinese medicine, *Shen Nong Ben Cao* [《神农本草经》, *Agriculture God's Canon of Materia Medica*] is actually the real classic where Chinese medicinal books descended from. Yi Yin of Yin Dynasty made decoction out of materia medica and Zhang Zhongjing of Han Dynasty held decoction as the main treatment method. Their practice was regarded as medical convention followed by later famous physicians without any change. Therefore, I collected their books and, based on the channel tropism of three yin and three yang channels, classified herbal medicinals into monarch, ministerial, assistant and conducting ones according to their major functions. The herbal categories are compiled in the order like this: jade and stone, grass and tree, insect and fish, with labels of first grade, second grade and third grade for each. For example, diseases on Taiyang meridian can be treated by Guizhi decoction and Mahuang decoction, with Guizhi [桂枝, cinnamon twig, Ramulus Cinnamomi], and Mahuang [麻黄, ephedra, Herba Ephedrae] as major medicinal followed by other herbs in the formula; diseases on Yangming meridian can be treated by Baihu Decoction, with Shigao [石膏, gypsum, Gypsum Fibrosum] as major medicinal followed by other herbs in the formula; diseases on Shaoyang meridian can be treated by Sanjin Decoction, with Chaihu [柴胡, bupleurum, Radix Bupleuri] as major medicinal followed by other herbs in the formula. Herbs heat in nature for treating diseases on Taiyin, Shaoyin and Jueyin meridian are all recorded in this way. As to the classical formulas in *Jin Gui Yao Lue* [《金匮要略》, *Essential Prescriptions of the Golden Cabinet*], this book followed and recorded in detail if they were practicable. Prescriptions for cold damage were sometimes adapted for miscellaneous diseases and expedient medicinal was sometimes used for normal diseases. Decoction was sometimes used as powder and powder as pill. Formulas were renamed or re-specialized when one or two ingredients were modified. *Tang Ye Ben Cao* [《汤液本草》, *Materia Medica for Decoctions*] summarized the medicinal administration methods in *Yi Lei Yuan Rong* [《医垒元戎》, *Medicinal Administration as Military Commander*], *Yin Zheng Lue Li* [《阴证略例》, *Treatise on Yin Syndrome with Medical Cases*], *Ban Lun Cui Ying* [《癍论萃英》, *Treatise on Macula and Measles*], *Qian Shi Bu Yi* [《钱氏补遗》, *Supplement of Master Qian*], and found they all originated from *Zhen Zhu Nang* [《珍珠囊》, *Pouch of Pearls*] written by Zhang Yuansu (also named Jiegu Laoren). Discussions and annotations from this book are innovative and particular, which are capable of making full use of the medicinals and treating diseases properly. It is believed that unnatural death can be avoided and longevity can be achieved with the use of the methods in *Tang Ye Ben Cao* [《汤液本草》, *Materia Medica for Decoctions*].

Wang Haogu
June, 1238

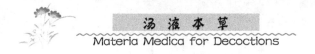

Preface Two

Shen Nong tasted all kinds of herbs and set nine positions for pulse-taking to know the changes of yin and yang and save people from unnatural deaths. For its ease and significance in practice, his methods have been respected as medical treatment ones for centuries. Yi Yin of Yin Dynasty followed and optimized Shen Nong's methods to get the gist and have faith in decoction; Zhang Zhongjing of Han Dynasty promoted and optimized Yi Yin's methods to get the gist and write treatise; Zhang Yuansu of Jin Dynasty schooled and optimized Zhang Zhongjing's methods to get the gist and annotate classics. The fact that Zhang Yuansu followed and optimized Zhang Zhongjing is just like that Zhang Zhongjing followed and optimized Yi Yin; the fact that Zhang Zhongjing followed and optimized Yi Yin is just like that Yi Yin followed and optimized Shen Nong. So it can be seen that their practice of following, promoting and schooling, though different in degree, all get the gist of treatment methods. People can know Zhang Zhongjing's words by reviewing Zhang Yuansu's theory and know Yi Yin's idea by reviewing Zhang Zhongjing's words, all deriving from Shen Nong's classic. Therefore, Ben Cao came out first, then Tang Ye Ben Cao [《汤液本草》, Materia Medica for Decoctions], then Shang Han Lun [《伤寒论》, On Cold Damage] and then Bao Ming Shu [《保命书》, Treatise on Safeguarding of Life], none of which is dispensable. Cheng Wuji said in his book Ming Li Fang Li [《明理方例》, Concise Exposition on Formulas], "It is hard to verify ancient formulas for the long time they experienced. Zhang Zhongjing's formulas can be regarded as formula ancestor." Zhang Zhongjing followed Yi Yin's treatment methods and Yi Yin followed Shen Nong's formulas. Among all the medical books, they are so meticulous and conventional, even making them like writings by great masters. Wen Lugong said in his book *Yao Zhun* [《药准》, *Criterion for Medicinal*], "Only Zhang Zhongjing can be called the ancestor of formulas." From Jin, Tang and Song dynasties, those who can be called physicians such as Wang Shuhe, Ge Hong, Sun Simiao, Fan Wang, Hu Qia, Zhu Fengyi, Wang Chaofeng, Qian Zhongyang, Cheng Wuji and Chen Wuze, all followed Zhang Zhongjing's theory of formulas, though with some modifications and variations sometimes. It has been more than 100 years since the beginning of Jin Dynasty when Zhang Yuansu met a great master who passed on priceless medical treatment methods to him. Later on, his son Zhang Bi and his student Li Gao got to know that those methods were actually decoctions by Zhang Zhongjing from Changsha. It is a pity that people seldom knew this point. Since I have ever been a student of Li Gao, I am confident to write the preface here.

Wang Haogu
June, 1246

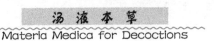

Preface Three

Liu Yuxi said: *Shen Nong Ben Jing* [《神农本经》, *Agriculture God's Canon of Materia Medica*] was written in red and *Ming Yi Bie Lu* [《名医别录》, *Miscellaneous Records of Famous Physicians*] was written in black. After long time of circulation, their copies were mixed with red and black texts and people in later generations were confused about whether the book was written by Shen Nong. As to *Su Wen* [《素问》, *Plain Conversation*], commentators thought that it was written in Warring States Period and put on several sections as "supplements", which were clearly not the original words of *Tai Su* [《太素》, *Grand Plain of Huangdi's Internal Classic*] and made it a book irrelative with Xuan Qi (referring to Xuan Yuan and Qi Bo, two ancestors of Chinese medicine). Chen Wuze said, Wang Shuhe's *Mai Jue* [《脉诀》, *The Pulse Secrets*] was plagiarized by Gao Yangsheng due to later supplements and confounding. How can I know this? In its annotated version by Liu Yuanbin, there are eight sentences lost after the part of "Life and Death Verses of Miscellaneous Diseases". How could people in later generation have no doubt about it since these sentences were not clear, coherent and overlapped with previous text? It is similar with the situation of *Shen Nong Ben Jing* [《神农本经》, *Agriculture God's Canon of Materia Medica*] and *Su Wen* [《素问》, *Plain Conversation*] whose content was mixed or confused due to the text color or random supplements. Certainly, the experts disagree and there would be debate ceaselessly. I have no idea as to the rightness of their views, such as Liu Yuanbin and Jie Gu [Zhang Yuansu] who did detailed research and declared to delete those questionable content, or those who talked about the original text instead of doing annotation. Is it unnecessary to discuss due to

Preface Three

their simpleness or is it to defend due to their not being from oracle? There must be one truth here. Another annotated version of *Su Wen* [《素问》, *Plain Conversation*] by Qi Xuanzi (another name for Wang Bing) was marked with red color in case there was place for improvement by future experts. However, it was copied and circulated by black color in later generations, resulting in inevitable errors. Take the chapter of "Ci Re Lun • Discussion on Acupuncture Treatment of Febrile Diseases" as an example. It was annotated that there were altogether 59 kinds of needling by Wang Bing, namely Qi Xuanzi, which is questionable because *Ling Shu* [《灵枢》, *Spiritual Pivot*] recorded that there were 89 kinds of needling. How do we judge which one is correct? Therefore, it is useless to learn if there are errors because the learners would be confused as to which one to follow. Take a look at *Jin Gui Yao Lue* [《金匮要略》, *Essential Prescriptions of the Golden Cabinet*]. It did not record any word if not addressed by Zhang Zhongjing, making the book consistent and doubtless. Lu Ruo discussed blood depletion and cited from *Tai Su* [《黄帝内经太素》, *Grand Plain of Huangdi's Internal Classic*]: It is due to the collapse from massive hemorrhage during childhood. He also cited that it is due to dead fetus not removed in the abdomen. He continued to cite that it is due to essence stagnation caused by the retention of the mixture of semen and menstrual blood from the conception vessel in the uterus if there was sexual intercourse in the menstrual period. During the period of Yuanfeng (1078 – 1085) and in the place of Xiongzhou, Chen Bangji collected a formula, which was similar with that recorded in *Nei Jing* [《黄帝内经》, *Yellow Emperor's Canon of Medicine*] and was effective to treat essence stagnation, extravasated blood retention and infertility due to cold uterus. Wuzeiyu Gu [乌贼鱼骨, cuttlefish bone, Sepiae Endoconcha] is used to treat vaginal bleeding and unceasing menstruation; Lüru [茼茹, Lüru medicinal, materia medica Lüru] is used to expel pus and blood stasis. These methods, used by ancient people, are all from *Ben Cao*. I noticed that this formula was annotated by the sentence "These methods used by ancient people are all from *Ben Cao*". How true it is! Medical science was originated from Shen Nong, so was Yi Yin's

Tang Ye [《汤液经法》, *Method and Canon of Decoctions*]. The word "all" here is extremely comprehensive, including the method of using Wuzeiyu Gu [乌贼鱼骨, cuttlefish bone, Sepiae Endoconcha] to treat unceasing menstruation but not limited to it at all. So Zhang Bozu learned medicine from *Tang Ye* [《汤液经法》, *Method and Canon of Decoctions*] and taught Zhang Zhongjing, who undertook the inheriting and spreading work to make it known till now. From the Jin, Tang and Song dynasties, all the physicians have learned and mastered it. During the period of Dading (1161 – 1189), there appeared three unprecedented physicians, namely Zhang Yuansu, Zhang Bi (son of Zhang Yuansu), and Li Gao. Why do I say this? The reason is that these three were the most outstanding ones though there were many others then.

Wang Haogu
May, 1248

Translation Specification

1. The translation of *Tang Ye Ben Cao* [《汤液本草》, *Materia Medica for Decoctions*] takes its Chinese photocopy from Wang Kentang's *Gu Jin Yi Tong Zheng Mai Quan Shu* [《古今医统正脉全书》, *Collection of Main Medical Books, Ancient and Modern*] collated by Wu Mianxue as the master copy, the version from *Si Ku Quan Shu* [《四库全书》, *Complete Library in the Four Branches of Literature*] as the checked copy, and also refers to many current versions.

2. For a better presentation and transmission of the content of *Tang Ye Ben Cao* [《汤液本草》, *Materia Medica for Decoctions*], this book is arranged in the order like this: Chinese text and English translation.

3. As to the translation of herbal names, the "Four Assurance Method" is adopted, namely every herbal name is translated in the way that its four forms are listed in the sequence of Pinyin, Chinese character, English and Latin. For instance, "防风" is translated as Fangfeng [防风, Divaricate Saposhnikovia Root, Radix Saposhnikoviae].

4. If a herbal name has three Chinese characters or less, its transliteration of Pinyin is put together; if a herbal name has four or more than four Chinese characters, its transliteration of Pinyin is divided into two parts according to its literal meaning for the convenience of easy reading.

5. The name of an ancient book is transliterated with its Chinese name and English version in brackets, every Chinese character being transliterated separately. For instance, 《汤液本草》is translated as *Tang Ye Ben Cao* [《汤液本草》, *Materia Medica for Decoctions*]. For the shortened book names, they are translated after the full names being complemented. For instance, 《珍》is

translated as *Zhen* [《珍珠囊》, *Pounch of Pearls*]. For the books whose names can not be confirmed after texal research, they are translaterated by Pinyin. For instance,《本草》is translated as *Ben Cao*,《经》is translated as *Jing*.

6. There are some Chinese herbal names from this book, even after textual research, hard to be exactly clarified and confirmed till now, so they are translated into English with Pinyin plus "medicinal" and into Latin with "materia medica" plus Pinyin.

7. For the simplified names of ancient doctors, they are made full and transliterated with Pinyin. For instance, "元宾" is transliterated as "Liu Yuanbin", "洁古" is transliterated as Jie Gu (Zhang Yuansu), "仲景" is transliterated as "Zhang Zhongjing"。

8. Traditional Chinese characters and variant Chinese characters in this book are changed into simplified and current Chinese characters according to today's publishing standards.

9. The names of formulas are translated with the method combining transliteration and literal translation. For instance, "桂枝汤" is translated as "Guizhi Decoction".

10. Traditional dose units involved in this book are translated with Pinyin. Refer to the table below:

Traditional dose unit	Metric dose unit	Pinyin
尺	0.3333333 meter	Chi
寸	0.0333333 meter	Cun
丈	3.3333333 meter	Zhang
升	200ml	Sheng
铢	1.303 gram	Zhu
分	7.818 gram	Fen
钱	3.125 gram	Qian
两	31.272 gram	Liang

目 录

卷 上

五脏苦欲补泻药味 …………… 1
脏腑泻火药 …………………… 4
东垣先生《药类法象》 ………… 5
　用药法象 ……………………… 5
　药性要旨 ……………………… 7
　升降者天地之气交 …………… 9
　用药升降浮沉补泻法 ………… 10
　五味所用 ……………………… 11
　药类法象 ……………………… 11
　标本阴阳论 …………………… 17
　五方之正气味(制方用药附) … 20
东垣先生《用药心法》 ………… 22
　随证治病药品 ………………… 22
　用药凡例 ……………………… 26
　东垣报使 ……………………… 30
　诸经向导 ……………………… 32
　制方之法 ……………………… 37
　用药各定分两 ………………… 40
　用药酒洗曝干 ………………… 40
　用药根梢身例 ………………… 41
　用丸散药例 …………………… 42
　升合分两 ……………………… 44
　君臣佐使法 …………………… 44

治法纲要 ……………………… 45
药味专精 ……………………… 47
汤药煎造 ……………………… 48
古人服药活法 ………………… 49
古人服药有法 ………………… 49
察病轻重 ……………………… 50
海藏老人《汤液本草》 ………… 50
　五宜 …………………………… 50
　五伤 …………………………… 52
　五走 …………………………… 53
　服药可慎 ……………………… 53
　论药所主 ……………………… 54
　天地生物有厚薄堪用不堪用
　　……………………………… 56
　气味生成流布 ………………… 76
　七方 …………………………… 77
　十剂 …………………………… 78

卷 中

草部 …………………………… 81
　防风 …………………………… 81
　升麻 …………………………… 83
　羌活 …………………………… 85
　独活 …………………………… 87
　柴胡 …………………………… 88

葛根	92	薏苡仁	136
威灵仙	94	甘草	136
细辛	95	白前	140
白芷	97	白薇	141
川芎	98	前胡	142
麻黄	100	木香	142
藁本	102	知母	144
桔梗	104	贝母	146
鼠黏子	106	黄芩	147
秦艽	106	黄连	150
天麻	107	大黄	153
黑附子	107	连翘	155
乌头	109	连轺	156
缩砂	110	人参	157
荜澄茄	111	沙参	160
荜茇	112	半夏	160
香附子	112	五味子	163
草豆蔻	113	甘遂	165
白豆蔻	114	大戟	166
延胡索	115	芫花	167
茴香	116	海藻	168
红蓝花	116	商陆根	168
良姜	117	旋覆花	169
黄芪	118	泽泻	169
苍术	121	红豆蔻	171
白术	123	肉豆蔻	172
当归	124	甘松	173
芍药	127	蜀漆	173
熟地黄	131	蒲黄	174
生地黄	133	天门冬	174
山药	134	麦门冬	176
麻仁	135	葳蕤	178

茵陈蒿 …… 178	胡芦巴 …… 205
艾叶 …… 179	马兜铃 …… 205
白头翁 …… 180	白及 …… 206
百合 …… 180	天南星 …… 207
苁蓉 …… 181	郁金 …… 207
玄参 …… 182	佛耳草 …… 208
款冬花 …… 183	蛇床 …… 209

卷 下

紫参 …… 184	
苦参 …… 185	
芦根 …… 186	木部 …… 210
射干(又名乌扇) …… 187	桂(桂心、肉桂、桂枝附) …… 210
败酱 …… 188	柏子仁 …… 214
败蒲 …… 188	侧柏叶 …… 215
苇叶 …… 189	柏皮 …… 216
防己 …… 189	槐实 …… 216
牵牛 …… 191	槐花 …… 217
三棱 …… 193	蔓荆子 …… 218
蓬莪术 …… 194	大腹子 …… 218
草龙胆 …… 194	酸枣 …… 219
栝楼根 …… 195	胡椒 …… 220
地榆 …… 196	川椒 …… 221
紫草 …… 197	吴茱萸 …… 222
茜根 …… 197	山茱萸 …… 223
菊花 …… 198	益智 …… 225
葶苈 …… 198	厚朴 …… 226
王不留行 …… 199	丁香 …… 228
通草 …… 200	沉香 …… 229
木通 …… 201	乳香 …… 229
瞿麦 …… 201	藿香 …… 230
车前子 …… 202	檀香 …… 231
石韦 …… 203	苏合香 …… 232
白附子 …… 204	槟榔 …… 232

栀子	233
黄柏	236
枳实	238
枳壳	240
牡丹皮	242
地骨皮	243
猪苓	244
茯苓	245
茯神	247
乌药	248
干漆	248
皂荚	249
竹叶	250
竹茹	251
淡竹叶	251
茗苦茶	252
秦皮	253
桑白皮	254
梓白皮	255
紫葳(即凌霄花)	255
诃黎勒	256
杜仲	257
琥珀	258
郁李仁	258
巴豆	259
芫花	260
苏木	262
川楝子	262
金铃子	263
没药	263
梧桐泪	264
桑东南根	264

果部 265
大枣 265
生枣 266
陈皮 266
青皮 268
桃仁 269
杏仁 270
乌梅 272
木瓜 273
甘李根白皮 274

菜部 275
荆芥穗 275
生姜 275
干姜 277
薄荷 280
葱白 280
韭白 281
薤白 282
瓜蒂 283
冬葵子 284
蜀葵花 284
香薷 285
炊单布 285

米谷部 285
粳米 285
赤小豆 286
黑大豆 287
大麦糵 288
小麦 289
神曲 290
酒 291
苦酒(一名醋,一名醯) 291

饴(即胶饴) ········· 292	牛黄 ············ 316
香豉 ············ 293	犀角 ············ 317
玉石部 ············ 294	阿胶 ············ 318
石膏 ············ 294	猪肤 ············ 319
滑石 ············ 296	猪胆汁 ·········· 320
朴硝 ············ 297	獭肝 ············ 321
盆硝(即芒硝) ····· 298	豭鼠粪 ·········· 321
硝石 ············ 299	人尿 ············ 321
玄明粉 ·········· 300	虫部 ············ 322
硫黄 ············ 301	牡蛎 ············ 322
雄黄 ············ 302	文蛤 ············ 325
赤石脂 ·········· 303	䗪虫 ············ 325
禹余粮 ·········· 304	水蛭(又名蚂蟥) ··· 326
代赭石 ·········· 305	䗪虫 ············ 326
铅丹 ············ 306	鼠妇 ············ 327
白粉 ············ 307	蜘蛛 ············ 328
紫石英 ·········· 308	蛴螬 ············ 328
伏龙肝 ·········· 309	蜜 ············· 329
白矾 ············ 310	蜣螂 ············ 330
朱砂 ············ 311	鳖甲 ············ 331
硇砂 ············ 312	蛇蜕 ············ 331
东流水 ·········· 313	蝉蜕 ············ 332
甘澜水 ·········· 313	白僵蚕 ·········· 332
禽部 ············ 314	斑蝥 ············ 333
鸡子黄 ·········· 314	乌蛇 ············ 333
兽部 ············ 314	五灵脂 ·········· 334
龙骨 ············ 314	绯帛 ············ 334
麝香 ············ 316	

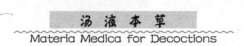

Contents

Volume 1

- Herbs That Treat Diseases of the Five Zang-organs　　　　　　　　　　/ 1
- Herbs That Purge the Fire of Zang-fu Organs　　　　　　　　　　　　/ 5
- Li Dongyuan's *Yao Lei Fa Xiang* [《药类法象》, *Rules for the Use of Medicinal Herbs*]　　/ 5

Rules for the Use of Medicinal Herbs　　　　　　　　　　　　　　　　/ 6
Essentials of Medicinal Properties　　　　　　　　　　　　　　　　　　/ 7
Actions of Ascending and Descending Being Qi-convergence of the Heaven and the Earth　　/ 9
Supplementing and Purging Actions of Medicinal Herbs Characterized by Ascending, Descending,
　　Floating and Sinking　　　　　　　　　　　　　　　　　　　　　/ 10
Actions of the Five Flavors　　　　　　　　　　　　　　　　　　　　　/ 11
Rules for the Use of Medicinal Herbs　　　　　　　　　　　　　　　　/ 12
Discussion on Manifestation, Root Cause, Yin and Yang　　　　　　　　/ 18
Properties and Flavors in the Five Orientations (Prescription Formulating and Drug Medications)　/ 21

- Li Dongyuan's *Yong Yao Xin Fa* [《用药心法》, *Gist for the Use of Medicinal Herbs*]　　/ 22

Medicinal Herbs for Disease Treatment According to the Syndromes　　　/ 23
Notes on Medication　　　　　　　　　　　　　　　　　　　　　　　　/ 27
Guiding Action of Medicinal Herbs by Li Dongyuan　　　　　　　　　　/ 30
Channel Entering　　　　　　　　　　　　　　　　　　　　　　　　　/ 34
Approaches of Prescription Formulating　　　　　　　　　　　　　　　/ 38
Dosage of Medication　　　　　　　　　　　　　　　　　　　　　　　/ 40
Wine-processing Herbs　　　　　　　　　　　　　　　　　　　　　　　/ 41
Examples for the Use of Different Medicinal Parts　　　　　　　　　　/ 42
Examples of Dosage Form　　　　　　　　　　　　　　　　　　　　　/ 42
Weights and Measures　　　　　　　　　　　　　　　　　　　　　　　/ 44
Monarch, Minister, Assistant and Guiding Medicinal Herbs　　　　　　/ 44
Essentials of Treatment　　　　　　　　　　　　　　　　　　　　　　/ 46
Specializations of Herbs　　　　　　　　　　　　　　　　　　　　　　/ 47
Decoction Methods　　　　　　　　　　　　　　　　　　　　　　　　　/ 49

Contents

Administration Rules	/ 49
Administration Methods	/ 49
Differentiation of Patient's Conditions	/ 50
● Haizang's *Tang Ye Ben Cao*［《汤液本草》, Materia Medica for Decoctions］	/ 50
Five Suitabilities	/ 51
Five Injuries	/ 52
Functional Tendencies of the Five Flavors	/ 53
Prohibition of Administration	/ 54
Medicinal Efficacy	/ 54
Usable or Unusable Medicinal Herbs	/ 66
Formation and Distribution of Qi and Flavor	/ 76
Seven Types of Prescriptions	/ 77
Ten Types of Formulas	/ 79

Volume 2

● Grass Herbs	/ 81
Fangfeng［防风, saposhnikovia, Radix Saposhnikoviae］	/ 81
Shengma［升麻, cimicifuga, Rhizoma Cimicifuga］	/ 83
Qianghuo［羌活, notopterygium, Notopterygii Rhizoma et Radix］	/ 86
Duhuo［独活, pubescent angelica, Radix Angelicae Pubescentis］	/ 87
Chaihu［柴胡, bupleurum, Radix Bupleuri］	/ 89
Gegen［葛根, pueraria, Radix Puerariae］	/ 92
Weilingxian［威灵仙, clematis, Clematidis Radix］	/ 94
Xixin［细辛, as arum, Herba Asari］	/ 95
Baizhi［白芷, dahurian angelicaroot, Radix Angelicae Dahuricae］	/ 97
Chuanxiong［川芎, Sichuan lovage rhizome, Rhizoma Ligustici Chuanxiong］	/ 99
Mahuang［麻黄, ephedra, Herba Ephedrae］	/ 101
Gaoben［藁本, Chinese Lovage, Rhizoma Ligustici］	/ 103
Jiegeng［桔梗, platycodon grandiflorum, Radix Platycodi］	/ 104
Shunianzi［鼠黏子, arctium, Arctium Lappa L.］	/ 106
Qinjiao［秦艽, largeleaf gentian root, Radix Gentianae Macrophyllae］	/ 106
Tianma［天麻, gastrodia, Gastrodiae Rhizoma］	/ 107
Heifuzi［黑附子, aconite, Radix Aconiti Praeparata］	/ 108
Wutou［乌头, common monkshood, Aconitum carmichaeli Debx.］	/ 109
Suosha［缩砂, Fructus Amomi Xanthioidis, Amomum villosum Lour. Var. xanthioides T. L. Wu et Senjen］	/ 110
Bichengqie［荜澄茄, cubeb, Litseae Fructus］	/ 111

Biba [荜茇, long pepper, Piper Longum L.] / 112
Xiangfuzi [香附子, cyperus, Cyperi Rhizoma] / 112
Caodoukou [草豆蔻, katsumada galangal seed, Semen Alpiniae Katsumadai] / 113
Baidoukou [白豆蔻, cardamom, Amomi Fructus Rotundus] / 114
Yanhusuo [延胡索, yanhusuo, Rhizoma Corydalis] / 115
Huixiang [茴香, fennel, Foeniculum Vulgare] / 116
Honglanhua [红蓝花, Tulipa, Carthamus Tinctorius L.] / 117
Liangjiang [良姜, lesser galangal rhizome, Rhizoma Alpiniae Officinarum] / 118
Huangqi [黄芪, milkvetch root, Radix Astragali seu Hedysari] / 119
Cangzhu [苍术, atractylodes rhizome, Rhizoma Atractylodis] / 122
Baizhu [白术, argehead atractylodes rhizome, Rhizoma Atractylodis Macrocephalae] / 123
Danggui [当归, Chinese angelica, Radix Angelicae Sinensis] / 125
Shaoyao [芍药, Chinese herbaceous peony, Paeonia Lactiflora Pall] / 128
Shudihuang [熟地黄, prepared rehmannia root, Radix Rehmanniae Preparata] / 131
Shengdihuang [生地黄, unprocessed rehmannia root, Radix Rehmanniae Recens] / 133
Shanyao [山药, common yam rhizome, Dioscorea opposita Thunb.] / 135
Maren [麻仁, cannabis fruit, Cannabis Fructus] / 135
Yiyiren [薏苡仁, coix, Semen Coicis] / 136
Gancao [甘草, liquorice root, Glycyrrhiza Uralensis Fisch.] / 137
Baiqian [白前, willowleaf rhizome, Rhizoma Cynanchi Stauntonii] / 140
Baiwei [白薇, blackend swallowwort root, Radix Cynanchi Atrati] / 141
Qianhu [前胡, hogfennel root, Radix Peucedani] / 142
Muxiang [木香, root of common aucklandia, Radix Aucklandiae] / 143
Zhimu [知母, rhizome of common anemarrhena, Rhizoma Anemarrhenae] / 144
Beimu [贝母, fritillaria, Bulbus Fritillariae Thunbergii] / 146
Huangqin [黄芩, baical skullcap root, Radix Scutellariae] / 147
Huanglian [黄连, golden thread, Rhizoma Coptidis] / 151
Dahuang [大黄, rhubarb, Radix et Rhizoma Rhei] / 153
Lianqiao [连翘, fruit of weeping forsythia, Fructus Forsythiae] / 156
Lianyao [连轺, the root of weeping forsythia capsule, Forsythia Suspensa (Thunb.) Vahl] / 156
Renshen [人参, ginseng, Radix Ginseng] / 157
Shashen [沙参, fourleaf ladybell root, Radix Adenophorae] / 160
Banxia [半夏, pinellia Tuber, Rhizoma Pinelliae] / 161
Wuweizi [五味子, Chinese magnoliavine fruit, Fructus Schisandrae Chinensis] / 163
Gansui [甘遂, kansui, Radix Euphorbiae Kansui] / 165
Daji [大戟, peking euphorbia root, Radix Euphorbiae Pekinensis] / 166

Contents

Raohua [莞花, flower of longflower stringbush, Wikstroemia Canescens (Wall.) Meisn.] / 167
Haizao [海藻, seaweed, Sargassum] / 168
Shanglugen [商陆根, pokeberry root, Radix Phytolaccae] / 168
Xuanfuhua [旋覆花, inula flower, Flos Inula Japonica] / 169
Zexie [泽泻, oriental waterplantain rhizome, Rhizoma Alismatis] / 170
Hongdoukou [红豆蔻, galanga galangal fruit, Fructus Alpiniae Galangae] / 172
Roudoukou [肉豆蔻, nutmeg, Semen Myristicae] / 172
Gansong [甘松, nardostachys root, Radix et Rhizoma Nardostachyos] / 173
Shuqi [蜀漆, dichroa, Ramulus et Folium Dichroae] / 173
Puhuang [蒲黄, cattail pollen, Pollen Typhae] / 174
Tianmendong [天门冬, asparagus, Radix Asparagi] / 175
Maimendong [麦门冬, radix ophiopogonis, Ophiopogon Japonicus Ker-Gawl] / 176
Weirui [葳蕤, stem of October clematis, Caulis Clematidis Apiifoliae] / 178
Yinchenhao [茵陈蒿, capillaries, Herba Artemisiae Scopariae] / 179
Aiye [艾叶, argy wormwood leaf, Folium Artemisiae Argyi] / 180
Baitouweng [白头翁, Chinese pulsatilla root, Radix Pulsatillae] / 180
Baihe [百合, lily bulb, Lilium Brownii var. Viridulum Baker] / 181
Congrong [苁蓉, desertliving cistanche herb, Herba Cistanches] / 181
Xuanshen [玄参, figwort root, Radix Scrophulariae] / 182
Kuandonghua [款冬花, immature flower of common coltsfoot, Flos Farfarae] / 183
Zishen [紫参, Chinese sage herb, Herba Salviae Chinesnsis] / 185
Kushen [苦参, flavescent sophora, Radix Sophorae Flavescentis] / 185
Lugen [芦根, reed rhizome, Rhizoma Phragmitis] / 186
Shegan (also named Wushan) [射干, blackberry lily rhizome, Rhizoma Belamcandae] / 187
Baijiang [败酱, patrinia, Herba Patriniae] / 188
Baipu [败蒲, cattail, Typha Angustifolia] / 189
Weiye [苇叶, reed, Phragmites Trins.] / 189
Fangji [防己, root of fourstamen stephania, Radix Stephaniae Tetrandrae] / 190
Qianniu [牵牛, morning glory, Pharbitis nil (L.) Choisy] / 191
Sanleng [三棱, common buried rubber, Rhizoma Sparganii] / 193
Peng'eshu [蓬莪术, zedoary, Curcuma Phaeocaulis Valeton] / 194
Caolongdan [草龙胆, Chinese gentian, Radix Gentianae] / 195
Gualougen [栝楼根, root of Mongolian snakegourd, Radix Trichosanthis] / 195
Diyu [地榆, root of garden burnet, Radix Sanguisorbae] / 196
Zicao [紫草, arnebia root, Radix Arnebiae seu Lithospermi] / 197
Qiangen [茜根, root of Indian madder, Radix Rubiae] / 197

Juhua [菊花, flower of florists chrysanthemum, Flos Chrysanthemi] / 198

Tingli [葶苈, Semen Lepidii, Semen Descurainiae] / 199

Wangbuliu Xing [王不留行, cowherb seed, Semen Vaccariae] / 200

Tongcao [通草, ricepaperplant pith, Medulla Tetrapanacis] / 200

Mutong [木通, akebia stem, Caulis Akebiae] / 201

Qumai [瞿麦, lilac pink herb, Herba Dianthi] / 201

Cheqianzi [车前子, seed of Asiatic plantain, Semen Plantaginis] / 202

Shiwei [石韦, shearer's pyrrosia leaf, Folium Pyrrosiae] / 203

Baifuzi [白附子, giant typhonium rhizome, Rhizoma Typhonii] / 204

Huluba [胡芦巴, fenugreek seed, Semen Trigonellae] / 205

Madouling [马兜铃, root of common aucklandia, Fructus Aristolochiae] / 205

Baiji [白及, Common Bletilla Rubber, Rhizoma Bletillae] / 206

Tiannanxing [天南星, Jackinthepulpit Tuber, Rhizoma Arisaematis] / 207

Yujin [郁金, Turmeric Root Tuber, Radix Curcumae] / 208

Fo'ercao [佛耳草, Longtube Ground Ivy, Glechoma Longituba (Nakai) Kupr.] / 208

Shechuang [蛇床, Common Cnidium Fruit, Fructus Cnidii] / 209

Volume 3

● Tree Herbs / 210

Gui [桂, Cinnamon bark, Cortex Cinnamomum Cassia] (also named Guixin, Rougui and Guizhifu) / 211

Baiziren [柏子仁, Chinese arborvitae kernel, Semen Platycladi] / 215

Cebaiye [侧柏叶, arborvitae leaf, Platycladi Cacumen] / 215

Baipi [柏皮, arborvitae root bark, Platycladi Radicis Cortex] / 216

Huaishi [槐实, sophora fruit, Sophorae Fructus] / 216

Huaihua [槐花, pagodatree flower, Flos Sophorae] / 217

Manjingzi [蔓荆子, vitex, Viticis Fructus] / 218

Dafuzi [大腹子, areca, Arecae Semen] / 219

Suanzao [酸枣, crataegus, Crataegi Fructus] / 219

Hujiao [胡椒, pepper, Piperis Fructus] / 220

Chuanjiao [川椒, zanthoxylum, Zanthoxyli Pericarpium] / 221

Wuzhuyu [吴茱萸, evodia, Fructus Evodiae] / 222

Shanzhuyu [山茱萸, cornus, Fructus Corni] / 224

Yizhi [益智, sharp-leaf glangal fruit, Fructus Alpiniae Oxyphyllae] / 225

Houpu [厚朴, magnolia bark, Cortex Magnoliae Officinalis] / 226

Dingxiang [丁香, clove, Flos Caryophylli] / 228

Chenxiang [沉香, aquilaria, Aquilariae Lignum Resinatum] / 229

Ruxiang [乳香, frankincense, Olibanum] / 230

Contents

Huoxiang [藿香, Wrinkled Gianthyssop Herb, Agastache Rugosa] / 230
Tanxiang [檀香, sandalwood, Santali Albi Lignum] / 231
Suhexiang [苏合香, storax, Styrax] / 232
Binlang [槟榔, areca seed, Semen Arecae] / 233
Zhizi [栀子, gardenia, Gardeniae Fructus] / 234
Huangbo [黄柏, bark of amur corktree, Cortex Phellodendri] / 237
Zhishi [枳实, immature orange fruit, Fructus Aurantii Immaturus] / 239
Zhiqiao [枳壳, orange fruit, Fructus Aurantii] / 241
Mudanpi [牡丹皮, tree peony root bark, Cortex Moutan Radicis] / 242
Digupi [地骨皮, Chinese wolfberry root-bark, Cortex Lycii] / 243
Zhuling [猪苓, zhuling, Polyporus Umbellatus] / 244
Fuling [茯苓, Indian bread, Poria] / 246
Fushen [茯神, root poria, Poria cum Pini Radice] / 247
Wuyao [乌药, lindera, Linderae Radix] / 248
Ganqi [干漆, Dried Lacquer, Resina Toxicodendri] / 249
Zaojia [皂荚, gymnocladus fruit, Gymnocladi Fructus] / 249
Zhuye [竹叶, bamboo leaf, Lophatheri Folium] / 251
Zhuru [竹茹, bamboo shavings, Bumbusae Caulis in Taenia] / 251
Danzhuye [淡竹叶, lophatherum, Lophatheri Herba] / 252
Mingkucha [茗苦茶, bitter tea, Camellia assamica (Mast.) Chang var. kucha Chang et Wang] / 252
Qinpi [秦皮, ash, Fraxini Cortex] / 253
Sangbaipi [桑白皮, white mulberry root-bark, Cortex Mori] / 254
Zibaipi [梓白皮, root-bark of ovate catalpa, Cortex Catalpae Ovatae Radicis] / 255
Ziwei [紫葳, campsis flower, Campsis Flos] (also called Lingxiaohua) / 255
Helile [诃黎勒, chebule, Terminalia Chebula Retz.] / 256
Duzhong [杜仲, eucommia, Eucommiae Cortex] / 257
Hupo [琥珀, Amber, Ambrum] / 258
Yuliren [郁李仁, bush cherry kernel, Pruni Semen] / 259
Badou [巴豆, croton, Crotonis Fructus] / 259
Yuanhua [芫花, genkwa, Genkwa Flos] / 261
Sumu [苏木, sappan wood, Lignum Sappan] / 262
Chuanlianzi [川楝子, szechwan chinaberry fruit, Fructus Meliae Toosendan] / 263
Jinlingzi [金铃子, toosendan, Toosendan Fructus] / 263
Moyao [没药, myrrh, Myrrha] / 263
Wutonglei [梧桐泪, tear of fermiana platanifolia, Firmiana Platanifolia (L. f.) Marsili] / 264
Sangdongnan Gen [桑东南根, root of white mulberry, Cortex Mori] / 265

- **Fruit Herbs** / 265

Dazao [大枣, Chinese date, Fructus Jujubae] / 265
Shengzao [生枣, fresh jujube, Fructus Ziziphi Jujubae] / 266
Chenpi [陈皮, dried tangerine peel, Pericarpium Citri Reticulatae] / 267
Qingpi [青皮, immature tangerine peel, Pericarpium Citri Reticulatae Viride] / 268
Taoren [桃仁, peach seed, Semen Persicae] / 269
Xingren [杏仁, bitter apricot seed, Semen Armeniacae Amarum] / 271
Wumei [乌梅, smoked plum, Fructus Mume] / 273
Mugua [木瓜, common floweringqince fruit, Fructus Chaenomelis] / 274
Ganligen Baipi [甘李根白皮, Root-bark of Japanese Plum, Prunus Salicina Lindl] / 274

- **Vegetable Herbs** / 275

Jingjiesui [荆芥穗, schizonepetae spica, Herba Schizonepetae] / 275
Shengjiang [生姜, fresh ginger, Rhizoma Zingiberis Recens] / 276
Ganjiang [干姜, dry ginger, Rhizoma Zingiberis] / 278
Bohe [薄荷, peppermint, Herba Menthae] / 280
Congbai [葱白, scallion white, Allii Fistulosi Bulbus Recens] / 281
Jiubai [韭白, Chinese chive stalk, Allium Tuberosum Rottb. ex Spreng] / 282
Xiebai [薤白, longstamen onion bulb, Bulbus Allii Macrostemonis] / 282
Guadi [瓜蒂, muskmelon fruit pedicel, Pediculus Melo] / 283
Dongkuizi [冬葵子, cluster mallow fruit, Fructus Malvae] / 284
Shukuihua [蜀葵花, Flower of Hollyhock, Althaea Rosea] / 284
Xiangru [香薷, Chinese mosla, Herba Moslae] / 285
Chuidanbu [炊单布, gauze, gaze] / 285

- **Rice and Grain Herbs** / 285

Jingmi [粳米, rice, Oryza Sativa L.] / 286
Chixiaodou [赤小豆, red phaseolus bean, Semen Phaseoli] / 287
Heidadou [黑大豆, black soybean, Glycine Max (L.) Merr.] / 288
Damainie [大麦蘖, barley sprout, Hordei Fructus Germinatus] / 288
Xiaomai [小麦, wheat, Triticum Aestivum] / 289
Shenqu [神曲, medicated leaven, Massa Medicata Fermentata] / 290
Jiu [酒, liquor, Vinum] / 291
Kujiu [苦酒, vinegar, Acetum] (also named Cu or Xi) / 291
Yi [饴, malt sugar, Maltosum] (also named Jiaoyi) / 292
Xiangchi [香豉, fermented soybean, Semen Sojae Preparatum] / 293

- **Jade Herbs** / 294

Shigao [石膏, gypsum, Gypsum Fibrosum] / 294

Contents

Huashi [滑石, talc, Talcum] / 296
Puxiao [朴硝, crystallized sodium sulfate, Natrii Sulfas] / 298
Penxiao [盆硝, crystallized sodium sulfate, Natrii Sulfas] (also named Mangxiao) / 298
Xiaoshi [硝石, niter, Sal Nitri] / 299
Xuanmingfen [玄明粉, sodium sulfate powder, Natrii Sulfas Exsiccatus] / 301
Liuhuang [硫黄, sulphur, Sulfur] / 301
Xionghuang [雄黄, realgar, Realgar] / 302
Chishizhi [赤石脂, red halloysite, Halloysitum Rubrum] / 303
Yuyuliang [禹余粮, limonite, Limonitum] / 305
Daizheshi [代赭石, hematite, Haematitum] / 306
Qiandan [铅丹, minium, Minium] / 306
Baifen [白粉, processed galenite, Galenitum Praeparatum] / 307
Zishiying [紫石英, fluorite, Fluoritum] / 308
Fulonggan [伏龙肝, oven earth, Terra Flava Usta] / 309
Baifan [白矾, alum, Alumen] / 310
Zhusha [朱砂, cinnabar, Cinnabaris] / 311
Naosha [硇砂, sal ammoniac, Sal Ammoniacum] / 312
Dongliushui [东流水, water running toward the east, Materia Medica Dongliushui] / 313
Ganlanshui [甘澜水, worked water, Aqua Manipulata] / 313

- **Fowl Herbs** / 314

Jizihuang [鸡子黄, egg yolk, Galli Vitellus] / 314

- **Beast Herbs** / 314

Longgu [龙骨, dragon bone, Mastodi Ossis Fossilia] / 315
Shexiang [麝香, musk, Moschus] / 316
Niuhuang [牛黄, bovine bezoar, Bovis Calculus] / 316
Xijiao [犀角, rhinoceros horn, Rhinoceros Unicornis L.] / 317
Ejiao [阿胶, ass hide glue, Colla Corii Asini] / 318
Zhufu [猪肤, pig skin, Suis Corium] / 319
Zhudanzhi [猪胆汁, pig bile, Suis Bilis] / 320
Tagan [獭肝, otter liver, Lutrae Iecur] / 321
Jiashufen [貑鼠粪, cornus, Corni Fructus] / 321
Renniao [人尿, human urine, Hominis Urina] / 321

- **Insect Herbs** / 322

Muli [牡蛎, oyster shell, Concha Ostreae] / 323
Wenge [文蛤, meretrix clam shell, Concha Meretricis] / 325
Mengchong [虻虫, tabanus, Tabanus] / 325

Shuizhi［水蛭, Leech, Hirudo］(also named Mahuang) / 326

Zhechong［䗪虫, ground beetle, Corydiidae］ / 327

Shufu［鼠妇, pillbug, Armadillidium］ / 327

Zhizhu［蜘蛛, spider, Aranea］ / 328

Qicao［蛴螬, June beetle grub, Holotrichiae Vermiculus］ / 328

Mi［蜜, honey, Mel］ / 329

Qianglang［蜣螂, dung beetle, Catharsius］ / 330

Biejia［鳖甲, turtle shell, Trionycis Carapax］ / 331

Shetui［蛇蜕, snake slough, Serpentis Periostracum］ / 331

Chantui［蝉蜕, cicada molting, Cicadae Periostracum］ / 332

Baijiangcan［白僵蚕, silkworm larva, Larva Bombycis］ / 332

Banmao［斑蝥, mylabris, Mylabris］ / 333

Wushe［乌蛇, black-striped snake, Zaocys］ / 333

Wulingzhi［五灵脂, squirrel's droppings, Trogopteri Faeces］ / 334

Feibo［绯帛, red silk, Rubei Serica］ / 334

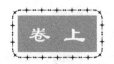

Volume 1

五脏苦欲补泻药味
Herbs That Treat Diseases of the Five Zang-organs

肝苦急,急食甘以缓之,甘草;欲散,急食辛以散之,川芎。以辛补之,细辛;以酸泻之,芍药。虚,以生姜、陈皮之类补之。《经》曰:虚则补其母。水能生木,肾乃肝之母。肾,水也。苦以补肾,熟地黄、黄柏是也;如无他证,钱氏地黄丸主之。实,则白芍药泻之;如无他证,钱氏泻青丸主之。实则泻其子,心乃肝之子,以甘草泻之。

心苦缓,急食酸以收之,五味子;欲软,急食咸以软之,芒硝。以咸补之,泽泻;以甘泻之,人参、黄芪、甘草。虚,以炒盐补之。虚则补其母,木能生火,肝乃心之母。肝,木也。以生姜补肝;如无他证,钱氏安神丸主之。实,则甘草泻之;如无他证,钱氏方中重则泻心汤,轻则导赤散。

脾苦湿,急食苦以燥之,白术;欲缓,急食甘以缓之,甘草。以甘补之,人参;以苦泻之,黄连。虚,则以甘草、大枣之类补之;如无他证,钱氏益黄散主之。心乃脾之母,以炒盐补心。实,则以枳实泻之;如无他证,以泻黄散泻之。肺乃脾之子,以桑白皮泻肺。

肺苦气上逆,急食苦以泻之,诃子皮(一作黄芩);欲收,急食酸以收之,白芍药。以辛泻之,桑白皮;以酸补之,五味子。虚,则五味子补之;如无他证,钱氏阿胶散补之。脾乃肺之母,以甘草补脾。实,则桑白皮泻之;如无他证,以泻白散泻之。肾乃肺之子,以泽泻泻之。

肾苦燥,急食辛以润之,知母、黄柏;欲坚,急食苦以坚之,知母。以苦补之,黄柏;以咸泻之,泽泻。虚,则熟地黄、黄柏补之。肾本无实,不可泻,钱氏止有补肾地黄丸,无泻肾之药。肺乃肾之母,以五味子补肺。

The liver tends to suffer from the rapid flow of qi which can be relieved by the herbs with sweet flavor, such as Gancao [甘草, liquorice root, Glycyrrhiza uralensis Fisch.]. Since the liver needs to be dissipated, the treatment of liver disease requires immediate use of the herbs with pungent flavor to dissipate such as Chuanxiong [川芎, Sichuan lovage rhizome, Ligusticum Chuanxiong Hort.]. The liver can be replenished with pungent flavor such as Xixin [细辛, asarum, Asarum sieboldii Miq.], and can be purged with sour flavor such as Shaoyao [芍药, Chinese herbaceous peony, Paeonia lactiflora Pall.]. If the liver is in deficiency, it can be supplemented by Shengjiang [生姜, fresh ginger, Rhizoma Zingiberis Recens], Chenpi [陈皮, dried tangerine peel, Pericarpium Citri Reticulatae], etc. *Nan Jing* [《难经》, *Canon of Difficult Issues*] says, "To reinforce the mother-organ in case of deficiency." Water can generate wood and kidney is the mother-organ of liver. The kidney pertains to water, so the treatment of kidney disease requires herbs with bitter flavor such as Shudihuang [熟地黄, prepared rehmannia root, Radix Rehmanniae Preparata] and Huangbo [黄柏, bark of amur corktree, Cortex Phellodendri]. It can be treated by Qianshi Dihuang Pill if there is no other complicatons. Baishao [白芍, white peony root, Radix Paeoniae Alba] can purge the excess syndrome. It can be treated by Qianshi Xieqing Pill if there are no other complications. Excess syndromes should be treated by purging the child-organ. Since the heart is the child-organ of liver, it can be purged by Gancao [甘草, liquorice root, Glycyrrhiza uralensis Fisch.].

The heart tends to suffer from the slackening of qi which can be astringed by the herbs with sour flavor such as Wuweizi [五味子, Chinese magnoliavine fruit, Fructus Schisandrae Chinensis]. Since the heart needs to be softened, the treatment of heart disease requires immediate use of the herbs with salty flavor such as Mangxiao [芒硝, crystallized sodium sulfate, Natrii Sulfas] to soften, the herbs with salty flavor such as Zexie [泽泻, oriental waterplantain rhizome, Rhizoma Alismatis] to supplement, and the herbs with sweet flavor to purge such as Renshen [人参, ginseng, Radix Ginseng], Huangqi [黄芪, milkvetch root, Radix Astragali seu Hedysari] and Gancao [甘草, liquorice root, Glycyrrhiza Uralensis Fisch.]. If the heart is in deficiency, it can be supplemented by stir-frying salt. The deficiency syndromes should be treated by reinforcing the mother-organ. Wood can generate fire and the liver is the mother-organ of the heart. The liver, pertaining to wood, can be supplemented by Shengjiang [生姜, fresh ginger, Rhizoma Zingiberis Recens]; it can be treated by Qianshi Xieqing Pill if there are no other complications. Gancao〔甘草, liquorice root, Glycyrrhiza uralensis Fisch.〕can be used to treat the excess syndrome of the heart. The liver can be treated by Xiexin Decoction for severe cases and Daochi Powder for mild cases if there are no other complications.

The spleen tends to suffer from dampness which can be relieved by the herbs with bitter flavor such as Baizhu〔白术, argehead atractylodes rhizome, Rhizoma Atractylodis Macrocephalae〕. Since the spleen needs to be moderated, the treatment of spleen disease requires immediate use of the herbs with sweet flavor to moderate such as Gancao〔甘草, liquorice root, Glycyrrhiza uralensis Fisch.〕, the herbs with bitter flavor to purge such as Huanglian〔黄连, golden thread, Rhizoma Coptidis〕and the herbs with sweet flavor to supplement such as Renshen〔人参, ginseng, Radix Ginseng〕. The herbs like Gancao〔甘草, liquorice root, Glycyrrhiza uralensis Fisch.〕and Dazao〔大枣, Chinese date, Fructus Jujubae〕can be used to supplement the deficiency syndrome of the spleen. The spleen can be treated by Qianshi Yihuang Powder if there are no other complications. The heart is the mother-organ of the spleen and can be supplemented by stir-frying salt. If the heart is in excess, it can be purged by Zhishi〔枳实, immature orange fruit, Fructus Aurantii Immaturus〕. The heart can be treated by Xiehuang Powder if there are no other complications. The lung is the child-organ of the spleen and can be purged by Sangbaipi〔桑白皮, white mulberry root-bark, Cortex Mori〕.

The lung tends to suffer from the adverse flow of qi which can be stopped by the herbs with bitter flavor such as Huangqin〔黄芩, baical skullcap root, Radix Scutellariae〕. Since the lung needs to be astringed, the treatment of lung disease requires the immediate use of the herbs with sour flavor to astringe such as Baishao〔白芍, white peony root, Radix Paeoniae Alba〕, the herbs with pungent flavor to purge such as Sangbaipi〔桑白皮, white mulberry root-bark, Cortex Mori〕, and the herbs with sour flavor to supplement such as Wuweizi〔五味子, Chinese magnoliavine fruit, Fructus Schisandrae Chinensis〕. If the lung is in deficiency, it can be treated by Wuweizi〔五味子, Chinese magnoliavine fruit, Fructus Schisandrae Chinensis〕; Qianshi Ejiao Powder can supplement the lung if there are no other complications. The spleen is the mother-organ of the lung and can be supplemented by Gancao〔甘草, liquorice root, Glycyrrhiza uralensis Fisch.〕. If the spleen is in excess, Sangbaipi [桑白皮, white mulberry root-bark, Cortex Mori] can be used to purge it. The lung can be treated by Xiebai Powder if there are no other complications. The kidney is the child-organ of the lung and can be purged by Zexie [泽泻, oriental waterplantain rhizome, Rhizoma Alismatis].

The kidney tends to suffer from dryness which can be moistened by herbs with pungent flavor such as Zhimu [知母, common anemarrhena rhizome, Rhizoma Anemarrhenae] and Huangbo [黄柏, bark of amur corktree, Cortex Phellodendri]. Since the kidney needs to be consolidated, the treatment of kidney diseases requires immediate use of herbs with bitter flavor to consolidate such as Zhimu [知母, common anemarrhena rhizome, Rhizoma Anemarrhenae] and to supplement such as Huangbo [黄柏, bark of amur corktree, Cortex Phellodendri], and the use of herbs with salty flavor to purge such as Zexie [泽泻, oriental waterplantain rhizome, Rhizoma Alismatis]. If the kidney is in deficiency, it can be supplemented by Shudihuang [熟地黄, prepared rehmannia root, Radix Rehmanniae Preparata] and Huangbo [黄柏, bark of amur corktree, Cortex Phellodendri]. Since the kidney has no excess syndrome and can not be purged, there are no kidney-purging herbs recorded. Dihuang Pill for supplementing the kidney was recorded in *Xiao Er Yao Zheng Zhi Jue* [《小儿药证直诀》, *Key to Therapeutics of Children's Diseases*]. The lung is the mother-organ of the kidney and can be supplemented by Wuweizi [五味子, Chinese magnoliavine fruit, Fructus Schisandrae Chinensis].

以上五脏补泻,《内经·脏气法时论》中备言之,欲究其精,详看本论。

The above theories of the supplementing and purging of five zang-organs are explicated in *Nei Jing · Zang Qi Fa Shi Lun* [《内经·脏气法时论》, *Internal Classic · Discussion on the Association of the Zang-qi with the Four Seasons*]. If the readers want to know more about it, see the details below.

脏腑泻火药

黄连泻心火,木通泻小肠火,黄芩泻肺火(栀子佐之),黄芩泻大肠火,柴胡泻肝火(黄连佐之),柴胡泻胆火(亦以黄连佐之),白芍药泻脾火,石膏泻胃火,知母泻肾火,黄柏泻膀胱火,柴胡泻三焦火(黄芩佐之)。以上诸药,各泻其火,

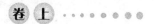

不惟止能如此，更有治病，合为君、合为臣处，详其所宜而用，勿执一也。

Herbs That Purge the Fire of Zang-fu Organs

Huanglian［黄连, golden thread, Rhizoma Coptidis］can purge the heart-fire. Mutong［木通, akebia stem, Caulis Akebiae］can purge the fire in the small intestine. Huangqin［黄芩, baical skullcap root, Radix Scutellariae］can purge the lung-fire assisted by Zhizi［栀子, capejasmine fruit, Gardenia Jasminoides Ellis］. Huangqin［黄芩, baical skullcap root, Radix Scutellariae］can purge the fire in the large intestine. Chaihu［柴胡, Chinese thorowax root, Radix Bupleuri］can purge the liver-fire and gallbladder-fire assisted by Huanglian［黄连, golden thread, Rhizoma Coptidis］. Baishao［白芍, white peony root, Radix Paeoniae Alba］can purge the spleen-fire. Shigao［石膏, gypsum, Gypsum Fibrosum］can purge the stomach-fire. Zhimu［知母, common anemarrhena rhizome, Rhizoma Anemarrhenae］can purge the kidney-fire. Huangbo［黄柏, bark of amur corktree, Cortex Phellodendri］can purge the bladder-fire. Chaihu［柴胡, Chinese thorowax root, Radix Bupleuri］can purge the fire in the triple energizer assisted by Huangqin［黄芩, baical skullcap root, Radix Scutellariae］. All the herbs mentioned above can purge the fire respectively. In treating diseases, if the monarch drug and the minister drug are not appropriate, they can be adjusted according to the different conditions.

东垣先生《药类法象》
Li Dongyuan's *Yao Lei Fa Xiang*［《药类法象》, *Rules for the Use of Medicinal Herbs*］

用药法象

天有阴阳，风寒暑湿燥火，三阴、三阳上奉之。温凉寒热，四气是也。温、热者，天之阳也；凉、寒者，天之阴也。此乃天之阴阳也。

地有阴阳，金木水火土，生长化收藏下应之。辛甘淡酸苦咸，五味是也，皆象于地。辛甘淡者,地之阳也;酸苦咸者,地之阴也。此乃地之阴阳也。

味之薄者,为阴中之阳,味薄则通,酸、苦、咸、平是也;味之厚者,为阴中之阴,味厚则泄,酸、苦、咸、寒是也。

气之厚者,为阳中之阳,气厚则发热,辛、甘、温、热是也;气之薄者,为阳中之阴,气薄则发泄,辛、甘、淡、平、凉、寒是也。

轻清成象(味薄,茶之类),本乎天者亲上;重浊成形(味厚,大黄之类),本乎地者亲下。

气味辛甘发散为阳,酸苦涌泄为阴。

清阳发腠理,清之清者也;清阳实四肢,清之浊者也;浊阴归六腑,浊之浊者也;浊阴走五脏,浊之清者也。

Rules for the Use of Medicinal Herbs

Wind, Cold, Summer-Heat, Dampness, Dryness and Fire represent yin and yang of the heavens, which are followed by three yin and three yang. Warm, cool, cold and heat are called four properties. Warm and heat stand for yang of the heaven; while cool and cold stand for yin of the heaven. These are the connotations of yin and yang in the heaven.

Metal, Wood, Water, Fire and Earth stand for yin and yang of the earth, which are followed by generation, growth, transformation, ripening and storage. The so-called five flavors are pungent, sweet, bland, sour, bitter and salty, and they all pertain to the earth. The flavors of pungent, sweet and bland represent yang of the earth; while sour, bitter and salty stand for yin of the earth. These are the connotations of yin and yang on the earth.

The thin flavors pertaining to yang within yin are effective for dredging, including sour, bitter, salty and mild. The thick flavors pertain to yin within yin and are helpful for purging, including sour, bitter, salty and cold.

The thick qi pertains to yang within yang and generates heat, including pungent, sweet, warm and hot. The thin qi belongs to yin within yang and has the function to disperse, which include pungent, sweet, bland, mild, cool and cold.

The lucid qi of thin flavor such as tea rises to the heavens and displays images. The turbid qi of thick flavor such as Dahuang [大黄, rhubarb root and rhizome, Radix et Rhizoma Rhei] descends to the earth and demonstrates forms.

The pungent and sweet flavors pertain to yang because they disperse; the sour and bitter flavors pertain to yin because they induce vomiting and purgation.

The lucid-yang permeates through muscular interstices and pertains to lucid within lucid. The lucid-yang fortifies the limbs and pertains to turbid within lucid. The turbid-yin enters the six fu-organs and pertains to turbid within turbid; while the turbid-yin enters the five zang-organs and pertains to lucid within turbid.

药性要旨

苦药平升,微寒平亦升。甘辛药平降,甘寒泻火。苦寒泻湿热,苦甘寒泻血热。

气味厚薄寒热阴阳升降图

```
    桂枝之甘                       白虎之甘
     附子                           茯苓
    阳中之阳                       阳中之阴
      心                             肺
      厚                             薄
      之                             之
           气    午   气
              夏至阴生
         血    卯   酉    气
              冬至阳生
           味    子   味
      之                             之
      薄                             厚
      肝                             肾
    阴中之阳                       阴中之阴
     麻黄                           大黄
    柴胡之甘                       调胃之甘
```

Essentials of Medicinal Properties

The herbs with bitter flavor have the action of ascending, so does the slightly cold and mild flavor. The herbs with sweet and pungent flavor have the action of descending, and the herbs with sweet and cold flavor can purge fire. The herbs with bitter and cold flavor can purge damp-heat, and the herbs with sweet and cold flavor can purge blood-heat.

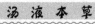
Materia Medica for Decoctions

Ascending and Descending Tendencies of Qi and Flavors Concerning Thick, Thin, Cold, Heat, Yin, Yang

sweet flavor of Guizhi		sweet flavor of Baihu Decoction
Fuzi		Fuling
yang within yang		yin within yang
thick		thin
qi		qi
of		of
the		the
heart	Wu*	lung

yin arising in summer solstice
blood   Mao*   You*   qi
yang arising in winter solstice

liver	Zi*	kidney
the		the
of		of
flavor		flavor
thin		thick
yang within yin		yin within yin
Mahuang		Dahuang
sweet flavor of Chaihu		sweet flavor of Tiaowei Chengqi Decoction

---

* Wu: the seventh of the twelve Earthly Branches

* Mao: the fourth of the twelve Earthly Branches

* You: the tenth of the twelve Earthly Branches

* Zi: the first of the twelve Earthly Branches

升降者天地之气交

茯苓淡，为在天之阳也。阳当上行，何谓利水而泄下？《经》云："气之薄者，乃阳中之阴"，所以茯苓利水而泄下。然而，泄下亦不离乎阳之体，故入手太阳；麻黄苦，为在地之阴也，阴当下行，何谓发汗而升上？《经》云："味之薄者，乃阴中之阳"，所以麻黄发汗而升上。然而，升上亦不离乎阴之体，故入手太阴；附子，气之厚者，乃阳中之阳，故《经》云：发热；大黄，味之厚者，乃阴中之阴，故《经》云：泄下；粥淡，为阳中之阴，所以利小便。茶苦，为阴中之阳，所以清头目。

Actions of Ascending and Descending Being Qi-convergence of the Heaven and the Earth

Fuling [茯苓, Indian bread, Poria] is bland in flavor and pertains to yang of the heaven. Being yang in nature, it has the action of going upward. Why does it have the functions of promoting urination and draining dampness downward? *Huang Di Nei Jing* [《黄帝内经》, *Yellow Emperor's Canon of Medicine*] says that the thin qi pertains to yin within yang, thus Fuling [茯苓, Indian bread, Poria] can promote urination and drain dampness downward. Since the function of draining downward can not be separated from its yang nature, Fuling [茯苓, Poria] enters into the small intestine meridian of hand-taiyang; Mahuang [麻黄, ephedra, Herba Ephedrae] is bitter in flavor and pertains to yin of the earth. Being yin in nature, it has the action of going downward. Why does it have the functions of inducing sweat and dispersing upward? It is also said in *Huang Di Nei Jing* [《黄帝内经》, *Yellow Emperor's Canon of Medicine*] that the thin flavor pertains to yang within yin, thus Mahuang [麻黄, ephedra, Herba Ephedrae] can induce sweat and disperse upward. Since the function of dispersing upward can not be separated from its yin nature, Mahuang [麻黄, ephedra, Herba Ephedrae] enters into the lung meridian of hand-taiyin. Fuzi [附子, aconite, Radix Aconiti Praeparata] pertains to yang within yang with thick qi and has the action of warming; Dahuang [大黄, rhubarb root and rhizome, Radix et Rhizoma Rhei] pertains to yin within yin with thick flavor and has the action of purging; rice porridge is bland in flavor and pertains to yin within yang and has the action of promoting urination. Tea is bitter in flavor and pertains to yang within yin, which can clear heat from the head and eyes.

用药升降浮沉补泻法

肝、胆：味，辛补酸泻；气，温补凉泻（肝胆之经，前后寒热不同，逆顺互换，人求责法）。

心、小肠：味，咸补甘泻；气，热补寒泻（三焦命门补泻同）。

脾、胃：味，甘补苦泻；气，温凉寒热补泻各从其宜（逆从互换，人求责法）。

肺、大肠：味，酸补辛泻；气，凉补温泻。

肾、膀胱：味，苦补咸泻；气，寒补热泻。

五脏更相平也，一脏不平，所胜平之，此之谓也。故云：安谷则昌，绝谷则亡。水去则荣散，谷消则卫亡。荣散卫亡，神无所居。又，仲景云：水入于经，其血乃成，谷入于胃，脉道乃行。故血不可不养，卫不可不温。血温卫和，荣卫将行，常有天命矣。

Supplementing and Purging Actions of Medicinal Herbs Characterized by Ascending, Descending, Floating and Sinking

Liver and gallbladder: As to flavor, pungent flavor can supplement and sour flavor can purge; as to qi, warm can reinforce and cool can reduce. (Since liver and gallbladder channel manifest different properties on the front and back, it should be seriously considered and applied in contrary treatment or routine treatment respectively.)

Heart and small intestine: As to flavor, salty flavor can supplement and sweet flavor can purge; as to qi, heat can reinforce and cold can reduce (the same as reinforcing and reducing the function of the triple energizer and Mingmen acupoint.)

Spleen and stomach: As to flavor, sweet flavor can supplement and bitter flavor can purge; as to qi, different properties of warm, cool, cold and heat should be used according to different conditions. (To apply proper treatment based on the serious consideration.)

Lung and large intestine: As to flavor, sour flavor can supplement and pungent flavor can purge; as to qi, cool can reinforce and warm can reduce.

Kidney and bladder: As to flavor, bitter flavor can supplement and salty flavor can purge; as to qi, cold can reinforce and heat can reduce.

The five zang-organs would be healthy in harmonious state, and the weakness of any of them will be counter-restricted by the one that normally dominates. So it is said that if the patient can eat food, he will be revived, otherwise he will die. The nutrient qi will disperse without water while the defense qi will exhaust without food. And thus spirit has no residence. Zhang Zhongjing says, "The body fluid infuses into the vessels and transforms into blood; the food nutrients enter into the stomach and begin to transform, thus the channels of the body are unimpeded." Blood should be nourished and qi should be warmed, which thus can ensure harmorious and smooth flow of the nutrient qi and the defense qi as well as a long life.

五味所用

苦泄,甘缓,酸收,咸软,淡渗泄,辛散。

Actions of the Five Flavors

Bitter flavor can purge, sweet flavor can relieve spasms and pain, sour flavor can induce astringency, salty flavor can soften hard masses, bland flavor can promote urination, and pungent flavor can disperse.

药类法象

风升生(味之薄者,阴中之阳,味薄则通,酸苦咸平是也):防风(纯阳,性温,味甘辛)、升麻(气平,味微苦)、柴胡(气平,味苦辛)、羌活(气微温,味苦甘平)、威灵仙(气温,味苦)、葛根(气平,味甘)、独活(气微温,味苦甘平)、细辛(气温,味大辛)、桔梗(气微温,味甘辛)、白芷(气温,味大辛)、藁本(气温,味大辛)、鼠黏子(气平,味辛)、蔓荆子(气清,味辛)、川芎(气温,味辛)、天麻(气平,味苦)、秦艽(气微温,味苦辛平)、麻黄(气温,味甘苦)、荆芥(气温,味苦辛)、前胡(气微寒,味苦)、薄荷(气温,味苦辛)。

热浮长(气之厚者,阳中之阳,气厚则发热,辛甘温热是也):黑附子(气热,味大辛)、乌头(气热,味大辛)、干姜(气热,味大辛)、干生姜(气温,味辛)、良姜(气热,味辛,本味甘辛)、肉桂(气热,味大辛)、桂枝(气热,味甘辛)、草豆蔻(气热,味大辛)、丁香(气温,味辛)、厚朴(气温,味辛)、木香(气热,味苦辛)、益智(气热,味大辛)、白豆蔻(气热,味大辛)、川椒(气热温,味大辛)、吴茱萸(气热,味苦辛)、茴香(气平,味辛)、延胡索(气温,味辛)、缩砂(气温,味辛)、红蓝花(气温,味辛)、神曲(气大暖,味甘)。

湿化成(戊,湿,其本气平,其兼气温凉寒热,在人以胃应之。己,土,其本味咸,其兼味辛甘咸苦,在人以脾应之):黄芪(气温平,味甘)、人参(气温,味甘)、甘草(气平,味甘)、当归(气温,味辛,一作味甘)、熟地黄(气寒,味苦)、半夏(气微寒,味辛平)、白术(气温,味甘)、苍术(气温,味甘)、陈皮(气温,味微苦)、青皮(气温,味辛)、藿香(气微温,味甘辛)、槟榔(气温,味辛)、莪术(气平,味苦辛)、京三棱(气平,味苦)、阿胶(气微温,味甘辛)、诃子(气温,味苦)、杏仁(气温,味甘苦)、大麦芽(气温,味咸)、桃仁(气温,味甘苦)、紫草(气寒,味苦)、苏木(气平,味甘咸,一作味酸)。

燥降收(气之薄者,阳中之阴,气薄则发泄,辛甘淡平寒凉是也):茯苓(气平,味甘)、泽泻(气平,味甘)、猪苓(气寒,味甘)、滑石(气寒,味甘)、瞿麦(气平,味甘)、车前子(气寒,味甘)、灯心草(气平,味甘)、五味子(气温,味酸)、桑白皮(气寒,味苦酸)、天门冬(气寒,味微苦)、白芍药(气微寒,味酸)、麦门冬(气寒,味微苦)、犀角(气寒,味苦酸)、乌梅(气平,味酸)、牡丹皮(气寒,味苦)、地骨皮(气寒,味苦)、枳壳(气寒,味苦)、琥珀(气平,味甘)、连翘(气平,味苦)、枳实(气寒,味苦酸)、木通(气平,味甘)。

寒沉藏(味之厚者,阴中之阴,味厚则泄,酸苦咸气寒是也):大黄(气寒,味苦)、黄柏(气寒,味苦)、黄芩(气寒,味苦)、黄连(气寒,味苦)、石膏(气寒,味辛)、草龙胆(气寒,味大苦)、生地黄(气寒,味苦)、知母(气寒,味大辛)、防己(气寒,味大苦)、茵陈(气微寒,味甘平)、朴硝(气寒,味苦辛)、栝楼根(气寒,味苦)、牡蛎(气微寒,味咸平)、玄参(气寒,味微苦)、山栀子(气寒,味微苦)、川楝子(气寒,味苦平)、香豉(气寒,味苦)、地榆(气微寒,味甘咸)。

Rules for the Use of Medicinal Herbs

The herbs with the action of dispersing upward and outward act as wind (the thin flavor pertains to yang within yin which is effective for dredging, sour, bitter, salty and bland in flavor): Fangfeng [防风, divaricate saposhnikovia root, Radix

Saposhnikoviae〕(with yang property, warm in nature and sweet and pungent in flavor), Shengma〔升麻, largetrifoliolious bugbane rhizome, Rhizoma Cimicifugae〕(mild in nature and slightly bitter in flavor), Chaihu〔柴胡, Chinese thorowax root, Radix Bupleuri〕(mild in nature, and bitter and pungent in flavor), Qianghuo〔羌活, incised notopterygium rhizome and root, Rhizoma et Radix Notopterygii〕(slightly warm in nature, and bitter, sweet and bland in flavor), Weilingxian〔威灵仙, Clematis Root, Radix Clematidis Chinese〕(warm in nature and bitter in flavor), Gegen〔葛根, kudzuvine root, Radix Puerariae〕(mild in nature and sweet in flavor), Duhuo〔独活, pubescent angelica, Radix Angelicae Pubescentis〕(slightly warm in nature and bitter and sweet in flavor), Xixin〔细辛, asarum, Asarum sieboldii Miq.〕(warm in nature and highly pungent in flavor), Jiegeng〔桔梗, platycodon root, Platycodon Grandiflorus A. DC.〕(slightly warm in nature and sweet and pungent in flavor), Baizhi〔白芷, root of dahurian angelica, Radix Angelicae Dahuricae〕(warm in nature and highly pungent in flavor), Gaoben〔藁本, Chinese lovage, Rhizoma Ligustici〕(warm in nature and highly pungent in flavor), Shunianzi〔鼠黏子, great burdock achene, Fructus Arctii〕(mild in nature and pungent in flavor), Manjingzi〔蔓荆子, shrub chastetree fruit, Fructus Viticis〕(cold in nature and pungent in flavor), Chuanxiong〔川芎, Sichuan lovage rhizome, Ligusticum Chuanxiong Hort.〕(warm in nature and pungent in flavor), Tianma〔天麻, gastrodia, Gastrodiae Rhizoma〕(mild in nature and bitter in flavor), Qinjiao〔秦艽, largeleaf gentian root, Radix Gentianae Macrophyllae〕(slightly warm in nature, and bitter, bland and pungent in flavor), Mahuang〔麻黄, ephedra, Herba Ephedrae〕(warm in nature, and sweet and bitter in flavor), Jingjie〔荆芥, fineleaf schizonepeta herb, Herba Schizonepetae〕(warm in nature, and bitter and pungent in taste), Qianhu〔前胡, radix peucedani, Peucedanum Praeruptorum Dunn〕(slightly cold in nature and bitter in taste), and Bohe〔薄荷, peppermint, Herba Menthae〕(warm in nature, and bitter and pungent in taste).

The herbs with the action of warming interior and flaring upward act as heat (the thick qi pertains to yang within yang and generates heat, pugent, sweet, warm and heat in flavor): Heifuzi〔黑附子, aconite, Radix Aconiti Praeparata〕(heat in nature and highly pungent in flavor), Wutou〔乌头, common monkshood, Aconitum carmichaeli Debx.〕(heat in nature and highly pungent in flavor), Ganjiang〔干姜, dried ginger, Rhizoma Zingiberis〕(heat in nature and highly pungent in flavor), Ganshengjiang〔干生姜, fresh ginger, Rhizoma Zingiberis Recens〕(warm in nature and pungent in flavor), Liangjiang〔良姜, lesser galangal rhizome, Rhizoma Alpiniae Officinarum〕(heat in nature, pungent in flavor, and sweet and pungent in taste), Rougui〔肉桂, cassia bark, Cortex Cinnamomi〕(heat in nature, and highly pungent in flavor), Guizhi〔桂枝, Cinnamon bark, Cortex Cinnamomum Cassia〕(heat in nature and sweet and pungent in flavor), Caodoukou〔草豆蔻, katsumada galangal seed, Semen Alpiniae Katsumadai〕(heat in nature and extremely pungent in flavor), Dingxiang〔丁香, clove, Flos Caryophylli〕(warm in nature and pungent in flavor), Houpu〔厚朴, magnolia bark, Cortex Magnoliae Officinalis〕(warm in nature and pungent in flavor), Muxiang〔木香, root of common aucklandia, Radix Aucklandiae〕(heat in nature, and bitter and pungent in flavor), Yizhi〔益智, sharp-leaf glangal fruit, Fructus Alpiniae oxyphyllae〕(heat in nature and highly pungent in flavor), Baidoukou〔白豆蔻, cardamon fruit, Fructus Ammomi Rotundus〕(heat in nature and extremely pungent in flavor), Chuanjiao〔川椒, zanthoxylum pipertum, Zanthoxylum bungeanum Maxim.〕(heat and warm in nature and highly pungent in flavor), Wuzhuyu〔吴茱萸, evodia, Fructus Evodiae〕(heat in nature and bitter and pungent in taste), Huixiang〔茴香, fennel, Foeniculum vulgare〕(mild in nature and pungent in flavor), Yanhusuo〔延胡索, yanhusuo, Rhizoma Corydalis〕(warm in nature and pungent in flavor), Suosha〔缩砂, Fructus Amomi Xanthioidis, Amomum Villosum Lour. Var. Xanthioides (Wwall. ex Bak.) T. L. Wu et Senjen〕(warm in nature and pungent in flavor), Honglanhua〔红蓝花, Tulipa, Carthamus tinctorius L.〕(warm in nature and pungent in flavor), and Shenqu〔神曲, medicated leaven, Massa Medicata Fermentata〕(extremely warm in nature and sweet in flavor).

The herbs with the action of transforming act as dampness (Wu pertains to dampness, corresponding to stomach, which is mild in nature, also accompanied by warm, cool, cold and heat property. Ji pertains to earth, corresponding to spleen, which is salty in flavor and accompanied by pungent, sweet, salty and bitter flavor): Huangqi〔黄芪, milkvetch root, Radix Astragali seu Hedysari〕

(warm and mild in nature, and sweet in flavor), Renshen [人参, ginseng, Radix Ginseng] (warm in nature and sweet in flavor), Gancao [甘草, liquorice root, Glycyrrhiza uralensis Fisch.] (mild in nature and sweet in flavor), Danggui [当归, Chinese angelica, Radix Angelicae Sinensis] (warm in nature, and pungent or sweet in flavor), Shudihuang [熟地黄, prepared rehmannia root, Radix Rehmanniae Preparata] (cold in nature and bitter in flavor), Banxia [半夏, pinellia tuber, Rhizoma Pinelliae] (slightly cold in nature and pungent in flavor), Baizhu [白术, argehead atractylodes rhizome, Rhizoma Atractylodis Macrocephalae] (warm in nature and sweet in flavor), Cangzhu [苍术, atractylodes rhizome, Rhizoma Atractylodis] (warm in nature and sweet in flavor), Chenpi [陈皮, dried tangerine peel, Pericarpium Citri Reticulatae] (warm in nature and slightly bitter in flavor), Qingpi [青皮, immature tangerine peel, Pericarpium Citri Reticulatae Viride] (warm in nature and pungent in flavor), Huoxiang [藿香, wrinkled gianthyssop herb, Agastache Rugosa] (slightly warm in nature, and sweet and pungent in flavor), Binlang [槟榔, areca seed, Semen Arecae] (warm in nature and pungent in flavor), Ezhu [莪术, zedoray rhizome, Rhizoma Curcumae] (mild in nature, and bitter and pungent in flavor), Jingsanleng [京三棱, common buried rubber, Rhizoma Sparganii] (mild in nature and bitter in flavor), Ejiao [阿胶, ass hide glue, Colla Corii Asini] (slightly warm in nature, and sweet and pungent in flavor), Kezi [诃子, medicine terminalia fruit, Fructus Chebulae] (warm in nature and bitter in flavor), Xingren [杏仁, bitter apricot seed, Semen Armeniacae Amarum] (warm in nature, and sweet and bitter in flavor), Damaiya [大麦芽, germinated barley, Fructus Hordei Germinatus] (warm in nature and salty in flavor), Taoren [桃仁, peach seed, Semen Persicae] (warm in nature, and sweet and bitter in flavor), Zicao [紫草, arnebia root, Radix Lithospermi] (cold in nature and bitter in flavor), and Sumu [苏木, sappan wood, Lignum Sappan] (mild in nature, sweet and salty in flavor, or sour in flavor).

The herbs with the action of drying and astringing downward act as dryness (the thin qi pertains to yin within yang and has the function of dispersing, pungent, sweet, bland, mild, cool and cold in flavor): Fuling [茯苓, Indian bread, Poria] (mild in nature and sweet in flavor), Zexie [泽泻, oriental waterplantain rhizome, Rhizoma Alismatis〕(mild in nature and sweet in flavor), Zhuling〔猪苓, zhuling, Polyporus Umbellatus〕(cold in nature and sweet in flavor), Huashi〔滑石, talc, Talcum〕(cold in nature and sweet in flavor), Qumai〔瞿麦, lilac pink herb, Herba Dianthi〕(mild in nature and sweet in flavor), Cheqianzi〔车前子, plantain seed, Semen Plantaginis〕(cold in nature and sweet in flavor), Dengxincao〔灯心草, common rush, Medulla Junci〕(mild in nature and sweet in flavor), Wuweizi〔五味子, Chinese magnoliavine fruit, Fructus Schisandrae Chinensis〕(warm in nature and sour in flavor), Sangbaipi〔桑白皮, white mulberry root-bark, Cortex Mori〕(cold in nature and bitter and sour in flavor), Tianmendong〔天门冬, cochinchinese asparagus root, Radix Asparagi〕(cold in nature and slightly bitter in flavor), Baishao〔白芍, white peony root, Radix Paeoniae Alba〕(slightly cold in nature and sour in flavor), Maimendong〔麦门冬, radix ophiopogonis, Ophiopogon Japonicus Ker-Gawl〕(cold in nature and slightly bitter in flavor), Xijiao〔犀角, rhinoceros horn, Rhinoceros unicornis L.〕(cold in nature, and bitter and sour in flavor), Wumei〔乌梅, smoked plum, Fructus Mume〕(mild in nature and sour in flavor), Mudanpi〔牡丹皮, tree peony root bark, Cortex Moutan Radicis〕(cold in nature and bitter in flavor), Digupi〔地骨皮, Chinese wolfberry root-bark, Cortex Lycii〕(cold in nature and bitter in flavor), Zhiqiao〔枳壳, orange fruit, Fructus Aurantii〕(cold in nature and bitter in flavor), Hupo〔琥珀, Amber, Ambrum〕(mild in nature and sweet in flavor), Lianqiao〔连翘, weeping forsythia capsule, Fructus Forsythiae〕(mild in nature and bitter in flavor), Zhishi〔枳实, immature orange fruit, Fructus Aurantii Immaturus〕(cold in nature, and bitter and sour in flavor), and Mutong〔木通, akebia stem, Caulis Akebiae〕(mild in nature and sweet in flavor).

The herbs with the action of storing and sinking inward act as cold (the thick flavor pertains to yin within yin and it is helpful for purgation, sour, bitter, salty and cold in flavor): Dahuang〔大黄, rhubarb root and rhizome, Radix et Rhizoma Rhei〕(cold in nature and bitter in flavor), Huangbo〔黄柏, bark of amur corktree, Cortex Phellodendri〕(cold in nature and bitter in flavor), Huangqin〔黄芩, baical skullcap root, Radix Scutellariae〕(cold in nature and bitter in flavor), Huanglian〔黄连, golden thread, Rhizoma Coptidis〕(cold in nature and bitter in flavor), Shigao [石膏, gypsum, Gypsum Fibrosum] (cold in nature and pungent in flavor), Caolongdan [草龙胆, Chinese gentian, Radix Gentianae] (cold in nature and extremely bitter in flavor), Shengdihuang [生地黄, unprocessed rehmannia root, Radix Rehmanniae Recens] (cold in nature and bitter in flavor), Zhimu [知母, common anemarrhena rhizome, Rhizoma Anemarrhenae] (cold in nature and extremely pungent in flavor), Fangji [防己, mealy fangji root, Stephania tetrandra] (cold in nature and extremely bitter in flavor), Yinchen [茵陈, virgate wormwood herb, Herba Artemisiae Scopariae] (slightly cold in nature, and sweet and bland in flavor), Puxiao [朴硝, crystallized sodium sulfate, Natrii Sulfas] (cold in nature, and bitter and pungent in flavor), Gualougen [栝楼根, snakegourd root, Radix Trichosanthis] (cold in nature and bitter in flavor), Muli [牡蛎, oyster shell, Concha Ostreae] (slightly cold in nature, and salty and bland in flavor), Xuanshen [玄参, figwort root, Radix Scrophulariae] (cold in nature and slightly bitter in flavor), Shanzhizi [山栀子, cape jasmine fruit, Fructus Gardeniae] (cold in nature and slightly bitter in flavor), Chuanlianzi [川楝子, szechwan chinaberry fruit, Fructus Meliae Toosendan] (cold in nature, and bitter and bland in flavor), Xiangchi [香豉, fermented soybean, Semen Sojae Preparatum] (cold in nature and bitter in flavor), and Diyu [地榆, garden burnet root, Radix Sanguisorbae] (slightly cold in nature, and sweet and salty in flavor).

标本阴阳论

天阳无圆，气上外升，生浮昼动，轻燥六腑。

地阴有方，血下内降，杀沉夜静，重湿五脏。

夫治病者，当知标本。以身论之，则外为标、内为本，阳为标、阴为本，故六腑属阳为标，五脏属阴为本，此脏腑之标本也。又，脏腑在内为本，各脏腑之经络在外为标，此脏腑经络之标本也。更，人身之脏腑阴阳、气血经络，各有标本也。以病论之，先受病为本，后传流病为标。凡治者，必先治其本，后治其标。若先治其标，后治其本，邪气滋甚，其病益畜。若先治其本，后治其标，虽病有十数证皆去矣。谓如先生轻病，后滋生重病，亦先治轻病，后治重病，如是则邪气乃伏，盖先治本故也。若有中满，无问标本，先治中满，谓其急也。若中满后有大小便不利，亦无问标本，先利大小便，次治中满，谓尤急也。除大小便不利及中满三者之外，皆治其本，不可不慎也。

从前来者，为实邪，从后来者为虚邪，此子能令母实，母能令子虚是也。治法云：虚则补其母，实则泻其子。假令肝受心火之邪，是从前来者，为实邪，当泻其子，火也。然非直泻其火，十二经中各有金木水火土，当木之分，泻其火也。故《标本论》云：本而标之，先治其本，后治其标。既肝受火邪，先于肝经五穴中泻荥心，行间穴是也。后治其标者，于心经五穴内泻荥火，少府穴是也。以药论之，入肝经药为之引，用泻心火药为君，是治实邪之病也。假令肝受肾邪，是从后来者，为虚邪，虚则当补其母。故《标本论》云：标而本之，先治其标，后治其本。既受水邪，当先于肾经涌泉穴中，补水，是先治其标。后于肝经曲泉穴中泻水，是后治其本。此先治其标者，推其至理，亦是先治其本也。以药论之，入肾经药为引，用补肝经药为君是也。

Discussion on Manifestation, Root Cause, Yin and Yang

The heaven yang pertains to qi and goes upward and outward, bearing the properties of being active and floating in the daytime, which slightly dries the six fu-organs.

The earth yin pertains to blood and flows downward and inward, bearing the properties of being static and sinking at night, which highly moistens the five zang-organs.

To treat the diseases, one must be clear about manifestation and root cause. For the human body, the exterior is manifestation and the interior is root cause, and yang belongs to manifestation while yin pertains to root cause. So the six fu-organs belong to yang and manifestation, and the five zang-organs attribute to yin and root cause. Furthermore, the viscera are in the interior and belong to root cause while the meridians are on the exterior and pertain to manifestation. So the viscera, qi, blood, meridians and collaterals of human beings have their own manifestation and root cause respectively. The disease that occurs first belongs to root cause and the one that occurs later attributes to manifestation. The treatment of the disease should concentrate on root cause first and then on manifestation. If the treatment concentrates on manifestation prior to root cause, the pathogenic factors will spread and aggravate the disease. If the treatment first concentrates on root cause and then on manifestation, the disease will be cured though it may be complicated. If the mild disease occurs first and the serious disease later, the treatment should concentrate on the mild first and then the serious, the pathogenic factors will be subdued for the treatment focusing on root cause. If the patient suffers fullness in the chest, the treatment should focus on the fullness first, whether it is manifestation or root cause because the emergency is a priority. If the disease is accompanied by difficulty in urinating and defecating after fullness in the chest, the treatment must concentrate on inducing urination and defecation, and then the fullness. This is also called "treating manifestation for emergency". Except for the three conditions above, the treatment should focus on root cause. It is very important.

The pathogenic factor coming from the front (the child-organ) is known as excess-pathogen; the pathogenic factor coming from the back (the mother-organ) is known as deficiency-pathogen. So reinforcing the child-organ can strengthen the mother-organ and reducing the mother-organ can weaken the child-organ. The treatment method says, "To reinforce the mother-organ in case of deficiency and to reduce the child-organ in case of excess." If the liver is affected by the heart-fire which comes from the front and belongs to excess-pathogen, it should be treated by purging the heart fire. The treatment does not always purge fire directly. According to the five elements in the twelve channels, it is effective to purge fire in case of wood diseases. So *Biao Ben Lun* [《黄帝内经·标本论》, *Yellow Emperor's Internal Canon of Medicine · Biaoben*] says, "A disease with excessive pathogenic factors may cause other diseases. The treatment should first concentrate on root cause and then on manifestation." Thus if the liver is attacked by pathogenic-fire, it should be treated by reducing the fire of Yingxin acupoint, also called Xingjian acupoint, among the five acupoints of the liver channel firstly, and then deals with its manifestation which is treated by reducing the fire of Ying acupoint, also called Shaofu acupoint, among the five acupoints of the heart channel. According to the medication, to treat excessive pathogenic factors, the herbs which can purge heart-fire should be used as the sovereign drug and the ones enter into the liver channel serve as the envoy drug. If the liver is attacked by the kidney-pathogen which comes from the back and belongs to deficient pathogenic factors, it should be treated by supplementing the kidney. So *Biao Ben Lun*［《黄帝内经·标本论》, *Yellow Emperor's Internal Canon of Medicine · Biaoben*］says, "A disease with insufficient healthy-qi may cause some other diseases. The treatment principle should first concentrate on manifestation and then on root cause. If the liver is attacked by kidney-pathogen, it should be treated by reinforcing the water of Yongquan acupoint on the kidney channel, the so-called treating manifestation firstly. And then, it deals with root cause by reducing the water of Ququan acupoint on the liver channel, the so-called treating root cause secondly. The treatment principle of concentration on manifestation first, on the other hand, is also treating root cause firstly. According to the medication, the herbs which can supplement the liver channel should be used as the sovereign drug and the ones enter into the kidney channel should serve as the envoy drug.

五方之正气味（制方用药附）

东方：甲风、乙木，其气温，其味甘，在人以肝、胆应之。
南方：丙热、丁火，其气热，其味辛，在人以心、小肠、三焦、包络应之。
中央：戊湿，其本气平，其兼气温凉寒热，在人以胃应之。
中央：己土，其本味咸，其兼味辛甘酸苦，在人以脾应之。
西方：庚燥、辛金，其气凉，其味酸，在人以肺、大肠应之。
北方：壬寒、癸水，其气寒，其味苦，在人以肾、膀胱应之。

人乃万物中之一也，独阳不生，独阴不长，须禀两仪之气而生化也。圣人垂世立教，不能浑说，必当分析。以至理而言，则阴阳相附不相离，其实一也。呼则因阳出，吸则随阴入。天以阳生阴长，地以阳杀阴藏，此上说止明补泻用药君之一也。故曰：主病者为君。用药之机会，要明轻清成象，重浊成形。本乎天者亲上，本乎地者亲下，则各从其类也。清中清者，清肺以助其天真；清中浊者，荣华腠理；浊中清者，荣养于神；浊中浊者，坚强骨髓。故《至真要大论》云：五味阴阳之用，辛甘发散为阳，酸苦涌泄为阴，淡味渗泄为阳，咸味涌泄为阴。六者或收或散，或缓或急，或燥或润，或软或坚，各以所利而行之，调其气使之平也。详见本论。

Properties and Flavors in Five Orientations

(Prescription Formulating and Drug Medications)

East: Jia (the first of the ten Heavenly Stems) wind and Yi (the second of the ten Heavenly Stems) wood, warm in nature, sweet in flavor, correspond to the liver and gallbladder in human body.

South: Bing (the third of the ten Heavenly Stems) heat and Ding (the fourth of the ten Heavenly Stems) fire, heat in nature, pungent in flavor, correspond to the heart and small intestine in human body.

Centre: Wu (the fifth of the ten Heavenly Stems) dampness, mild in nature, combining warm, cool, cold and heat, corresponds to the stomach in human body.

Centre: Ji (the sixth of the ten Heavenly Stems) earth, originally salty, and sometimes pungent, sweet, sour and bitter in flavor, corresponds to the spleen in human body.

West: Geng (the seventh of the ten Heavenly Stems) dryness and Xin (the eighth of the ten Heavenly Stems) metal, cool in nature, sour in flavor, correspond to the lung and large intestine in human body.

North: Ren (the ninth of the ten Heavenly Stems) cold and Gui (the tenth of the ten Heavenly Stems) water, cold in nature, bitter in flavor, correspond to the kidney and bladder in human body.

The human being is one of the creatures on the earth, who is transformed from yin and yang. Neither yin nor yang can ever exist without the other. The sages known to the world as the advisers must fully analyze all things, otherwise they may mislead the people. For the theory of everything, yin and yang are interdependent and can not be separated. They constitute the wholeness. When a person breathes out, the waste air goes out from the yang phase; when a person breathes in, the fresh air inhaled comes deep into the yin phase. Yang ensures growth while yin promotes development in the heaven. Yang is responsible for killing and yin for storing on the earth. So the herbs which can treat the main diseases are called sovereign drugs. For the drug use, one should be clear about the rule that "the lucid forms image while the turbid produces shape". If the herb pertains to the heaven, it has the action of going upward; if it pertains to the earth, it has the action of going downward. All the herbs ought to be attributed to their own category. The herbs with light and clear properties can clear the lung to promote its natural energy; the herbs with light and turbid properties can nourish muscular interstices; the herbs with heavy and clear properties can replenish spirit; the herbs with heavy and turbid properties can strengthen the bones and marrows. So *Zhi Zhen Yao Da Lun* [《至真要大论》, *Discussion on the Most Important and Abstruse Theory*] says, "The use of herbs with the attributes of the five flavors that pertain to either yin or yang, pungent and sweet flavors pertain to yang for dispersing, sour and bitter flavors pertain to yin for inducing vomiting and purgation, bland flavor pertains to yang for discharging fluid and dampness, salty flavor pertains to yin for inducing vomiting and purgation. The actions of these six flavors are either astringent or dispersing, either moderate or drastic, either drying or moistening, either softening or solidifying. They should be used according to their effects to regulate qi in harmony." See it in the discussion below.

东垣先生《用药心法》
Li Dongyuan's *Yong Yao Xin Fa* [《用药心法》, *Gist for the Use of Medicinal Herbs*]

随证治病药品

如头痛,须用川芎。如不愈,各加引经药:(太阳,川芎;阳明,白芷;少阳,柴胡;太阴,苍术;少阴,细辛;厥阴,吴茱萸)。

如顶巅痛,须用藁本,去川芎;如肢节痛,须用羌活,去风湿亦宜用之;如腹痛,须用芍药,恶寒而痛,加桂,恶热而痛,加黄柏;如心下痞,须用枳实、黄连;如肌热及去痰者,须用黄芩,肌热,亦用黄芪;如腹胀,用姜制厚朴。如虚热,须用黄芪,止虚汗,亦用;如胁下痛,往来潮热,日晡潮热,须用柴胡;如脾胃受湿,沉困无力,怠惰好卧,去痰,用白术;如破滞气,用枳壳,高者用之,夫枳壳者,损胸中至高之气,二三服而已;如破滞血,用桃仁、苏木;如补血不足,须用甘草;如去痰,须用半夏,热痰加黄芩,风痰加南星,胸中寒痰痞塞,用陈皮、白术,多用则泻脾胃；如腹中窄狭，须用苍术；如调气，须用木香；如补气，须用人参；如和血，须用当归，凡血受病者，皆宜用当归也；如去下焦湿肿及痛，并膀胱有火邪者，必须酒洗防己、草龙胆、黄柏、知母；如去上焦湿及热，须用黄芩，泻肺火故也；如去中焦湿与痛热，用黄连，能泻心火故也；如去滞气用青皮，勿多服，多则泻人真气；如渴者，用干葛、茯苓，禁半夏；如嗽者，用五味子；如喘者，用阿胶；如宿食不消，须用黄连、枳实；如胸中烦热，须用栀子仁；如水泻，须用白术、茯苓、芍药；如气刺痛，用枳壳，看何部分，以引经药导使之行则可；如血刺痛，用当归，详上下，用根梢；如疮痛不可忍者，用寒苦药，如黄柏、黄芩；详上下，用根梢，及引经药则可；如眼痛不可忍者，用黄连、当归身，以酒浸煎；如小便黄者，用黄柏；数者、涩者，或加泽泻；如腹中实热，用大黄、芒硝；如小腹痛，用青皮；如茎中痛，用生甘草梢；如惊悸恍惚，用茯神；如饮水多，致伤脾，用白术、茯苓、猪苓；如胃脘痛，用草豆蔻。凡用纯寒、纯热药，必用甘草，以缓其力也；寒热相杂，亦用甘草，调和其性也。中满者禁用，《经》云：中满者勿食甘。

Medicinal Herbs for Disease Treatment According to the Syndromes

The symptom of headache should be treated with Chuanxiong [川芎, Sichuan lovage rhizome, Ligusticum Chuanxiong Hort]. If it is not cured, the channel ushering drug should be added: Chuanxiong [川芎, Sichuan lovage rhizome, Ligusticum Chuanxiong Hort] is usually applied for Taiyang headache, Baizhi [白芷, root of dahurian angelica, Radix Angelicae Dahuricae] for Yangming headache, Chaihu [柴胡, Chinese thorowax root, Radix Bupleuri] for Shaoyang disease, Cangzhu [苍术, atractylodes rhizome, Rhizoma Atractylodis] for Taiyin headache, Xixin [细辛, asarum, Asarum sieboldii Miq.] for Shaoyin headache, Wuzhuyu [吴茱萸, evodia, Fructus Evodiae] for Jueyin headache.

If the parietal headache exists, Gaoben [藁本, Chinese lovage, Rhizoma Ligustici] should be used to replace Chuanxiong [川芎, Sichuan lovage rhizome, Ligusticum Chuanxiong Hort.]. If the arthrodynia of the limbs exists, Qianghuo [羌活, notopterygium, Notopterygii Rhizoma et Radix] should be used, and it is also applied in dispelling the wind dampness syndrome. If the abdominal pain exists, Shaoyao [芍药, Chinese herbaceous peony, Paeonia lactiflora Pall.] should be used. Guizhi [桂枝, Cinnamon bark, Cortex Cinnamomum Cassia] can be added when it manifests the aversion to cold and pain, and Huangbo [黄柏,

bark of amur corktree, Cortex Phellodendri] is added while it manifests the aversion to heat and pain. If there is fullness below the heart, Zhishi [枳实, immature orange fruit, Fructus Aurantii Immaturus] and Huanglian [黄连, golden thread, Rhizoma Coptidis] should be used. If the patients suffer from the scorching heat in muscles, Huangqin [黄芩, baical skullcap root, Radix Scutellariae] and Huangqi [黄芪, milkvetch root, Radix Astragali seu Hedysari] can be applied, and the former can also dispel phlegm. If the abdominal distension exists, Houpu [厚朴, magnolia bark, Cortex Magnoliae Officinalis] processed by ginger juice should be used. Huangqi [黄芪, milkvetch root, Radix Astragali seu Hedysari] can be used to treat the deficiency heat syndrome and sweating due to debility. If the patients suffer from hypochondriac pain, alternation of cold and heat, tidal fever in the late afternoon, Chaihu [柴胡, Chinese thorowax root, Radix Bupleuri] should be used. If the spleen and stomach suffer from dampness and manifest heaviness and weakness, lassitude and somnolence, Baizhu [白术, argehead atractylodes rhizome, Rhizoma Atractylodis Macrocephalae] should be used to expel phlegm. Zhiqiao [枳壳, orange fruit, Fructus Aurantii] can be used to break the stagnant qi in the upper portion, for it is the herb which can resolve the stagnant qi in the chest, and 2 or 3 doses of it are enough. Taoren [桃仁, peach seed, Semen Persicae] and Sumu [苏木, sappan wood, Lignum Sappan] can be used to break the blood stasis, while Gancao [甘草, liquorice root, Glycyrrhiza uralensis Fisch.] can tonify the blood. If phlegm exists, Banxia [半夏, pinellia, Rhizoma Pinelliae] should be used, and Huangqin [黄芩, baical skullcap root, Radix Scutellariae] can be added for heat-phlegm and Nanxing [南星, jackinthepulpit tuber, Rhizoma Arisaematis] for wind-phlegm. If there is cold phlegm and fullness in the chest, it can be treated with Chenpi [陈皮, Tangerine Peel, Pericarpium Citri Reticulatae] and Baizhu [白术, argehead atractylodes rhizome, Rhizoma Atractylodis Macrocephalae] which can purge the spleen and stomach with large doses. Cangzhu [苍术, atractylodes rhizome, Rhizoma Atractylodis] should be used if there is fullness in the abdomen. Muxiang [木香, root of common aucklandia, Radix Aucklandiae] should be used to regulate qi, and Renshen [人参, ginseng, Radix Ginseng] can be applied for tonifying qi and Danggui [当归, Chinese angelica, Radix Angelicae Sinensis] for harmonizing blood. Danggui〔当归, Chinese angelica, Radix Angelicae Sinensis〕can be used for all the blood syndromes. If there exist dampness-edema and pain in the lower energizer accompanied by the pathogenic fire in the bladder, Fangji〔防己, mealy fangji root, Stephania tetrandra〕, Caolongdan〔草龙胆, Chinese gentian, Radix Gentianae〕, Huangbo〔黄柏, bark of amur corktree, Cortex Phellodendri〕and Zhimu〔知母, common anemarrhena rhizome, Rhizoma Anemarrhenae〕processed by wine should be applied. If there is dampness fire in the upper energizer, Huangqin〔黄芩, baical skullcap root, Radix Scutellariae〕should be used to purge the lung fire. When dampness, fire and pain exist in the middle energizer, Huanglian〔黄连, golden thread, Rhizoma Coptidis〕should be used to purge the heart fire. Qingpi〔青皮, immature tangerine peel, Pericarpium Citri Reticulatae Viride〕can be used to break the stagnant qi, but it should not be overdosed for it can damage the genuine qi. Gegen〔葛根, kudzuvine root, Radix Puerariae〕and Fuling〔茯苓, Indian bread, Poria〕can be applied when thirst exists, and it is forbidden to use Banxia〔半夏, pinellia, Rhizoma Pinelliae〕. Patients can use Wuweizi〔五味子, Chinese magnoliavine fruit, Fructus Schisandrae Chinensis〕for the treatment of cough, Ejiao〔阿胶, ass hide glue, Colla Corii Asini〕for asthma, Huanglian〔黄连, golden thread, Rhizoma Coptidis〕and Zhishi〔枳实, immature orange fruit, Fructus Aurantii Immaturus〕for indigestion, and Shanzhizi〔山栀子, cape jasmine fruit, Fructus Gardeniae〕for irritable feverish sensation in chest. Baizhu〔白术, argehead atractylodes rhizome, Rhizoma Atractylodis Macrocephalae〕, Fuling〔茯苓, Indian bread, Poria〕and Shaoyao〔芍药, Chinese herbaceous peony, Paeonia lactiflora Pall.〕are applied to deal with the watery diarrhea. The stabbing pain due to qi stagnation can be treated with Zhiqiao〔枳壳, orange fruit, Fructus Aurantii〕, accompanied by the use of channel ushering drugs according to the disease location. For the stabbing pain due to blood stasis, the root tubers or tips of Danggui〔当归, Chinese angelica, Radix Angelicae Sinensis〕can be applied respectively according to different locations. If there are severe sores with unbearable pain, it should be treated by the herbs with cold and bitter nature such as Huangbo〔黄柏, bark of amur corktree, Cortex Phellodendri〕and Huangqin〔黄芩, baical skullcap root, Radix Scutellariae〕. According to different locations, different medicinal parts of drugs and different channel ushering drugs, herbs are selected. For the case of unbearable eye pain, the wine-processed root tubers of Huanglian〔黄连, golden thread, Rhizoma Coptidis〕and Danggui〔当归, Chinese angelica, Radix Angelicae Sinensis〕should be applied. Huangbo〔黄柏, bark of amur corktree, Cortex Phellodendri〕is used to treat yellowish urine, combined with Zexie〔泽泻, oriental waterplantain rhizome, Rhizoma Alismatis〕for the frequent urination and dysuria. If there is excess heat in the abdomen, Dahuang〔大黄, rhubarb root and rhizome, Radix et Rhizoma Rhei〕and Mangxiao〔芒硝, crystallized sodium sulfate, Natrii Sulfas〕can be used. Qingpi〔青皮, immature tangerine peel, Pericarpium Citri Reticulatae Viride〕is used to treat the lower abdominal pain, and the raw root tips of Gancao〔甘草, liquorice root, Glycyrrhiza uralensis Fisch.〕are used to treat the pain in penis and Fushen〔茯神, poria with hostwood; Poria cocos(Schw.) Wolf.〕for palpitating with fear. For the case of profuse drinking damaging spleen, it can be treated with Baizhu〔白术, argehead atractylodes rhizome, Rhizoma Atractylodis Macrocephalae〕, Fuling〔茯苓, Indian bread, Poria〕and Zhuling〔猪苓, zhuling, Polyporus Umbellatus〕. Caodoukou〔草豆蔻, katsumada galangal seed, Semen Alpiniae Katsumadai〕is used to deal with the epigastric pain. When applying the herbs with pure cold or pure heat properties, they should be combined with Gancao〔甘草, liquorice root, Glycyrrhiza uralensis Fisch.〕to moderate the efficacy, or to harmonize the drug properties. In the case of abdominal fullness, Gancao〔甘草, liquorice root, Glycyrrhiza uralensis Fisch.〕is forbidden to use. *Huang Di Nei Jing*〔《黄帝内经》, *Yellow Emperor's Internal Canon of Medicine*〕says, "The herbs with sweet property are forbidden to apply on the abdominal fullness."

用药凡例

凡解利伤风，以防风为君；甘草、白术为佐。《经》云：辛甘发散为阳。风宜辛散，防风味辛及治风通用，故防风为君，甘草、白术为佐。

凡解利伤寒，以甘草为君，防风、白术为佐，是寒宜甘发也。或有别证，于前随证治病药内选用。分两以君臣论。

凡眼暴发赤肿，以防风、黄芩为君，以泻火；以黄连、当归身和血，为佐。兼以各经药用之。

凡眼久病昏暗,以熟地黄、当归身为君;以羌活、防风为臣;甘草、甘菊之类为佐。

凡痢疾腹痛,以白芍药、甘草为君;当归、白术为佐。便血先后,以三焦热论。

凡水泻,以茯苓、白术为君;芍药、甘草为佐。

凡诸风,以防风为君,随治病为佐。

凡嗽,以五味子为君;有痰者,以半夏为佐;喘者,以阿胶为佐;有热、无热,以黄芩为佐,但分两多寡不同耳。

凡小便不利,黄柏、知母为君;茯苓、泽泻为佐。

凡下焦有湿,草龙胆、防己为君;甘草、黄柏为佐。

凡痔漏,以苍术、防风为君;甘草、芍药为佐。详别证加减。

凡诸疮,以黄连、当归为君;甘草、黄芩为佐。

凡疟,以柴胡为君,随所发时所属经,分用引经药佐之。

已上皆用药之大要。更详别证于前,随证治病药内,逐旋加减用之。

Notes on Medication

In treating wind diseases, Fangfeng [防风, divaricate saposhnikovia root, Radix Saposhnikoviae] serves as the sovereign drug, and Gancao [甘草, liquorice root, Glycyrrhiza uralensis Fisch.] and Baizhu [白术, argehead atractylodes rhizome, Rhizoma Atractylodis Macrocephalae] serve as assistant drugs. *Huang Di Nei Jing* [《黄帝内经》, *Yellow Emperor's Canon of Medicine*] says, "Pungent and sweet flavors pertain to yang because they disperse." As the wind syndrome should be dispersed by pungent herbs and Fangfeng [防风, divaricate saposhnikovia root, Radix Saposhnikoviae] is pungent in nature and indicates to the wind syndrome, it is the sovereign drug. Gancao [甘草, liquorice root, Glycyrrhiza uralensis Fisch.] and Baizhu [白术, argehead atractylodes rhizome, Rhizoma Atractylodis Macrocephalae] are assistant drugs.

In treating cold diseases, Gancao [甘草, liquorice root, Glycyrrhiza uralensis Fisch.] usually serves as the sovereign drug, and Fangfeng [防风, divaricate saposhnikovia root, Radix Saposhnikoviae] and Baizhu [白术, argehead atractylodes rhizome, Rhizoma Atractylodis Macrocephalae] serve as assistant drugs, which is consistent with the rule of "the cold syndrome should be dispersed with herbs with sweet nature". If it is accompanied with other syndromes, one should select the herbs in the group which deal with the former syndromes and classify them into sovereign and assistant drugs.

In the case of acute inflamed eye diseases, Fangfeng [防风, divaricate saposhnikovia root, Radix Saposhnikoviae] and Huangqin [黄芩, baical skullcap root, Radix Scutellariae] serve as sovereign drugs to purge fire, and Huanglian [黄连, golden thread, Rhizoma Coptidis] and Danggui [当归, Chinese angelica, Radix Angelicae Sinensis] serve as assistant drugs to harmonize blood, combined with ushering drugs of each channel.

In treating chronic eye diseases, Shudihuang [熟地黄, prepared rehmannia root, Radix Rehmanniae Preparata] and Danggui [当归, Chinese angelica, Radix Angelicae Sinensis] are used as sovereign drugs, Qianghuo [羌活, notopterygium, Notopterygii Rhizoma et Radix] and Fangfeng [防风, divaricate saposhnikovia root, Radix Saposhnikoviae] as minister drugs, and Gancao [甘草, liquorice root, Glycyrrhiza uralensis Fisch.] as the assistant drug.

In the case of dysentery and abdominal pain, Baishao [白芍, white peony root, Radix Paeoniae Alba] and Gancao [甘草, liquorice root, Glycyrrhiza uralensis Fisch.] usually serve as sovereign drugs, and Danggui [当归, Chinese angelica, Radix Angelicae Sinensis] and Baizhu [白术, argehead atractylodes rhizome, Rhizoma Atractylodis Macrocephalae] serve as assistant drugs. The manifestations of early or late arrival of hemafecia are treated according to the location of heat in the triple energizer.

For those with watery diarrhea, Fuling [茯苓, Indian bread, Poria] and Baizhu [白术, argehead atractylodes rhizome, Rhizoma Atractylodis Macrocephalae] serve as sovereign drugs, and Shaoyao [芍药, Chinese herbaceous peony, Paeonia lactiflora Pall.] and Gancao [甘草, liquorice root, Glycyrrhiza uralensis Fisch.] serve as assistant drugs.

For those with wind syndromes, Fangfeng [防风, divaricate saposhnikovia root, Radix Saposhnikoviae] always acts as the sovereign drug, other herbs dealing with the syndromes act as the assistant drugs.

In treating cough, Wuweizi [五味子, Chinese magnoliavine fruit, Fructus

Schisandrae Chinensis] serves as the sovereign drug. Banxia [半夏, pinellia tuber, Rhizoma Pinelliae] serves as the assistant drug if it is accompanied with phlegm. With asthma, Ejiao [阿胶, ass hide glue, Colla Corii Asini] always acts as the assistant drug. With heat or not, Huangqin [黄芩, baical skullcap root, Radix Scutellariae] can serve as the assistant drug with different doses according to different conditions.

If difficult urination exists, Huangbo [黄柏, bark of amur corktree, Cortex Phellodendri] and Zhimu [知母, common anemarrhena rhizome, Rhizoma Anemarrhenae] are chosen to be the sovereign drugs, while Fuling [茯苓, Indian bread, Poria] and Zexie [泽泻, oriental waterplantain rhizome, Rhizoma Alismatis] as assistant drugs.

For those with dampness in lower energizer, Caolongdan [草龙胆, Chinese gentian, Radix Gentianae] and Fangji [防己, mealy fangji root, Stephania tetrandra] are used to be the sovereign drugs, and Gancao [甘草, liquorice root, Glycyrrhiza uralensis Fisch.] and Huangbo [黄柏, bark of amur corktree, Cortex Phellodendri] are the assistant drugs.

In treating anal fistula, Cangzhu [苍术, atractylodes rhizome, Rhizoma Atractylodis] and Fangfeng [防风, divaricate saposhnikovia root, Radix Saposhnikoviae] serve as sovereign drugs, and Gancao [甘草, liquorice root, Glycyrrhiza Uralensis Fisch.] and Shaoyao [芍药, Chinese herbaceous peony, Paeonia lactiflora Pall.] serve as assistant drugs. It is modified according to other syndromes.

To treat all the sore syndromes, Huanglian [黄连, golden thread, Rhizoma Coptidis] and Danggui [当归, Chinese angelica, Radix Angelicae Sinensis] serve as sovereign drugs, and Gancao [甘草, liquorice root, Glycyrrhiza uralensis Fisch.] and Huangqin [黄芩, baical skullcap root, Radix Scutellariae] serve as assistant drugs.

In treating malaria, Chaihu [柴胡, Chinese thorowax root, Radix Bupleuri] always serves as the sovereign drug, and channel ushering drugs act as assistant drugs in accordance with different channel diseases.

All the above are the essentials of medication. One should modify the herbs according to the different syndromes while making further syndrome differentiation.

东垣报使

太阳:羌活,下黄柏。
阳明:白芷、升麻,下石膏。
少阳:柴胡,下青皮。
太阴:白芍药。
少阴:知母。
厥阴:青皮,柴胡。
小腹膀胱属太阳,藁本羌活是本方。
三焦胆与肝包络,少阳厥阴柴胡强。
阳明大肠兼足胃,葛根白芷升麻当。
太阴肺脉中焦起,白芷升麻葱白乡。
脾经少与肺经异,升麻芍药白者详。
少阴心经独活主,肾经独活加桂良。
通经用此药为使,更有何病到膏肓。

Guiding Action of Medicinal Herbs by Li Dongyuan

Taiyang channel: Qianghuo [羌活, notopterygium, Notopterygii Rhizoma et Radix] is the channel ushering drug, and Huangbo [黄柏, bark of amur corktree, Cortex Phellodendri] is applied for lower portion.

Yangming channel: Baizhi [白芷, root of dahurian angelica, Radix Angelicae Dahuricae] and Shengma [升麻, largetrifoliolious bugbane rhizome, Rhizoma Cimicifugae] are channel ushering drugs, and Shigao [石膏, gypsum, Gypsum Fibrosum] is always indicated for lower portion.

Shaoyang channel: Chaihu [柴胡, Chinese thorowax root, Radix Bupleuri] is the channel ushering drug, while Qingpi [青皮, immature tangerine peel, Pericarpium Citri Reticulatae Viride] is applied for lower portion.

Taiyin channel: Baishao [白芍, white peony root, Radix Paeoniae Alba] is the channel ushering drug.

Shaoyin channel: Zhimu [知母, common anemarrhena rhizome, Rhizoma Anemarrhenae] is the channel ushering drug.

Jueyin channel: Qingpi [青皮, immature tangerine peel, Pericarpium Citri Reticulatae Viride] and Chaihu [柴胡, Chinese thorowax root, Radix Bupleuri] are the channel ushering drugs.

Lower abdomen and bladder belong to Taiyang channel, and Gaoben [藁本, Chinese lovage, Rhizoma Ligustici] and Qianghuo [羌活, notopterygium, Notopterygii Rhizoma et Radix] enter this channel.

The triple energizer, gallbladder and liver belong to Shaoyang channel, and Chaihu [柴胡, Chinese thorowax root, Radix Bupleuri] is the channel ushering drug.

The large intestine and stomach belong to Yangming channel, Gegen [葛根, kudzuvine root, Radix Puerariae], Baizhi [白芷, root of dahurian angelica, Radix Angelicae Dahuricae] and Shengma [升麻, largetrifoliolious bugbane rhizome, Rhizoma Cimicifugae] enter Yangming channel.

The lung and middle energizer belong to Taiyin channel, and Baizhi [白芷, root of dahurian angelica, Radix Angelicae Dahuricae], Shengma [升麻, largetrifoliolious bugbane rhizome, Rhizoma Cimicifugae] and Congbai [葱白, fistular onion stalk, Allium fislulosum L.] are their channel ushering drugs.

The spleen also belongs to Taiyin channel, and Shengma [升麻, largetrifoliolious bugbane rhizome, Rhizoma Cimicifugae] and Baishao [白芍, white peony root, Radix Paeoniae Alba] are the channel ushering drugs.

Duhuo [独活, pubescent angelica, Radix Angelicae Pubescentis] is the channel ushering drug of hand-shaoyin channel, and Duhuo [独活, pubescent angelica, Radix Angelicae Pubescentis] and Rougui [肉桂, cassia bark, Cortex Cinnamomi] usually enter the channel of foot-shaoyin.

If the disease is treated properly by these channel ushering drugs, it will not deteriorate.

诸经向导

寅手太阴肺经 向导图　脾足巳	南星　款冬花　升麻　桔梗　檀香 山药　粳米　白茯苓　五味子　天门冬 阿胶　麦门冬　桑白皮　杏仁　葱白 麻黄　丁香　益智　白豆蔻　知母 缩砂（檀香豆蔻为使）　栀子　黄芩　石膏	升麻　芍药 木瓜 藿香
	防风　当归 草豆蔻　茱萸　缩砂（人参益智为使） 益智　黄芪　苍术　白术　胶饴 代赭石　赤茯苓　麻仁　甘草　半夏	白芍药（酒浸） 延胡索 缩砂

卯手大肠阳明经 向导图　胃足辰	升麻　白芷　麻仁　秦艽　薤白 白石脂　缩砂（白石脂为使）　肉豆蔻　石膏	麻黄 大黄 连翘 升麻　白芷　葛根
	丁香　草豆蔻　缩砂　防风　石膏 知母　白术　神曲　葛根　乌药 半夏　苍术　升麻　白芷　葱白	石膏 白术 檀香（佐以他药下） 白芷　升麻 石膏

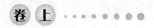

亥三焦手少阳经 向导图 足胆子	川芎　柴胡　青皮　白术　熟地黄 黄芪　地骨皮　石膏　细辛　附子	青皮　川芎 柴胡
	半夏　草龙胆　柴胡	连翘 柴胡　下青皮

戌心包手厥阴经 向导图 足肝五	沙参　白术　柴胡　熟地黄　牡丹皮　败酱	青皮　柴胡 熟地黄
	草龙胆　蔓荆子　阿胶　瞿麦　桃仁 山茱萸　代赭石　紫石英　当归　甘草 青皮　羌活　吴茱萸　白术	柴胡 川芎 皂角 桃仁 茗苦茶

未小肠手太阳经 向导图 足膀胱申	白术　生地黄　赤茯苓　羌活　赤石脂 缩砂（赤石脂为使）	防风　羌活 藁本　蔓荆 茴香　黄柏
	蔓荆子　滑石　茵陈　白茯苓 猪苓　泽泻　桂枝　黄柏 羌活　麻黄	白术　泽泻 防己 大黄（酒浸） 藁本　羌活 羌活下　黄柏

午心手少阴经　向导图　足肾酉右肾附	麻黄　桂心　当归　生地黄　黄连 代赭石　紫石英　栀子　独活　赤茯苓	细辛 熟地黄 五味子 泽泻 地榆 附子 知母 白术
	知母　黄柏　地骨皮　阿胶　猪肤 牡丹皮　玄参　败酱　牡蛎　乌药 山茱萸　天门冬　猪苓　泽泻　白茯苓 檀香　甘草　五味子　茱萸　益智	
	丁香　独活（或用梢）　桔梗（或用梢）　豉 　缩砂（黄柏、茯苓为使）	
	附子　沉香　益智　黄芪	

Channel Entering

Yin (the third of the twelve Earthly Branches) The Lung Meridian of Hand-Taiyin Guiding Chart The Spleen Meridian of Foot-Taiyin Si (the sixth of the twelve Earthly Branches)	Nanxing　Kuandonghua　Shengma　Jiegeng Tanxiang　Shanyao　Jingmi　Baifuling　Wuweizi Tianmendong　Ejiao　Maimendong　Sangbaipi Xingren　Congbai　Mahuang　Dingxiang　Yizhi Baidoukou　Zhimu　Suosha（Tanxiang and Doukou serving as the assistant）　Zhizi　Huangqin　Shigao	Shengma Shaoyao Mugua Huoxiang
	Fangfeng　Danggui Caodoukou　Zhuyu　Suosha（Renshen and Yizhi serving as the assistant） Yizhi　Huangqi　Cangzhu　Baizhu　Jiaoyi Daizheshi　Chifuling　Maren　Gancao　Banxia	Baishaoyao (soaked with wine) Yanhusuo Suosha

Mao (the fourth of the twelve Earthly Branches) The Large Intestine Meridian of Hand-Yangming Guiding Chart The Stomach Meridian of Foot-Yangming Chen (the fifth of the twelve Earthly Branches)	Shengma Baizh Maren Qinjiao Xiebai Baishizhi Suosha (Baishizhi serving as the envoy) Roudoukou Shigao	Mahuang Dahuang Lianqiao Shengma Baizhi Gegen
	Dingxiang Caodoukou Suosha Fangfeng Shigao Zhimu Baizhu Shenqu Gegen Wuyao Banxia Cangzhu Shengma Baizhi Congbai	Shigao Baizhu Tanxiang (assisted by other drugs) Baizhi Shengma Shigao

Hai (the last of the twelve Earthly Branches) The Triple Energizer Meridian of Hand-Shaoyang Guiding Chart The Gallbladder Meridian of Hand-Shaoyang Zi (the first of the twelve Earthly Branches)	Chuanxiong Chaihu Qingpi Baizhu Shudihuang Huangqi Digupi Shigao Xixin Fuzi	Qingpi Chuanxiong Chaihu
	Banxia Caolongdan Chaihu	Lianqiao Chaihu Lower Qingpi

Xu (the eleventh of the twelve Earthly Branches) The Pericardium Meridian of Hand-Jueyin Guiding Chart	Shashen Baizhu Chaihu Shudihuang Mudanpi Baijiang	Qingpi Chaihu Shudihuang
The Liver Meridian of Foot-Jueyin Chou (the second of the twelve Earthly Branches)	Caolongdan Manjingzi Ejiao Qumai Taoren Shanzhuyu Daizheshi Zishiying Danggui Gancao Qingpi Qianghuo Wuzhuyu Baizhu	Chaihu Chuanxiong Zaojiao Taoren Mingkucha

Wei (the eighth of the twelve Earthly Branches) The Small Intestine Meridian of Hand-Taiyang Guiding Chart	Baizhu Shengdihuang Chifuling Qianghuo Chishizhi Suosha (Chishizhi serving as the envoy)	Fangfeng Qianghuo Gaoben Manjing Huixiang Huangbo
The Bladder Meridian of Foot-Taiyang Shen (the ninth of the twelve Earthly Branches)	Manjingzi Huashi Yinchen Baifuling Zhuling Zexie Guizhi Huangbo Qianghuo Mahuang	Baizhu Zexie Fangji Dahuang (soaked with wine) Gaoben Qianghuo Lower Qianghuo Huangbo

Wu (the seventh of the twelve Earthly Branches) The Heart Meridian of Hand-Shaoyin Guiding Chart The Kidney Meridian of Foot-Shaoyin You (the tenth of the twelve Earthly Branches)	Mahuang　Guixin　Danggui　Shengdihuang Huanglian　Daizheshi　Zishiying　Zhizi　Duhuo Chifuling	Xixin Shudihuang Wuweizi Zexie
	Zhimu　Huangbo　Digupi　Ejiao　Zhufu Mudanpi　Xuanshen　Baijiang　Muli　Wuyao Shanzhuyu　Tianmendong　Zhuling　Zexie Baifuling　Tanxiang　Gancao　Wuweizi　Zhuyu Yizhi	Diyu Fuzi Zhimu Baizhu
	Fuzi　Chenxiang　Yizhi　Huangqi	

制方之法

夫药有寒热温凉之性，酸苦辛咸甘淡之味。各有所能，不可不通也。药之气味，不比同时之物，味皆咸，其气皆寒之类是也。凡同气之物必有诸味，同味之物必有诸气。互相气味，各有厚薄，性用不等。制其方者，必且明其为用。经曰：味为阴，味厚为纯阴，味薄为阴中之阳；气为阳，气厚为纯阳，气薄为阳中之阴。然味厚则泄，薄则通；气薄则发泄，厚则发热。又曰：辛甘发散为阳，酸苦涌泄为阴；咸味涌泄为阴，淡味渗泄为阳。凡此之味，各有所能。然辛能散结、润燥；苦能燥湿泄热；咸能软坚；酸能收缓收散；甘能缓急；淡能利窍。故经曰：肝苦急，急食甘以缓之；心苦缓，急食酸以收之；脾苦湿，急食苦以燥之；肺苦气上逆，急食苦以泄之；肾苦燥，急食辛以润之，开腠理、致津液、通其气也。肝欲散，急食辛以散之；心欲软，急食咸以软之；脾欲缓，急食甘以缓之；肺欲收，急食酸以收之；肾欲坚，急食苦以坚之。凡此者，是明其气味之用也。若用其味，必明其气之可否；用其气，必明其味之所宜。识其病之标本、脏腑、寒热、虚实、微甚、缓急而用其药之气味，随其证而制其方也。是故方有君臣、佐使、轻重、缓急、大小、反正、逆从之制也。

主治病者为君，佐君者为臣，应臣者为使。用此随病之所宜，而又赞成方而用之。

君一臣二,奇之制也,君二臣四,偶之制也;君二臣三,奇之制也;君二臣六,偶之制也。去咽嗌近者奇之,远者偶之。汗者不奇,下者不偶。补上治上,制之以缓;补下治下,制之以急。急者气味厚也,缓者气味薄也;薄者少服而频食,厚者多服而顿食。

又当明五气之郁:木郁达之,谓吐,令条达也;火郁发之,谓汗,令疏散也;土郁夺之,谓下,无壅滞也;金郁泄之,谓解表、泄小便也;水郁折之,谓制其冲逆也。通此五法,乃治病之大要也。

Approaches of Prescription Formulating

Each herb has its own nature (cold, heat, warm and cold), flavor (sour, bitter, acrid, salty, sweet and light) and indications, and one should know it clearly. In contrast to other things which only have their single nature and flavor such as salty flavor or cold nature, the herbs are completely different. Those herbs with the same nature may have different flavors, and those with the same flavor are likely to have different natures. The different natures and flavors of herbs give rise to different properties and efficacy. One who wants to write a prescription should be familiar with them. *Huang Di Nei Jing* [《黄帝内经》, *Yellow Emperor's Canon of Medicine*] says, "Flavor belongs to yin. The thick flavor pertains to pure yin and the thin flavor pertains to yang within yin. Nature belongs to yang. The thick qi pertains to pure yang while the thin qi pertains to yin within yang. The thick flavor is helpful for purgation while the thin flavor is effective for dredging. The thin qi functions to disperse while the thick qi generates heat." It also says, "The herbs with pungent and sweet flavors pertain to yang because they disperse; the herbs with sour and bitter flavors pertain to yin because they induce vomiting and purgation; the herbs with salty flavor pertain to yin because they induce vomiting and purgation, the herbs with bland flavor pertain to yang because they discharge fluid and dampness." The herbs with different flavors have their correspondent efficacy. The herbs with pungent flavor can disperse stagnation and moisten dryness; the herbs with bitter flavor can dry dampness and purge fire; the herbs with salty flavor can soften hard masses; the herbs with sour flavor can induce astringency; the herbs with sweet flavor can relieve spasms; and the herbs with bland flavor can promote urination. So *Huang Di Nei Jing* [《黄帝内经》,

Yellow Emperor's Canon of Medicine] says, "The liver tends to suffer from rapid flow of qi which can be relieved by sweet flavor. The heart tends to suffer from the slackening of qi which can be astringed by sour flavor. The spleen tends to suffer from dampness which can be relieved by bitter flavor. The lung tends to suffer from the adverse flow of qi which can be stopped by bitter flavor. The kidney tends to suffer from dryness which can be moistened by pungent flavor. In this way, the muscular interstice is opened, the flow of body fluid is promoted and the activity of qi is activated." Since the liver needs to be dissipated, the treatment of liver diseases requires immediate use of pungent flavor to dissipate. Since the heart needs to be softened, the treatment of heart diseases requires immediate use of salty flavor to soften. Since the spleen needs to be moderated, the treatment of spleen diseases requires immediate use of sweet flavor to moderate. Since the lung needs to be astringed, the treatment of lung diseases requires immediate use of sour flavor to astringe. Since the kidney needs to be consolidated, the treatment of kidney diseases requires immediate use of bitter flavor to consolidate." All the treatments are based on the knowledge about the theory of herbal properties. If one wants to use the herbal flavor, he or she should know well about its nature, and vice versa. According to the natures and flavors of herbs and on the basis of identifying the manifestation or root cause, zang or fu, deficiency or excess, mild or severe, acute or chronic of the disease, one can formulate the prescription in accordance with the syndromes. Thus the prescriptions usually include the sovereign, minister, assistant and envoy drugs, which are formulated according to the mild or severe, moderate or drastic, large or small, routine treatment or contrary treatment.

The herbs for treating diseases are called sovereign drugs; the herbs for assisting sovereign drugs are called minister drugs; and the herbs for corresponding to minister drugs are called envoy drugs. Medicinal herbs can be modified in accordance with the syndrome, and thus to formulate prescriptions.

The odd prescription is composed of one sovereign drug and two minister drugs; the even prescription is composed of two sovereign drugs and four minister drugs; the odd prescription is composed of two sovereign drugs and three minister drugs; the even prescription is composed of two sovereign drugs and six minister drugs. That is why it is said that adjacently located diseases should be treated with the odd prescription; distally located diseases should be treated with the even prescription. The odd prescription can not be used to induce sweating; the even prescription can not be used for purgation. The prescription for supplementing the upper and treating the upper portion should be moderate, while the prescription for supplementing the lower and treating the lower portion should be drastic. The drugs with drastic effects are thick in flavor; the drugs with mild effects are thin in flavor. The thin ones are usually taken with a small dose and high frequency while the thick ones are taken with a large dose and administered at draught.

One should fully understand the stagnation of five qi. The stagnation of wood should be treated by out-thrust, and vomiting can make it act freely; the stagnation of fire should be treated by dispersing, and sweating can make it dispersing; the stagnation of earth should be treated by attacking, and purging can make it run smoothly; the stagnation of metal should be treated by dredging, that is, relieving the exterior and inducing urination; the stagnation of water should be treated by inhibiting, which is the way to regulate the adverse flow of qi. These five approaches are the essentials of treatment.

用药各定分两

为君者最多,为臣者次之,佐者又次。药之于证,所主同者则等分。

Dosage of Medication

As to the dosage, the sovereign drug occupies the most, the minister drug comes the second, and the assistant drug takes the third. If the drugs indicate the same syndrome, the doses may be the same.

用药酒洗曝干

黄芩、黄连、黄柏、知母,病在头面及手梢皮肤者,须用酒炒之。借酒力以上腾也。咽之下、脐之上,须酒洗之。在下生用。大凡生升、熟降。大黄须煨,恐寒则损胃气,至于川乌、附子,须炮,以制毒也。黄柏、知母,下部药也,久弱之人,须合用之者,酒浸、曝干,恐寒伤胃气也。熟地黄,酒洗亦然。当归,酒浸,助发之意也。

Liquor-processing Herbs

If the disease is located on the head, face, extremities and skin, Huangqin [黄芩, baical skullcap root, Radix Scutellariae], Huanglian [黄连, golden thread, Rhizoma Coptidis], Huangbo [黄柏, bark of amur corktree, Cortex Phellodendri] and Zhimu [知母, common anemarrhena rhizome, Rhizoma Anemarrhenae] should be stir-frying with liquor to improve the ascending efficacy. If the disease is located below the throat and above the navel, the herbs should be washed with liquor. If the disease is located below the navel, unprepared herbs should be used. Usually, the unprepared herbs have the ascending action while the prepared ones have the descending action. Dahuang [大黄, rhubarb root and rhizome, Radix et Rhizoma Rhei] should be liquor-roasted because its cold property can damage the stomach qi. Chuanwu [川乌, monkshood, Radix Aconiti] and Fuzi [附子, aconite, Radix Aconiti Praeparata] should be dry-fried to reduce the toxicity. Both Huangbo [黄柏, bark of amur corktree, Cortex Phellodendri] and Zhimu [知母, common anemarrhena rhizome, Rhizoma Anemarrhenae] are the lower portion drugs which should be used for the invalid persons. They should be steeped in liquor and dried by solarizing to avoid their cold property damaging the stomach qi, so should Shudihuang [熟地黄, prepared rehmannia root, Radix Rehmanniae Preparata]. Danggui [当归, Chinese angelica, Radix Angelicae Sinensis] should be steeped in liquor to improve its efficacy.

用药根梢身例

凡根之在上者,中半以上,气脉之上行也,以生苗者为根;中半以下,气脉之下行也,入土以为梢。病在中焦与上焦者,用根;在下焦者,用梢。根升而梢降。大凡药根有上中下:人身半以上,天之阳也,用头;在中焦用身;在身半以下,地之阴也,用梢。述类象形者也。

Examples for the Use of Different Medicinal Parts

Those roots located on the upper part which serve as seedling can promote the upward flow of qi and blood; the ones located on the lower part which enter the soil can guide the downward flow of qi and blood. The diseases located on the upper and middle energizer can be treated with root body, while the diseases located on the lower energizer should be treated with root tip. Usually the root body has the ascending action while the root tip has the descending action. In general, the root can be divided into three parts. To treat the upper portion of the human body, which belongs to the heaven yang, the root head should be used; to treat the middle energizer portion, the root body can be used; the root tip is usually applied on the lower portion of human body which belongs to the earth yin. All these rules attribute to the theory of analogy.

用丸散药例

仲景言:锉如麻豆大,与㕮咀同意。夫㕮咀,古之制也。古者无铁刃,以口咬细,令如麻豆,为粗药。煎之,使药水清,饮于腹中则易升易降也,此所谓㕮咀也。今人以刀器挫如麻豆大,此㕮咀之易成也。若一概为细末,不分清浊矣。《经》云:清阳发腠理,浊阴走五脏,果何谓也? 又曰:清阳实四肢,浊阴归六腑。㕮咀之药,取汁易行经络也。若治至高之病,加酒煎。去湿,以生姜;补元气,以大枣;发散风寒,以葱白;去膈上痰,以蜜。细末者,不循经络,止去胃中及脏腑之积。气味厚者白汤调,气味薄者煎之,和渣服。去下部之疾,其丸极大而光且圆;治中焦者,次之;治上焦者,极小。稠面糊,取其迟化,直至下焦。或酒、或醋,取其收其散之意也。犯半夏、南星,欲去湿者,以生姜汁。稀糊为丸,取其易化也;水浸宿,炊饼,又易化;滴水丸,又易化。炼蜜丸者,取其迟化而气循经络也。蜡丸者,取其难化,而旋旋取效也。大抵汤者"荡"也,去大病用之;散者"散"也,去急病用之;丸者"缓"也,不能速去之,其用药之舒缓而治之意也。

Examples of Dosage Form

Zhang Zhongjing said, "These ingredients are grated to the size of hemp seeds which has the same meaning of Fuju." Fuju is an ancient term which means that the herbs are usually chewed into pieces as the size of hemp seeds because there is no iron knife in ancient times. The rough herbs are decocted with the removal of foams and dregs. So the clear decoction can be absorbed easily. This process is called Fuju. At present, people always easily finish Fuju by cutting herbs to the size of hemp seeds by knives. The lucid can not be separated from the turbid if the herbs are ground into small pieces. *Huang Di Nei Jing* [《黄帝内经》, *Yellow Emperor's Canon of Medicine*] says, "The lucid yang permeates through striae and interstice while the turbid yin enters the five zang-organs." It also says, "The lucid yang fortifies the limbs while the turbid yin enters the six fu-organs." If the herbs are processed with Fuju method, the extracted juice can enter the meridians easily. In treating the diseases on the upper head, the herbs should be decocted with liquor. Shengjiang [生姜, fresh ginger, Rhizoma Zingiberis Recens] can be used to remove the dampness and Dazao [大枣, Chinese date, Fructus Jujubae] for tonifying the primordial qi. Congbai [葱白, fistular onion stalk, Allium fislulosum L.] is used to disperse the wind-cold and honey to remove the phlegm above diaphragm. The fine powder herbs can be used to remove the mass in stomach and viscera without entering the channels. The herbs with thick flavor are taken with Baitang, and the herbs with thin flavor are decocted and taken with dregs. In treating the diseases in lower-energizer, the bolus should be very big and smooth. The size of the herbal form used to treat the middle-energizer diseases come the second. The smallest pills are used for the upper-energizer diseases. The herbs which are processed by thick paste can directly enter the lower-energizer, for they are difficult to dissolve. The pills can also be processed by liquor or vinegar for dispersing or astringing effect. Banxia [半夏, pinellia, Rhizoma Pinelliae] and Nanxing [南星, jackinthepulpit tuber, Rhizoma Arisaematis] are usually processed by fresh ginger juice to remove dampness. These medicinal forms such as thin paste pills, steamed cakes and drop pills are easiy to dissolve. The honey bolus is usually difficult to dissolve and enter the channels. Also the wax pills are difficult to dissolve with sustained release. In general, the decoction with cleansing function can be used to treat serious diseases, the powder with dispersing function is used to treat urgent diseases, and the pill with moderating function can deal with chronic diseases.

升合分两

古之方剂,锱铢分两,与今不同。谓如㕮咀者,即今锉如麻豆大是也。云一升者,即今之大白盏也。云铢者,六铢为一分,即二钱半也;二十四铢为一两也;云三两者,即今之一两;云二两,即今之六钱半也。料例大者,只合三分之一足矣。

Weights and Measures

For the weights and measures, there is a big difference between the past and the present. For example, Fuju in ancient times indicates the size of hemp seeds at present. The so-called one Sheng refers to the volume of big cup liquor. Zhu is an ancient unit of weight, which is equal to 1/24 Liang. Six Zhu is equal to one Fen which is 2.5 Qian; Three Liang in ancient times is equal to one Liang at present, and two Liang is equal to 6.5 Qian. That means the labeled weight in ancient books only indicates its 1/3 weight today.

君臣佐使法

帝曰:方制君臣何谓也? 岐伯曰:主病之谓君,佐君之谓臣,应臣之谓使,非上中下三品之谓也。帝曰:三品何谓? 曰:所以明善恶之殊贯也。

凡药之所用者,皆以气味为主。补泻在味,随时换气。主病者为君,假令治风者,防风为君;治上焦热,黄芩为君;治中焦热,黄连为君;治湿,防己为君;治寒,附子之类为君。兼见何证,以佐使药分治之。此制方之要也。《本草》说,上品药为君,各从其宜也。

Monarch, Minister, Assistant and Guiding Medicinal Herbs

Huangdi said, "Why are the drugs in a prescription divided into the categories of the monarch and the minister?" Qibo answered, "The drugs for treating diseases are called monarch drugs, the drugs for assisting monarch drugs are called minister drugs, and the drugs for corresponding to minister drugs are called guiding drugs. These three categories of drugs in a prescription are not the so-called upper, medium and lower grades of drugs." Huangdi asked, "What do those three grades mean?" Qibo answered, "Those three grades are used for differentiating good and poor qualities of drugs."

The application of drugs is based on their natures and flavors. Tonifying or purging function is determined by the drug nature with different flavors. The monarch drug always treats the main disease. To treat the wind syndrome, Fangfeng [防风, divaricate saposhnikovia root, Radix Saposhnikoviae] acts as the monarch drug. In treating the heat syndrome in the upper energizer, Huangqin [黄芩, baical skullcap root, Radix Scutellariae] serves as the monarch drug, so does Huanglian [黄连, golden thread, Rhizoma Coptidis] for the middle-energizer heat syndrome. Fangji [防己, mealy fangji root, Stephania tetrandra] will be the monarch drug to deal with the dampness syndrome, while Fuzi [附子, aconite, Radix Aconiti Praeparata] can be used for the cold syndrome. The accompanied syndromes are treated by assistant drugs and guiding drugs respectively. They are the essentials of prescription formulating. *Ben Cao* says that the herbs in the first grade should serve as monarch drugs, and the second and third grades would follow to be the assistant drugs and guiding drugs.

治法纲要

《气交变论》云：夫五运之政，犹权衡也。高者抑之，下者举之，化者应之，变者复之。此生长化成收藏之理，气之常也。失常则天地四塞矣。失常之理，则天地四时之气，无所运行。故动必有静，胜必有复，乃天地阴阳之道也。假令高者抑之，非高者固当抑也，以其本下，而失之太高，故抑之而使下。若本高，何抑之有？假令下者举之，非下者固当举之也，以其本高，而失之太下，故举而使之高。若本下，何举之有？

如仲景治表虚，制桂枝汤方：桂枝，味辛热，发散，助阳，体轻，本乎天者亲上，故桂枝为君，芍药、甘草为佐。阳脉涩、阴脉弦，法当腹中急痛，制小建中汤方：芍药，味酸寒，主收，补中，本乎地者亲下，故芍药为君，桂、甘草佐之。一则治表虚，一则治里虚，各言其主用也。后之用古方者，触类而长之，不致差误矣。

Essentials of Treatment

Qi Jiao Bian Lun [《气交变论》, *Discussion on the Changes of Qi-Convergence*] says, "The movement of five-motions is just like the relationship between the steelyard and the sliding weight. If it is excessive, it should be inhibited; if it is insufficient, it should be supplemented. If it is transformed normally, it should be responded; if it has changed abnormally, it should be adjusted. This is the law of generation, growth, transformation, reaping and storage. And this is the normal condition of qi. The abnormal change of qi will give rise to the stagnation of the heaven and the earth. These abnormalities will cause the qi of heaven and the earth in the four seasons to fail to move. Thus there will be motion accompanied by quietness, and excessiveness accompanied by inhibition, which is the law of yin and yang in the heaven and on the earth. For the adverse upward flow of qi, whether in its upper location or not, it should flow downward but move adversely. So it must be inhibited to guide downward. If the qi moves upward normally, it does not need to be inhibited. If the qi adversely descends, it should be lifted. It is not because of its downward flow, but because it should have gone upward and now downward on the contrary, so the treatment must be the lifting method. If the qi should flow downward, it does not need to be lifted.

For example, Zhang Zhongjing uses Guizhi Decoction to treat the exterior deficiency syndrome: Guizhi [桂枝, Cinnamon bark, Cortex Cinnamomum Cassia], pugent in flavor, dispersing, supporting yang, light in weight, ascending toward the heaven, serves as the sovereign drug. Shaoyao [芍药, Chinese herbaceous peony, Paeonia lactiflora Pall] and Gancao [甘草, liquorice root, Glycyrrhiza uralensis Fisch.] act as assistant drugs. If it manifests rough yang pulse, taut yin pulse and acute abdominal pain, it can be treated by Xiao Jianzhong Decoction: Shaoyao [芍药, Chinese herbaceous peony, Paeonia lactiflora Pall], sour and cold in nature, can astringe yin and strengthen the spleen and stomach with descending action. Thus Shaoyao [芍药, Chinese herbaceous peony, Paeonia lactiflora Pall] is the sovereign drug, while Guizhi [桂枝, Cinnamon bark, Cortex Cinnamomum Cassia] and Gancao [甘草, liquorice root, Glycyrrhiza Uralensis

Fisch.] are assistant drugs. As Guizhi Decoction indicates the exterior deficiency syndrome and Xiao Jianzhong Decoction indicates the interior deficiency syndrome, the sovereign drugs of each are different. Those who later apply the ancient prescriptions should fully understand how to follow the way and further develop the formulas, thus to avoid making mistakes.

药味专精

至元庚辰六月，许伯威年五十四，中气本弱，病伤寒八九日，医者见其热甚，以凉药下之，又食梨三四枚，痛伤脾胃，四肢冷，时发昏愦。予诊其脉，动而中止，有时自还，乃结脉也。心亦悸动，吃噫不绝，色变青黄，精神减少，目不欲开，倦卧，恶人语笑，以炙甘草汤治之。成无己云：补可去弱。人参、大枣之甘，以补不足之气；桂枝、生姜之辛，以益正气。五脏痿弱，荣卫涸流，湿剂所以润之。麻仁、阿胶、麦门冬、地黄之甘，润经益血，复脉通心是也。加以人参、桂枝，急扶正气，生地黄减半，恐伤阳气。锉一两剂，服之不效。予再候之，脉证相对，莫非药有陈腐者，致不效乎？再市药之气味厚者，煎服，其证减半，再服而安。

凡药之昆虫草木，产之有地；根叶花实，采之有时。失其地，则性味少异矣；失其时，则气味不全矣。又况新陈之不同，精粗之不等，倘不择而用之，其不效者，医之过也。《内经》曰：司岁备物，气味之精专也。修合之际，宜加谨焉。

Specializations of Herbs

In June 1280, Xu Bowei was 54 years old, manifested as the deficiency of middle qi, eight or nine days after suffering from the cold damage. The doctor diagnosed him as the extreme heat syndrome and prescribed him cold herbs to purge the fire. Then he ate 3 or 4 pears and developed abdominal pain, cold limbs and occasional dizziness. The pulse manifested as alternate ceasing and beating which indicated Jiemai (slow pulse with irregular intervals). Also there were other clinical manifestations such as palpitation, hoarseness and hiccup, bluish yellow complexion, reduced energy, unwillingness to open eye, lassitude, aversion to noise. He was treated by Zhigancao Decoction. Cheng Wuji said, "Tonic can be used to treat the deficiency syndrome." Renshen [人参, ginseng, Radix Ginseng] and Dazao [大枣, Chinese date, Fructus Jujubae] can tonify the qi due to their sweet flavor; Guizhi [桂枝, Cinnamon bark, Cortex Cinnamomum Cassia] and Shengjiang [生姜, fresh ginger, Rhizoma Zingiberis Recens] can support the vital energy because of their pungent flavor. The defense qi and nutrient qi are exhausted because of the weakness of viscera, which can be treated with moist formula. Maren [麻仁, hemp seed, Fructus Cannabis], Ejiao [阿胶, ass hide glue, Colla Corii Asini], Maimendong [麦门冬, radix ophiopogonis, Ophiopogon Japonicus Ker-Gawl] and Dihuang [地黄, unprocessed rehmannia root, Rehmannia glutinosa Libosch. ex Fisch. et Mey.] can nourish the blood and channels, and normalize the beating of heart because of their sweet flavor. Renshen [人参, ginseng, Radix Ginseng] and Guizhi [桂枝, Cinnamon bark, Cortex Cinnamomum Cassia] can be added to strengthen the body resistance, but the dose of Shengdihuang [生地黄, unprocessed rehmannia root, Radix Rehmanniae Recens] should be reduced to a half to avoid damaging the yang qi. It took no effect after taking two doses. I examined him again and found a coincidence of pulse and syndrome. Was it possible that some herbs were mouldy and affected the curative effects? So I went to buy herbs with good quality and decocted again. After a dose of the new ones was taken, the syndrome was halved, and the patient was cured after taking the second dose.

Chinese drugs usually have their genuine producing areas and optimal collection time. The drugs may be poor in quality if they are not grown in their original area, and also may be lack of some natures or flavors if they are not collected at the right time. Also there are differences in curative effect, regarding their being old or new, crude or fine. It is the doctor's fault if he does not care about the factors above, which will lead to the failure of treatment. *Huang Di Nei Jing* [《黄帝内经》, *Yellow Emperor's Canon of Medicine*] says, "To prepare drugs according to the qi that dominates in the year will make the drug properties more pure." The processing method should be more strictly considered as well.

汤药煎造

病人服药，必择人煎药。能识煎熬制度，须令亲信恭诚至意者煎药。铫器除油垢腥秽，必用新净甜水为上，量水大小，斟酌以慢火煎熬分数。用纱滤去渣,取清汁服之,无不效也。

Decoction Methods

Before taking the medicine, the patient should select the right person to make decoction for him. The people who make the decoction should know the rules clearly and have a loyal and respectful attitude. Clean the clingage and foul fishy smell of the pot, use fresh and clean water with proper volume and apply slow fire to decoct several times. Filter the decoction with gauze, remove the dregs and take the settled liquid, and the medicine will always be effective.

古人服药活法

在上不厌频而少,在下不厌顿而多,少服则滋荣于上,多服则峻补于下。

Administration Rules

The disease that is located on the upper part of the body should be treated by taking the herbal medicine in small doses with short intervals, while the disease that is located in the lower part should be cured by taking at draught in large doses. Small doses would nourish the upper part and large doses would powerfully tonify the lower part.

古人服药有法

病在心上者,先食而后药;病在心下者,先药而后食。病在四肢者,宜饥食而在旦;病在骨髓者,宜饱食而在夜。

Administration Methods

If the disease is located in the chest and diaphragm, the patient should eat food first and then take the medicine; if the disease is located below the heart, the patient should take medicine first and eat the meal later. If the disease is located at the limbs, one should take the medicine in the morning with empty stomach; if the disease is located in the marrow, one should take the medicine at night with satiation.

察病轻重

凡欲疗病,先察其源,先候其机。五脏未虚,六腑未竭,血脉未乱,精神未散,服药必效。若病已成,可得半愈;病势已过,命将难存。自非明医,听声察色,至于诊脉,孰能知未病之病乎?

Differentiation of Patient's Conditions

To treat a disease, one must be clear about its origin and pathogenesis first. If the five zang-organs are not in deficiency, the six fu-organs are not exhausted, blood vessels are not in disorder, and the essence and spirit are not dispersed, the disease certainly can be cured after the drugs are taken. If the disease is serious, there is half possibility to cure it. If the disease is very serious, it is difficult to be cured. The ordinary doctors usually listen to the voice, inspect the complexion and take the pulse. How can they predict the potential diseases?

海藏老人《汤液本草》
Haizang's *Tang Ye Ben Cao* [《汤液本草》, *Materia Medica for Decoctions*]

五 宜

肝色青,宜食甘,粳米、牛肉、枣、葵皆甘。
心色赤,宜食酸,犬肉、麻、李、韭皆酸。
肺色白,宜食苦,小麦、羊肉、杏、薤皆苦。
脾色黄,宜食咸,大豆、豕肉、栗、藿皆咸。
肾色黑,宜食辛,黄黍、鸡肉、桃、葱皆辛。
毒药攻邪,五谷为养,五果为助,五畜为益,五菜为充。
气味合而服之,以补精益气。此五者,有辛酸甘苦咸,各有所利:或散、或收、或缓、或急、或坚、或软,四时五脏,病随五味所宜也。
大毒治病,十去其六;常毒治病,十去其七;小毒治病,十去其八;无毒治病,十去其九。谷肉果菜,食养尽之,无使过之,伤其正也。盖阴之所生,本在五味,阴之五宫,伤在五味。是故味过于酸,肝气以津,脾气乃绝。味过于咸,大骨气劳,短肌,心气抑。味过于甘,心气喘满,色黑,肾气不衡。味过于苦,脾气不濡,胃气乃厚。味过于辛,筋脉沮弛,精神乃央。是故谨和五味,骨正筋柔,气血以流,腠理以密,如是则气骨以精,谨道如法,长有天命。

Five Suitabilities

The liver corresponds to the blue color, and the patient suffering from liver diseases should eat food with sweet flavor, such as polished round-grained rice, beef, jujube and cluster mallow.

The heart corresponds to the red color, and the patient suffering from heart diseases should eat food with sour flavor, such as dog meat, sesame, plum and Chinese chives.

The lung corresponds to the white color, and the patient suffering from lung diseases should eat food with bitter flavor, such as wheat, mutton, apricots and leeks.

The spleen corresponds to the yellow color, and the patient suffering from spleen diseases should eat food with salty flavor, such as soy beans, pork, chestnuts and leaves of pulse plants.

The kidney corresponds to the black color, and the patient suffering from kidney diseases should eat food with acrid flavor, such as millets, chicken, peaches and scallions.

The medicinal herbs with toxicity can be used to attack pathogenic factors, while the five kinds of grains can be used to nourish the body. The five kinds of fruits can be used as the assistant to nourish the body, the five kinds of domestic animals can be used to supplement the viscera and the five kinds of vegetables can be used to enrich the viscera.

The harmonic mixture of proper tastes and flavors can supplement essence and nourish qi. The five flavors are acrid, sour, sweet, bitter and salty, and they can benefit certain zang or fu organ by means of dispersing or astringing, moderating or urgent processing, hardening or softening respectively. In treating diseases, the five flavors should be applied in accordance with the change of the four seasons and the state of the zang and fu organs.

When patients use the drugs with great toxicity to treat a disease, the rule is to stop the use of them when 60% of the disease is cured; when patients use the drugs with moderate toxicity to treat a disease, the rule is to stop using them when 70% of the disease is cured; when patients use the drugs with mild toxicity to treat a disease, the rule is to stop using them when 80% of the disease is cured; when patients use nontoxic drugs to treat a disease, they should be stopped when 90% of the disease is cured. Then patients should take food, meat, fruit and vegetables to cultivate the health. Patients should prevent excessive use of drugs, otherwise the healthy qi will be damaged. Yin is transformed from the five flavors. The five zang-organs that store yin can be damaged by the five flavors. Excessive taking of sour flavor makes the liver qi hyperactive and the spleen qi exhausted. Excessive taking of salty flavor damages the bones, makes muscles atrophic and inhibits heart qi. Excessive taking of sweet flavor makes the heart qi stuffy, the complexion blackish and the kidney qi imbalanced. Excessive taking of bitter flavor makes the spleen qi stagnant and the stomach qi thick. Excessive taking of pungent flavor makes the tendons and vessels flaccid and spirit weary. So only when the five flavors are well balanced can the bones be straightened, the tendon be softened, the qi and blood flow smoothly, the striae and intersticebe compact, and thus the bone and the qi can be strengthened. Following the way of cultivating health will enable one to enjoy a long life span.

五 伤

多食咸,则脉凝涩而变色。多食苦,则皮槁而毛拔。多食辛,则筋急而爪枯。多食酸,则肉胝胎而唇揭。多食甘,则骨痛而发落。

Five Injuries

Excessive taking of salty food will stagnate the blood vessels and change the colors. Excessive taking of bitter food can make the skin dry and the body hair bald. Excessive taking of acrid food will cause tendon spasm and nails dry. Excessive taking of sour food can lead to wrinkled muscles and chapped lips.

Excessive taking of sweet food will result in the pain of bones and the loss of hair.

五 走

咸走血，血病毋多食咸。苦走骨，骨病毋多食苦。辛走气，气病毋多食辛。酸走筋，筋病毋多食酸。甘走肉，肉病毋多食甘。

夫五味入胃，各归所喜所攻，故酸先入肝，苦先入心，甘先入脾，辛先入肺，咸先入肾。久而增气，物化之常也；气增而久，夭之由也。

Functional Tendencies of the Five Flavors

The salty flavor travels to the blood, so if the disease is in the blood, the patient should avoid eating the food of salty flavor. The bitter flavor travels to the bones, so if the disease is in the bones, the patient should avoid eating the food of bitter flavor. The acrid flavor travels to qi, so if the disease is related to qi, the patient should avoid eating the food of acrid flavor. The sour flavor travels to the tendons, so if the disease is in the tendons, the patient should avoid eating the food of sour flavor. The sweet flavor travels to the muscles, so if the disease is in the muscles, the patient should avoid eating the food of sweet flavor.

The five flavors enter into the stomach and then go to different zang organs they prefer respectively. Thus the sour flavor enters the liver first, the bitter flavor enters the heart first, the sweet flavor enters the spleen first, the acrid flavor enters the lung first and the salty flavor enters the kidney first. When getting into the viscera for a long time, the five flavors can increase the qi of the viscera. This is the common way to transform things. After the viscera qi has been increased for a long time, it becomes superabundant and causes calamities.

服药可慎

热中、消中，不可服膏粱、芳草、石药。夫芳草之气美，石药之气悍，二者其气急疾坚劲，故非缓心和人，不可以服此。夫热气慓悍，药气亦然，二者相遇，恐内伤脾。脾者，土也，而恶木。服此药者，至甲乙日更论。

Prohibition of Administration

The patient with Rezhong (a disease marked by polydipsia and frequent urination) and Xiaozhong (a disease marked by polyphagia and frequent urination) can not eat rich food and can not be treated by fragrant and mineral drugs because fragrant drugs are aromatic and mineral drugs are drastic. These two kinds of drugs are swift and violent in action. So they can not be used to treat those who are not gentle in disposition. The heat qi is swift and violent, and so is the property of the drugs. The combination of them may impair the spleen. The spleen pertains to earth and counter-restricting wood. The use of such drugs will lead to aggravation in the days of jia and yi.

论药所主

海藏云：汤液要药，最为的当，其余方论所著杂例，比之汤液稍异，何哉？盖伊尹、仲景取其治之长也。其所长者，神农之所注也。何以知之？《本草》云：一物主十病，取其偏长为本。又当取洁古《珍珠囊》断例为准则，其中药之所主，不必多言，只一两句，多则不过三四句。非务简也，亦取其所主之偏长，故不为多也。

故治病者，必明六化分治，五味五色所生，五脏所宜，乃可以言盈虚病生之绪也。谨候气宜，无失病机。其主病何如，言采药之岁也。司岁备物，则无遗生矣。先岁物何也，天地之专精也，专精之气，药物肥浓，又于使用，当其正气味也。五运主岁，不足则物薄，有余则物精，非专精则散气，散气则物不纯。是以质同而异等，形质虽同，力用则异也。气味有厚薄，性用有躁静，治化有多少，力化有浅深，此之谓也。

Medicinal Efficacy

Haizang (Wang Haogu) said, "The basic characteristics of medicinal herbs are listed in this book, and some cases recorded in other books are usually a little different from it. How does it happen?" The reason may be that Yiyin and Zhang Zhongjing always made the best use of the strong traits of each medicinal herb. The strong traits of each drug were recorded by *Ben Cao*, "One drug can be used to treat many diseases, but in clinical practice it is usually applied on the disease which it excels in." Take Zhang Yuansu's *Zhen Zhu Nang* [《珍珠囊》, *Pouch of Pearls*] as an example. The indications of each medicinal herb are very brief, which is usually elucidated with one or two sentences, and no more than three or four sentences. These compact expositions focus on the predominant indications. That's why they are so succinct.

To treat diseases, one should understand the transformation managed by six qi, the generation of five flavors and five colors as well as the preference of five zang-organs respectively. Only by doing so can he be clear about the excess and insufficiency of qi transformation and their relationship with the occurrence of diseases. The change of qi must be carefully monitored to avoid missing the pathogenesis of diseases. The indications of drugs always correspond to their collection time. To prepare drugs according to qi that dominates in the year will prevent any omission. Why do people collect and prepare drugs that are transformed by qi dominating in the year? Because they have absorbed the essence from the heaven and the earth. The drugs with essential qi have the genuine thick flavors and good qualities for clinical application. For the drugs that are transformed by the five motions of the dominating qi in the year, the ones in insufficiency usually have thin flavor while the ones in excess always have thick pure flavor. The qi of drugs with thin flavor is usually scattered and the property is also not pure. They are similar to the drugs transformed by qi dominating the year in texture, but different in gradation and clinical application. Also they are different in flavor which is either thin or thick, different in property which is either drastic or mild, curative effect which is either remarkable or slight and potency which is either shallow or deep. The differences are just like these aspects.

天地生物有厚薄堪用不堪用				
酸				
苦				
甘	司地气故物化从			
苦				
辛				
咸				
酸化木		在泉		
苦化火				
甘化土				
苦化火				
辛化金				
咸化水				
风化				
热化				
湿化		司天		
火化				
燥化				
寒化				
厥阴	少阴	太阴	少阳	阳明	太阳

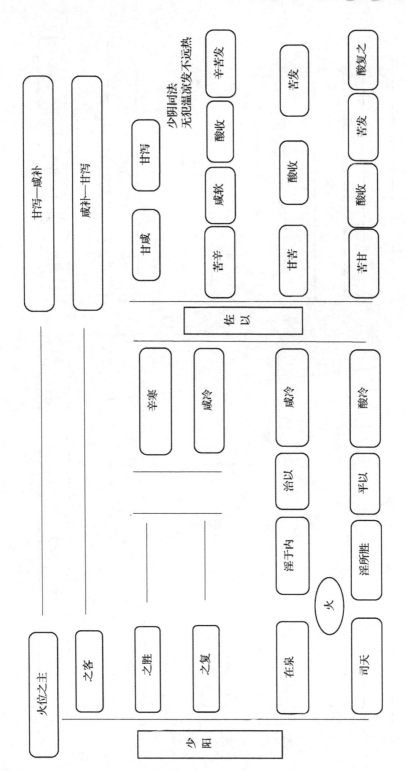

汤液本草

MATERIA MEDICA for Decoctions

木位之主：酸泻—辛补
之客：辛补—酸泻—甘缓

酸泻
苦辛

甘缓
甘辛

酸泻
甘缓
苦甘

辛散
甘缓
苦甘

酸泻
甘缓
苦甘

佐以

甘清
酸寒
辛凉
辛凉

治以
平以

淫于内
淫所胜

之胜
之复
在泉（风）司天

厥阴

```
                                        酸收        苦发

                 甘泻       甘泻       咸软       酸收       酸收
  甘泻—咸朴  咸朴—甘泻—酸收
                 甘咸       苦辛      辛苦发      苦甘       苦甘

                              ┌─────────┐
                              │  佐  以  │
                              └─────────┘

                  辛寒      咸寒       咸寒                咸寒


                                       治以       平以


                                      淫于内      淫所胜
                                                ○
                                                热
  火位之主  之客  之胜  之复       在泉                 司天

                              ┌─────────┐
                              │  少  阴  │
                              └─────────┘
```

汤液本草

```
                    ┌─────────┐
                    │ 以和为利 │
                    └────┬────┘
                         │
        ┌─────────┬──────┴──────┐
        │ 咸平之  │  酸平之     │  苦平之
        └─────────┴─────────────┘

   ┌────┐  ┌────┐  ┌────┐   ┌────┐  ┌────┐  ┌────┐
   │咸甘│  │苦甘│  │甘辛│   │苦酸│  │苦甘│  │苦辛│
   └────┘  └────┘  └────┘   └────┘  └────┘  └────┘

         ┌──────┐              ┌──────┐
         │ 佐以 │              │ 佐以 │
         └──────┘              └──────┘

   ┌────┐ ┌────┐ ┌────┐   ┌────┐ ┌────┐ ┌────┐
   │苦冷│ │平寒│ │咸冷│   │苦寒│ │辛寒│ │咸寒│
   └────┘ └────┘ └────┘   └────┘ └────┘ └────┘
   ─────────────────────────────────────────────
            ┌──────┐            ┌──────┐
            │ 洽以 │            │ 洽以 │
            └──────┘            └──────┘

                    ┌─────────┐
                    │ 热反胜之 │
                    └─────────┘
   ─────────────────────────────────────────────
           ┌──────┐            ┌──────┐
           │ 司地 │            │ 化天 │
           └──────┘            └──────┘

                 ┌───────────────┐
                 │   湿 燥 寒    │
                 └───────────────┘
```

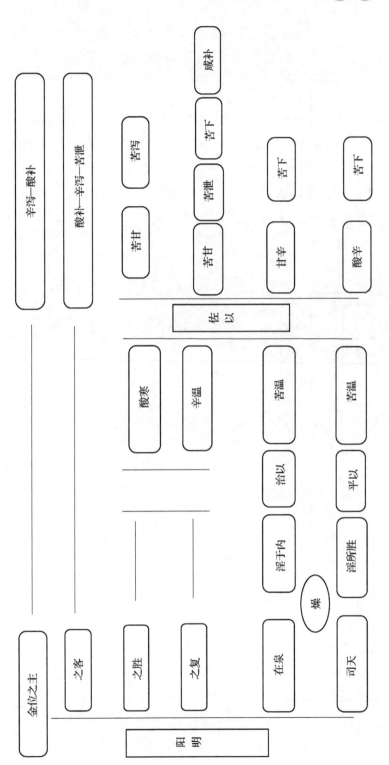

汤液本草
Materia Medica for Decoctions

```
                    ┌─────┐
                    │ 辛平 │
                    └─────┘
              ┌─────┐     ┌─────┐
              │ 苦甘 │     │ 苦甘 │
              └─────┘     └─────┘
                    ┌─────┐
                    │  佐  │
                    └─────┘
              ┌─────┐     ┌─────┐
              │ 酸温 │     │ 酸温 │
              │     │     │     │
              └─────┘     └─────┘
                    ┌─────┐
                    │ 以治 │
                    └─────┘
                    ┌─────┐
                    │清反胜之│
                    └─────┘
              ┌─────┐     ┌─────┐
              │ 司地 │     │ 化天 │
              └─────┘     └─────┘
              ┌───────────────┐
              │       风       │
              └───────────────┘
```

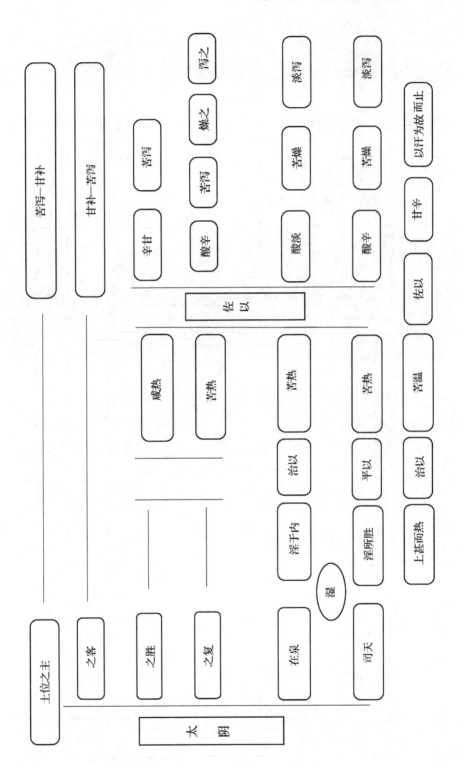

汤液本草

MATERIA MEDICA for Decoctions

```
                                                    苦坚

                                                    辛润
                              咸泻        苦坚
                                                    咸泻        咸泻
                              辛酸        甘辛
       咸泻─苦补  苦补─咸泻                            苦辛       苦甘

                                        佐以

                                                    甘热
                              甘热        咸热                  辛热

                                                    泄以        平以

                                                    淫于内      淫所胜
                                                         寒
        水位之主  之客      之胜      之复      在泉       司天

                                    太  阳
```

卷 上

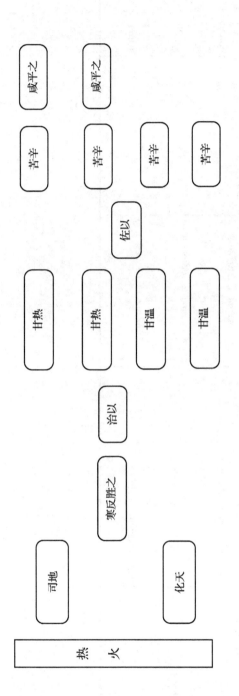

Usable or Unusable Medicinal Herbs

			domination in the heaven		in the spring		domination and transformation on the earth	
Jueyin		transformation of wind		transformation of sourness into wood		sourness		
Shaoyin		transformation of heat		transformation of bitterness into fire		bitterness		
Taiyin		transformation of dampness		transformation of sweetness into earth		sweetness		
Shaoyang		transformation of fire		transformation of bitterness into fire		bitterness		
Yangming		transformation of dryness		transformation of acridity into metal		acridity		
Taiyang		transformation of cold		transformation of saltiness into water		saltiness		

卷 上

```
                                                                    ┌──────────────┐
                                                                    │ sour to      │
                                                                    │ restore      │
                                                                    └──────────────┘
                                                    ┌──────────────┐
                                                    │ pungent      │
                                                    │ and bitter   │
                                                    │ to           │
                                    ┌──────────────┐└──────────────┘┌──────────────┐
                                    │The disease   │                │ bitter to    │
                                    │caused by     │                │ disperse     │
                                    │retaliation of│┌──────────────┐└──────────────┘
                                    │shaoyin can   ││ sour to      │
                                    │also be       ││ astringe     │┌──────────────┐
┌──────────────────────┐            │treated with  │└──────────────┘│ bitter to    │
│drugs sweet in flavor │            │the same      │                │ disperse     │
│can be used to reduce │            │method. Drugs │┌──────────────┐└──────────────┘
│and drugs salty in    │            │warm and cool ││ sour to      │
│flavor can be used to │            │in property   ││ astringe     │┌──────────────┐
│supplement            │            │should not be │└──────────────┘│ sour to      │
└──────────────────────┘┌──────────┐│used, drugs   │                │ astringe     │
                        │sweet to  ││hot in        │┌──────────────┐└──────────────┘
┌──────────────────────┐│reduce    ││property can  ││ salty to     │
│using drugs salty in  │└──────────┘│be used.      ││ soften       │
│flavor to supplement  │            └──────────────┘└──────────────┘
│and drugs sweet in    │┌──────────┐┌──────────────┐┌──────────────┐┌──────────────┐
│flavor to reduce      ││sweet and ││ bitter and   ││ sweet and    ││ bitter and   │
└──────────────────────┘│salty     ││ pungent      ││ bitter       ││ sweet        │
                        └──────────┘└──────────────┘└──────────────┘└──────────────┘

                                          ┌──────────────────────┐
                                          │      assisted by     │
                                          └──────────────────────┘

                        ┌──────────────┐┌──────────────┐┌──────────────┐┌──────────────┐
                        │pungent in    ││salty in      ││salty in      ││sour in flavor│
                        │flavor and    ││flavor and    ││flavor and    ││and cool in   │
                        │cold in nature││cool in nature││cool in nature││nature        │
                        └──────────────┘└──────────────┘└──────────────┘└──────────────┘

                                                        ┌──────────┐┌──────────┐
                                                        │treated by││balanced  │
                                                        │          ││with      │
                                                        └──────────┘└──────────┘

                                                        ┌──────────┐┌──────────┐
                                                        │interior  ││predomin- │
                                                        │excess    ││ance      │
                                                        └──────────┘└──────────┘
                                                              ( fire )
┌──────────────┐┌──────────┐┌──────────┐┌──────────┐┌──────────┐┌──────────┐
│fire is in    ││guest qi  ││in excess ││in        ││in the    ││dominating│
│domination    ││          ││          ││retaliation││spring   ││the heaven│
└──────────────┘└──────────┘└──────────┘└──────────┘└──────────┘└──────────┘

                                  ┌──────────────────────┐
                                  │       Shaoyang       │
                                  └──────────────────────┘
```

67

MATERIA MEDICA for DECOCTIONS

```
                                                                sour to          pungent to       sour to
                                                                reduce           disperse         reduce

                                               sour to          sweet to         sweet to         sweet to
                                               reduce           moderate         moderate         moderate

    drugs sour in flavor can be used to reduce and
    drugs pungent in flavor can be used to
    supplement

    using drugs pungent in flavor to supplement, drugs
    sour in flavor to reduce and sweet to moderate

                                               bitter and       sweet and        bitter and       bitter and
                                               pungent          pungent          sweet            sweet

                                                    assisted by

                              sweet in flavor and              pungent in flavor    pungent in flavor
                              lubricious in nature             and cool in nature   and cool in nature

                              sour in flavor and               treated              balanced
                              cold in nature                   by                   with

                                                               interior excess      Predominance

                                                                    wind

    guest qi      in excess      in retaliation                in the spring        dominating the
                                                                                    heaven

    wood is in domination

                                                    Jueyin
```

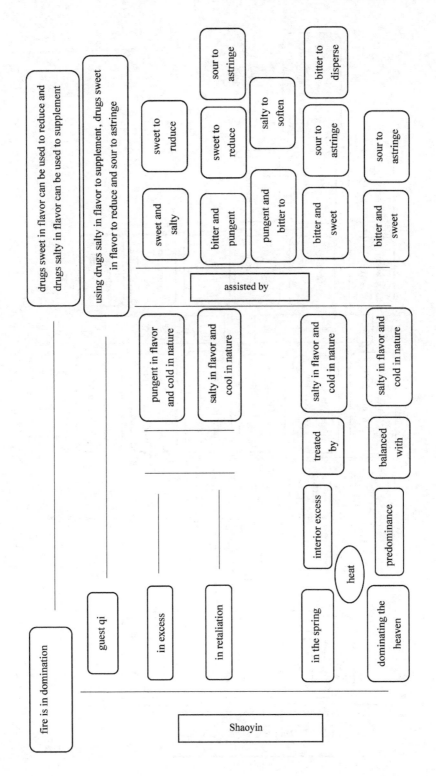

汤液本草
MATERIA MEDICA for Decoctions

```
                    ┌─────────────────────┐
                    │ the drugs should be │
                    │ used to harmonize   │
                    └─────────────────────┘

   ┌──────────┐    ┌──────────┐    ┌──────────┐
   │ salty to │    │ sour to  │    │ bitter to│
   │ balance  │    │ balance  │    │ balance  │
   └──────────┘    └──────────┘    └──────────┘

 ┌───────┐ ┌───────┐ ┌───────┐ ┌───────┐ ┌───────┐ ┌───────┐
 │salty  │ │bitter │ │sweet  │ │bitter │ │bitter │ │bitter │
 │and    │ │and    │ │and    │ │and    │ │and    │ │and    │
 │sweet  │ │sweet  │ │pungent│ │sour   │ │sweet  │ │pungent│
 └───────┘ └───────┘ └───────┘ └───────┘ └───────┘ └───────┘

         assisted by              assisted by

 ┌────────┐┌────────┐┌────────┐ ┌────────┐┌────────┐┌────────┐
 │bitter  ││mild in ││salty in│ │bitter  ││pungent ││salty in│
 │in flav-││flavor  ││flavor  │ │in flav-││in flav-││flavor  │
 │or and  ││and cold││and cool│ │or and  ││or and  ││and cold│
 │cool in ││in nat- ││in nat- │ │cold in ││cold in ││in nat- │
 │nature  ││ure     ││ure     │ │nature  ││nature  ││ure     │
 └────────┘└────────┘└────────┘ └────────┘└────────┘└────────┘

              ┌────────┐              ┌────────┐
              │treated │              │treated │
              │by      │              │by      │
              └────────┘              └────────┘

                      ┌──────────────┐
                      │ heat is      │
                      │ predominant  │
                      └──────────────┘

      ┌──────────┐                    ┌──────────┐
      │dominating│                    │dominating│
      │the earth │                    │the heaven│
      └──────────┘                    └──────────┘

              ┌──────────────────────────────┐
              │  Dampness Dryness Coldness   │
              └──────────────────────────────┘
```

```
metal is in domination
 ├─ guest qi
 ├─ in excess
 ├─ in retaliation
 │    ├─ sour in flavor and cold in nature
 │    └─ pungent in flavor and warm in nature
 └─ dryness
      ├─ in the spring ── interior excess ── treated by ── bitter in flavor and warm in nature
      └─ dominating the heaven ── predominance ── balanced with ── bitter in flavor and warm in nature
                              Yangming
```

assisted by:
- bitter and sweet — bitter to reduce
- bitter and sweet — bitter to reduce / bitter to purge / salty to supplement
- sweet and pungent — bitter to purge
- sour and pungent — bitter to purge

drugs pungent in flavor can be used to reduce and drugs sour in flavor can be used to supplement

using drugs sour in flavor to supplement, drugs pungent and bitter in flavor to reduce

71

MATERIA MEDICA FOR DECOCTIONS

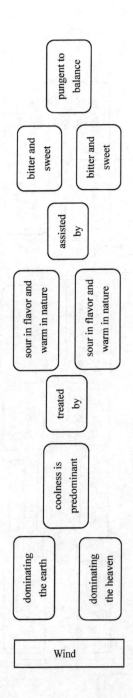

Taiyin

- earth is in domination
  - guest qi
    - in excess
    - in retaliation
    - in the spring
    - dominating the heaven
  - dampness
  - interior excess — treated by — salty in flavor and heat in nature / bitter in flavor and heat in nature
  - predominance — balanced with — bitter in flavor and heat in nature / bitter in flavor and heat in nature
  - excessive earth giving rise to heat — treated by — bitter in flavor and warm in nature

assisted by

- pungent and sweet — bitter to reduce
- sour and pungent — bitter to reduce / to dry
- sour and bland — bitter to dry / bland to reduce
- sour and pungent — bitter to dry / bland to reduce

assisted by

- sweet and pungent — to stop sweating

- drugs bitter in flavor can be used to reduce and drugs sweet in flavor can be used to supplement
- using drugs sweet in flavor to supplement and drugs bitter in flavor to reduce

Materia Medica for Decoctions

Taiyang

- water is in domination
- guest qi
  - in excess
  - in retaliation
- in the spring
- coldness
  - interior excess — treated by
    - sweet in flavor and heat in nature
    - salty in flavor and heat in nature
  - predominance
  - dominating the heaven — balanced with
    - sweet in flavor and heat in nature
    - pungent in flavor and heat in nature

assisted by

- drugs salty in flavor can be used to reduce and drugs bitter in flavor can be used to supplement
- using drugs bitter in flavor to supplement and drugs salty in flavor to reduce
  - salty to reduce
  - bitter to consolidate
  - pungent and sour
  - sweet and pungent
- bitter to consolidate
- pungent to moisten
- salty to reduce
- salty to reduce
- bitter and pungent
- bitter and sweet

74

```
                    ┌──────────┐   ┌──────────┐
                    │ salty to │   │ salty to │
                    │ balance  │   │ balance  │
                    └──────────┘   └──────────┘

    ┌──────────┐  ┌──────────┐  ┌──────────┐  ┌──────────┐
    │bitter and│  │bitter and│  │bitter and│  │bitter and│
    │  acrid   │  │ pungent  │  │ pungent  │  │ pungent  │
    └──────────┘  └──────────┘  └──────────┘  └──────────┘

                        ┌──────────┐
                        │ assisted │
                        │    by    │
                        └──────────┘

  ┌──────────┐  ┌──────────┐  ┌──────────┐  ┌──────────┐
  │sweet in  │  │sweet in  │  │sweet in  │  │sweet in  │
  │flavor and│  │flavor and│  │flavor and│  │flavor and│
  │heat in   │  │heat in   │  │warm in   │  │warm in   │
  │nature    │  │nature    │  │nature    │  │nature    │
  └──────────┘  └──────────┘  └──────────┘  └──────────┘

                        ┌──────────┐
                        │ treated  │
                        │    by    │
                        └──────────┘

                        ┌──────────┐
                        │coldness is│
                        │predominant│
                        └──────────┘

   ┌──────────┐                      ┌──────────┐
   │dominating│                      │dominating│
   │the earth │                      │the heaven│
   └──────────┘                      └──────────┘

          ┌───────────────────────────────┐
          │        Heat and Fire          │
          └───────────────────────────────┘
```

气味生成流布

阳为气,阴为味;味归形,形归气;气归精,精归化;精食气,形食味;化生精,气生形;味伤形,气伤精;精化为气,气伤于味。

阴味出下窍,阳气出上窍。味厚者为阴,薄为阴中之阳,厚则泄,薄则通;气厚者为阳,薄为阳中之阴,薄则发泄,厚则发热。

壮火之气衰,少火之气壮;壮火食气,气食少火;壮火散气,少火生气。天食人以五气,地食人以五味。五气入鼻,藏于心肺,上使五色修明,音声能彰;五味入口,藏于肠胃,味有所藏,以养五气,气和而生,津液相成,神乃自生。

Formation and Distribution of Qi and Flavor

Yang pertains to qi while yin pertains to flavor. The flavor nourishes the body, and the body depends on the qi. The qi nourishes the essence and the essence transforms into primordial qi. The essence absorbs the qi of food and the body takes the flavor of food. The transformation of primordial qi promotes the production of essence and the qi nourishes the body. Excessive flavor damages the body and excessive qi impairs the essence. The essence can transform into qi and the qi can be consumed by excessive flavor.

Yin flavor is discharged from the lower orifices and yang qi disperses from the upper orifices. The thick flavor pertains to yin and the thin flavor is yang within yin. The thick flavor is effective for purgation while the thin flavor is helpful for dredging. The thick qi pertains to yang and the thin qi is yin within yang. The thin qi functions to disperse while the thick qi generates heat.

The strong fire reduces qi while the mild fire strengthens qi. The strong fire consumes the primordial qi while the mild fire warms and promotes the primordial qi. The strong fire disperses qi while the mild fire supplements qi. The heaven provides man with five kinds of qi and the earth provides man with five kinds of flavors. When the five kinds of qi are inhaled through the nose and stored in the heart and the lung, they tend to rise and make the complexion ruddy and the voice sonorous. When the five kinds of flavors are taken through the mouth and stored in the intestines and the stomach, their essence infuses into the viscera to nourish the five kinds of qi. The harmony of visceral qi ensures the production of the body fluid and thus the spirit comes into being.

七　方

大:君一,臣三,佐九,制之大也。远而奇偶,制大其服也。大则数少,少则二之。肾肝位远,服汤散,不厌顿而多。

小:君一,臣二,制之小也。近而奇偶,制小其服也。小则数多,多则九之。心肺位近,服汤散,不厌频而少。

缓:补上治上,制以缓,缓则气味薄。治主以缓,缓则治其本。

急:补下治下,制以急,急则气味厚。治客以急,急则治其标。

奇:君一臣二,奇之制也;君二臣三,奇之制也。阳数奇。

偶:君二臣四,偶之制也;君二臣六,偶之制也。阴数偶。

复:奇之不去,则偶之。是为重方也。

Seven Types of Prescriptions

Big prescription: one sovereign drug, three minister drugs, nine assistant drugs. It is of high dosage. When the odd or even prescription is used to treat the disease that is distally located, the dosage should be large. The big prescription means fewer ingredients and may contain ingredients as few as two. The kidney and liver are distally located which should be treated with decoction which is taken at a draught with large doses.

Small prescription: one sovereign drug, two minister drugs. It is of low dosage. When the odd or even prescription is used to treat the disease that is proximate-located, the dosage should be small. The small prescription means more ingredients and may contain ingredients as many as nine. The heart and the lung are proximate-located which should be treated with decoction which is taken in small doses with short intervals.

Mild prescription: The prescription for supplementing the upper and treating the diseases on the upper part should be mild. The drugs with mild effect are thin in flavor. The primary disease should be treated mildly, by using the mild treatment to deal with the root causes of disease.

Drastic prescription: The prescription for supplementing the lower and treating the diseases in the lower part should be drastic. The drugs with drastic effect are thick in flavor. The visiting pathogens should be removed at once, by using the drastic treatment to deal with symptoms.

Odd prescription: The odd prescription is composed of one sovereign drug and two minister drugs, or two sovereign drugs and three minister drugs, being odd formulas. Yang belongs to odd.

Even prescription: The even prescription is composed of two sovereign drugs and four minister drugs, or two sovereign drugs and six minister drugs, being even formulas. Yin belongs to even.

Compound prescription: An even prescription is applied if an odd prescription fails to cure diseases. Such a way of using drugs is called double prescription.

十　剂

宣：可以去壅,姜、橘之属是也。

通：可以去滞,木通、防己之属是也。

补：可以去弱,人参、羊肉之属是也。

泻：可以去闭,葶苈、大黄之属是也。

轻：可以去实,麻黄、葛根之属是也。

重：可以去怯,磁石、铁浆之属是也。

滑：可以去著,冬葵子、榆白皮之属是也。

涩：可以去脱,牡蛎、龙骨之属是也。

燥：可以去湿,桑白皮、赤小豆之属是也。

湿：可以去枯,白石英、紫石英之属是也。

只如此体,皆有所属。凡用药者,审而详之,则靡所失矣。陶隐居云：药有宣、通、补、泻、轻、重、滑、涩、燥、湿。此十剂,今详之,惟寒、热二种,何独见遗,今补二种,以尽厥旨。

寒：可以去热,石膏、朴硝之属是也。

热：可以去寒,附子、官桂之属是也。

Ten Types of Formulas

Diffusing formula: This type of formula can expel the stagnation which consists of Shengjiang [生姜, fresh ginger, Rhizoma Zingiberis Recens], Jupi [橘皮, orange peel, Pericarpium Citri Reticulatae] and the drugs with the same properties.

Obstruction-removing formula: This type of formula can remove the stasis which consists of Mutong [木通, akebia stem, Caulis Akebiae], Fangji [防己, mealy fangji root, Stephania tetrandra] and the drugs with the same properties.

Tonifying formula: This type of formula can supplement the weakness which consists of Renshen [人参, ginseng, Radix Ginseng], mutton and the drugs with the same properties.

Purgative formula: This type of formula can discharge the obstruction which consists of Tinglizi [葶苈子, semen lepidii, Draba nemorosa L.], Dahuang [大黄, rhubarb root and rhizome, Radix et Rhizoma Rhei] and the drugs with the same properties.

Light formula: This type of formula can disperse the exterior excess syndrome which consists of Mahuang [麻黄, ephedra, Herba Ephedrae], Gegen [葛根, kudzuvine root, Radix Puerariae] and the drugs with the same properties.

Heavy formula: This type of formula can calm fright and tranquilize the mind which consists of Cishi [磁石, magnet, Magnetitum], Tiejiang [铁浆, iron solution, Ferrum] and the drugs with the same properties.

Lubricating formula: This type of formula can promote urination to relieve stranguria which consists of Dongkuizi [冬葵子, cluster mallow fruit, Fructus Malvae], Yubaipi [榆白皮, siberian elm bark, Ulmus pumila L.] and the drugs with the same properties.

Astringent formula: This type of formula can arrest the excessive discharge which consists of Muli [牡蛎, oyster shell, Concha Ostreae], Longgu [龙骨, bone fossil of big mammals, Os Draconis] and the drugs with the same properties.

Dry formula: This type of formula can drain the dampness which consists of Sangbaipi [桑白皮, white mulberry root-bark, Cortex Mori], Chixiaodou [赤小豆, rice bean, Semen Phaseoli] and the drugs with the same properties.

Moist formula: This type of formula can moisten the dryness which consists of Baishiying [白石英, quartz, Quartz Album], Zishiying [紫石英, fluorite, Fluoritum] and the drugs with the same properties.

Such classification of formulas ensures all the medicinal herbs attributing to certain category. The one who wants to make prescriptions should thoroughly know the properties of each drug and the conditions of patients to avoid mistakes. Tao Hongjing said, "There are ten kinds of formulas as diffusing, dredging, tonifying, purging, light, heavy, lubricious, astringent, dry and moist. These ten formulas can be divided into cold and heat types simply, and now I will add another two types for supplementing."

Cold formula: This type of formula can clear the heat which consists of Shigao [石膏, gypsum, Gypsum Fibrosum], Puxiao [朴硝, crystallized sodium sulfate, Natrii Sulfas] and the drugs with the same properties.

Heat formula: This type of formula can disperse the coldness which consists of Fuzi [附子, aconite, Radix Aconiti Praeparata], Guangui [官桂, cassia bark, Cortex Cinnamomi] and the drugs with the same properties.

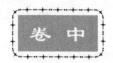

Volume 2

草 部
Grass Herbs

防 风

纯阳,性温,味甘、辛。无毒。

足阳明胃经、足太阴脾经,乃二经之行经药,太阳经本经药。

《象》云:治风通用,泻肺实,散头目中滞气,除上焦风邪之仙药也。误服,泻人上焦元气。去芦并钗股用。

《珍》云:身,去身半已上风邪;梢,去身半已下风邪。

《心》云:又去湿之仙药也,风能胜湿尔。

《本草》云:主大风头眩痛,恶风,风邪目盲无所见。风行周身,骨节疼痹。烦满,胁痛胁风。头面去来,四肢挛急,字乳,金疮内痉。

东垣云:防风能制黄芪,黄芪得防风,其功愈大。又云:防风乃卒伍卑贱之职,随所引而至,乃风药中润剂也。虽与黄芪相制,乃相畏而相使者也。

《本草》又云:得泽泻、藁本,疗风;得当归、芍药、阳起石、禹余粮,疗妇人子脏风。杀附子毒。恶干姜、藜芦、白蔹、芫花。

Fangfeng [防风, saposhnikovia, Radix Saposhnikoviae]

It is of yang property, warm in nature, sweet and pungent in taste and nontoxic.

It enters the stomach meridian of foot-yangming and the spleen meridian of foot-taiyin, helping to promote the circulation of the two meridians. It is regarded as the medicinal herb of the meridian of taiyang.

Xiang [《药类法象》, *Rules for the Use of Medicinal Herbs*] says: It is commonly used in treating wind diseases and proved effective in dispelling the lung excess, dispersing the stagnant qi in the head and eyes and driving out the wind pathogen in the upper energizer. If taken by mistake, it may cause loss of the original qi in the upper energizer. It is used in the clinical practice with its root removed.

Zhen [《珍珠囊》, *Pouch of Pearls*] says: The plant of Fangfeng [防风, saposhnikovia, Radix Saposhnikoviae] can eliminate the upward wind pathogen. The top part can eliminate the downward wind pathogen.

Xin [《用药心法》, *Gist for the Use of Medicinal Herbs*] says: It is also an effective medicinal herb to eliminate dampness, the reason being that wind dominates dampness.

Ben Cao says: It is mainly used to treat great wind, dizziness, headache, aversion to wind and blindness. It can treat the wind going through the body and joint paralysis, vexation and fullness, rib-side pain and wind, wind in the head and face, hypertonicity of limbs, delivering babies and internal injury caused by metallic tool.

Li Dongyuan said: Fangfeng [防风, saposhnikovia, Radix Saposhnikoviae] can generate Huangqi [黄芪, astragalus, Astragali Radix]. The effect of Huangqi [黄芪, astragalus, Astragali Radix] will be enhanced when it is taken together with Fangfeng [防风, saposhnikovia, Radix Saposhnikoviae]. It is also said that Fangfeng [防风, saposhnikovia, Radix Saposhnikoviae] is a medicinal herb similar to a private and its effectiveness depends on the conduct medicines. It is a medicinal herb with moistening function classified as the wind medicinal herb. There is inhibition and generation between Fangfeng [防风, saposhnikovia, Radix Saposhnikoviae] and Huangqi [黄芪, astragalus, Astragali Radix] and there are also mutual restraint and mutual enhancement beween them.

Ben Cao also says: Fangfeng [防风, saposhnikovia, Radix Saposhnikoviae], taken with Zexie [泽泻, alsma, Rhizoma Alismatis] and Gaoben [藁本, Chinese Lovage, Rhizoma Ligustici], will treat wind diseases. Taken with Danggui [当归, Chinese angelica, Radix Angelicae Sinensis], Shaoyao [芍药, peony, Radix Paeoniae], Yangqishi [阳起石, actinolite, Actinolitum] and Yuyuliang [禹余粮, limonite, Limonitum], it can treat uterine wind diseases. Fangfeng [防风,

saposhnikovia, Radix Saposhnikoviae] can eliminate the toxin of Fuzi [附子, aconite, Radix Aconiti Praeparata]. It is averse to Ganjiang [干姜, dry ginger, Rhizoma Zingiberis], Lilu [藜芦, root and rhizome of black falsehellebore, Radix et Rhizoma Veratri], Bailian [白蔹, ampelopsis, Radix Ampelopsis] and Yuanhua [芫花, immature flower of lilac daphne, Flos Genkwa].

升 麻

气平,味苦、甘。微苦,微寒,味薄气厚,阳中之阴也。无毒。

阳明经本经药,亦走手阳明经、太阴经。

《象》云:能解肌肉间热,此手足阳明经伤风之的药也。去黑皮并腐烂者用。若补脾胃,非此为引用不能补。若得葱白、白芷之类,亦能走手足阳明、太阴。

《心》云:发散本经风邪,元气不足者,用此于阴中升阳气上行。

《珍》云:脾痹,非此不能除。

《本草》云:主解百毒,杀百精老物殃鬼,辟瘟疫瘴气,邪气,蛊毒入口皆吐出,中恶腹痛,时气毒疠,头痛寒热,风肿诸毒,喉痛口疮。

东垣云:升麻入足阳明,若初病太阳证便服升麻、葛根,发出阳明经汗,或失之过,阳明经燥,太阳经不可解,必传阳明矣。投汤不当,非徒无益,而又害之也。

朱氏云:瘀血入里,若衄血吐血者,犀角地黄汤,乃阳明经圣药也。如无犀角,以升麻代之。升麻、犀角,性味相远,不同,何以代之?盖以升麻止是引地黄及余药,同入阳明耳。

仲景云:太阳病,若发汗,若利小便,重亡津液,胃中干燥,因转属阳明。其害不可胜言。又云:太阳几几,无汗者,葛根汤发之。若几几自汗者,表虚也,不宜用此。朱氏用升麻者,以表实无汗也。

《诀》云:主肺痿咳唾脓血,能发浮汗。

Shengma [升麻, cimicifuga, Rhizoma Cimicifuga]

It is mild in property, and bitter and sweet in taste. It is slightly bitter and slightly cold. Its taste is light and the flavor is strong, pertaining to yin within yang. It is nontoxic.

It is regarded as the medicinal herb of yangming meridian. It also enters the meridian of hand-yangming and the meridian of taiyin.

Xiang〔《药类法象》, *Rules for the Use of Medicinal Herbs*〕says: It can eliminate the heat in muscles caused by pathogenic qi. It is a crucial medicinal herb to treat the meridian of hand and foot yangming. The black peel and the rotten part should be removed before use. To tonify the spleen and the stomach, it must be used as the guiding herb. If it is combined with Congbai〔葱白, scallion white, Allii Fistulosi Bulbus Recens〕and Baizhi〔白芷, root of dahurian angelica, Radix Angelicae Dahuricae〕, it also enters the meridian of hand and foot yangming and taiyin.

Xin〔《用药心法》, *Gist for the Use of Medicinal Herbs*〕says: It can dissipate the wind pathogen of the meridian yangming. It can ascend the yang qi of patients who suffer from insufficiency of the original qi.

Zhen〔《珍珠囊》, *Pouch of Pearls*〕says: The spleen impediment can not be treated without Shengma〔升麻, cimicifuga, Rhizoma Cimicifuga〕.

Ben Cao says: It is mainly used to remove various toxins, kill various ghost-like evils that cause various diseases, eliminate scourge epidemic, miasmic qi and pathogenic qi to prevent warm diseases and stagnation. It is used to treat plague, headache due to cold and heat, sore throat and oral ulcer.

Li Dongyuan said: Shengma〔升麻, cimicifuga, Rhizoma Cimicifuga〕enters the meridian of foot yangming. If the location of a disease is in the meridian of Taiyang, it is called taiyang disease. Shengma〔升麻, cimicifuga, Rhizoma Cimicifuga〕and Gegen〔葛根, pueraria, Radix Puerariae〕will promote sweating in the meridian of yangming meridian. Too much sweat may cause overheat of yangming meridian. If the disease is located in the meridian of taiyang, it can not be treated. It may enter the meridian of yangming. It has no curing effect and may even do harm if the decoction is not taken properly.

Zhu Zuo said: If patients have internal blood stasis who spit blood or have nosebleed, Xijiao Dihuang Decoction can be very effective. If there is no Xijiao〔犀角, horn of Asiatic rhinoceros, Cornu Rhinocerotis Asiatici〕, it can be replaced by Shengma〔升麻, cimicifuga, Rhizoma Cimicifuga〕. Shengma〔升麻, cimicifuga, Rhizoma Cimicifuga〕and Xijiao〔犀角, horn of Asiatic rhinoceros, Cornu Rhinocerotis Asiatici〕have different properties and tastes.

Why can Shengma〔升麻, cimicifuga, Rhizoma Cimicifuga〕replace Xijiao

[犀角, horn of Asiatic rhinoceros, Cornu Rhinocerotis Asiatici]? The reason is that Shengma [升麻, cimicifuga, Rhizoma Cimicifuga] acts as a meridian conductor which can conduct Dihuang [地黄, rehmannia, Rehmanniae Radix] to the meridian of yangming.

Zhang Zhongjing said: Taiyang disease, if treated by promoting sweat or disinhibiting urine, may consume fluids and cause dryness in the stomach, turn into yangming disease and bring about severe damage. Zhang Zhongjing also said: Patients with Taiyang disease, unable to turn head flexibly and to sweat normally, can take Gegen Decoction to promote sweat. The reason why the patient can not turn his head flexibly with spontaneous perspiration is exterior deficiency. It is not proper to use Gegen Decoction in this case. Zhu Zuo used Shengma [升麻, cimicifuga, Rhizoma Cimicifuga] because the patients have exterior excessive syndromes without sweat.

Jue [《主治秘诀》, *Key to the Major Functions of Chinese Herbal Medicine*] says: It is mainly used to treat the lung atrophy, expectoration of saliva, purulent blood. It can help spit pus and blood phlegm and promote sweat.

羌 活

气微温,味苦、甘,平。苦、辛,气味俱轻,阳也。无毒。

足太阳经、厥阴经药,太阳经本经药也。

《象》云:治肢节痛,利诸节,手足太阳经风药也。加川芎,治足太阳、少阴头痛,透关节。去黑皮并腐烂者用。

《心》云:气温,湿风。

《珍》云:骨节痛,非此不能除。

《液》云:君药也,非无为之主,乃却乱反正之主。太阳经头痛,肢节痛,一身尽痛,非此不治。又云:是治,足太阳、厥阴、少阴药也。与独活不分二种,后人用羌活,多用鞭节者;用独活,多用鬼眼者。羌活则气雄,独活则气细,故雄者入足太阳,细者入足少阴也。又钱氏泻青丸用此,壬乙同归一治也。或问:治痛者何? 答曰:巨阳经从头走足,惟厥阴与督脉会于巅,逆而上行,诸阳不得下,故令头痛也。

Qianghuo [羌活, notopterygium, Notopterygii Rhizoma et Radix]

It is slightly warm, bitter and sweet in taste and mild in property. It is bitter and pungent, being light in flavor and property and pertaining to yang. It is nontoxic.

It enters the meridian of foot taiyang and jueyin. It is regarded as the medicinal herb of the meridian of taiyang.

Xiang [《药类法象》, *Rules for the Use of Medicinal Herbs*] says: It can be used to treat the joint pain and enhance the agility of coax joints. It is the wind herb of the meridian of hand and foot taiyang. If used together with Chuanxiong [川芎, Chuanxiong, Chuanxiong Rhizoma], it may treat the headache of the meridian of foot taiyang, shaoyin and free the joints. The black peel and the rotten part should be removed before use.

Xin [《用药心法》, *Gist for the Use of Medicinal Herbs*] says: It is warm in property and can treat rheumatic diseases.

Zhen [《珍珠囊》, *Pouch of Pearls*] says: The joints can not be relieved without Qianghuo [羌活, notopterygium, Notopterygii Rhizoma et Radix].

Ye [《汤液本草》, *Materia Medica for Decoctions*] says: Qianghuo [羌活, notopterygium, Notopterygii Rhizoma et Radix] is a monarch herb. It is helpful to make other herbs more effective. Qianghuo [羌活, notopterygium, Notopterygii Rhizoma et Radix] can be used to treat the headache of the taiyang meridian, pain of joints, aches and pains all over the body. *Ye* [《汤液本草》, *Materia Medica for Decoctions*] also says: Qianghuo [羌活, notopterygium, Notopterygii Rhizoma et Radix] is used to treat the diseases of the meridian of foot taiyang, the meridian of foot jueyin, the meridian of foot shaoyin. Qianghuo [羌活, notopterygium, Notopterygii Rhizoma et Radix] and Duhuo [独活, pubescent angelica, Radix Angelicae Pubescentis] are the same type of herbs. People prefer to use the jont parts of Qianghuo [羌活, notopterygium, Notopterygii Rhizoma et Radix] and the part which looks like the ghost eyes of Duhuo [独活, pubescent angelica, Radix Angelicae Pubescentis]. The property of Qianghuo [羌活, notopterygium, Notopterygii Rhizoma et Radix] is strong while the property of Duhuo [独活, pubescent angelica, Radix Angelicae Pubescentis] is mild. Qianghuo [羌活,

notopterygium, Notopterygii Rhizoma et Radix] enters the meridian of foot taiyang while Duhuo [独活, pubescent angelica, Radix Angelicae Pubescentis] enters the meridian of foot shaoyin. Qianghuo [羌活, notopterygium, Notopterygii Rhizoma et Radix] in Xieqing Pill can treat the diseases in the bladder and the liver. Why can it be used to relieve pains? The reason is that the meridian of foot taiyang starts from the head to the foot. The jueyin meridian and the governor vessel meet at vertex and then flow upward, making yang qi hard to flow downward and causing headache.

独 活

气味与羌活同。无毒。气厚味薄,升也,苦辛。

足少阴肾经行经之药。(肾足少阴)

《本草》云:主风寒所击,金疮止痛,贲豚痫痓,女子疝瘕,疗诸贼风,百节痛风,无久新者。

《液》云:独活细而低,治足少阴伏风,而不治太阳。故两足寒湿痹,不能动止,非此不能治。

《象》云:若与细辛同用,治少阴经头痛。一名独摇草,得风不摇,无风自摇。去皮净用。

《心》云:治风须用,又能燥湿。《经》云:风能胜湿。

《珍》云:头眩目晕,非此不能除。

Duhuo [独活, pubescent angelica, Radix Angelicae Pubescentis]

The smell of Duhuo [独活, pubescent angelica, Radix Angelicae Pubescentis] is the same as that of Qianghuo [羌活, notopterygium, Notopterygii Rhizoma et Radix]. It is nontoxic. Its property is strong and its flavor is thin. Its functional tendency is ascending. It is bitter and pungent in taste.

It promotes the circulation of kidney meridian of foot shaoyin.

Ben Cao says: It is mainly used to treat the wind cold attack, relieve the pain caused by metal injury, treat the palpitation underneath the navel similar to a running pig, epilepsy and hernia-conglomeration in woman, various diseases due to the pathogenic qi, relive the joint pain, treat the disease of recent onset.

Ye [《汤液本草》, *Materia Medica for Decoctions*] says: Duhuo [独活, pubescent angelica, Radix Angelicae Pubescentis] is thin and grows in low places. It is used to treat the latent wind in the meridian of shaoyin, instead of diseases in the meridian of taiyang. The cold and dampness impediment of feet can not be treated without it.

Xiang [《药类法象》, *Rules for the Use of Medicinal Herbs*] says: If used together with Xixin [细辛, as arum, Herba Asari], it can treat the headache of the meridian shaoyin. It is also called Duyaocao which remains still when there is wind blowing and spontaneously swings when there is no wind. The peel should be removed and it should be made clean before use.

Xin [《用药心法》, *Gist for the Use of Medicinal Herbs*] says: It is used to treat wind diseases and dry dampness. *Jing* [《黄帝内经》, *Yellow Emperor's Canon of Medicine*] says: Wind dominates over dampness.

Zhen [《珍珠囊》, *Pounch of Pearls*] says: Dizziness can not be treated without Duhuo [独活, pubescent angelica, Radix Angelicae Pubescentis].

柴 胡

气平、味微苦,微寒。气味俱轻,阳也,升也,纯阳。无毒。

少阳经、厥阴经行经之药(三焦手、胆足少阳,胞络手、肝足厥阴)

《象》云:除虚劳定热,解肌热,去早晨潮热,妇人产前后必用之药。善除本经头痛,非他药能止。治心下痞,胸膈痛。去芦用。

《心》云:少阳经分之药,引胃气上升,苦寒以发表热。

《珍》云:去往来寒热,胆痹,非此不能除。

《本草》云:主心腹,去肠胃中结气,饮食积聚,寒热邪气,推陈致新,除伤寒心下烦热,诸痰热结实,胸中邪逆,五脏间游气,大肠停积水胀及湿痹拘挛。亦可作浴汤。久服轻身,明目益精。半夏为之使,恶皂荚,畏藜芦、藜芦。入足少阳,主东方分也。在经主气,在脏主血。证前行则恶热,却退则恶寒,虽气之微寒,味之薄者,故能行经。若佐以三棱、广术、巴豆之类,故能消坚积,是主血也。妇人经水适来适断,伤寒杂病,易老俱用小柴胡汤主之,加以四物之类,并秦艽、牡丹皮辈,同为调经之剂。

《衍义》云:柴胡,《本经》并无一字治劳,今人治劳方中鲜有不用者,凡此误世甚多。尝原病劳,有一种真脏虚损,复受邪热,因虚而致劳,故曰劳者,牢也;须当斟酌用之。如《经验方》治劳热,青蒿煎丸,用柴胡正合宜耳,服之无不效。

《日华子》云:味甘,补五劳七伤,除烦止惊,益气力。《药性论》亦谓治劳乏羸瘦。若此等病,苟无实热,医者取而用之,不亡何待。注释本草,一字亦不可忽,盖后世所误无穷也。苟有明哲之士,自可处制,中下之士,不肯考究,枉致沦没,可不谨哉,可不戒哉。如张仲景治寒热往来如疟,用柴胡,正合其宜。

《图经》云:治伤寒有大小柴胡汤、柴胡加龙骨牡蛎、柴胡加芒硝等汤,故后人治伤寒热,此为最要之药。

东垣云:能引清气而行阳道,伤寒外诸药所加,有热则加之,无热则不加。又能引胃气上行升腾,而行春令是也。欲其如此,又何加之。

海藏云:能去脏腑内外俱乏,既能引清气上行而顺阳道,又入足少阳盖以少阳之气,初出地之皮为嫩阳,故以少阳当之。

Chaihu [柴胡, bupleurum, Radix Bupleuri]

Chaihu [柴胡, bupleurum, Radix Bupleuri] is mild in property, slightly bitter in taste and slightly cold in nature. Both of its property and taste are light. It is yang in property and nontoxic.

It promotes the circulation of the meridian of shaoyang and jueyin [triple energizer meridian of hand shaoyang, gallbladder meridian of foot-shaoyang, uterine vessels of hand jueyin, liver meridian of foot-jueyin].

Xiang [《药类法象》, *Rules for the Use of Medicinal Herbs*] says: Chaihu [柴胡, bupleurum, Radix Bupleuri] can relieve the consumptive disease. It clears the heat in the muscle. It can eliminate the tidal heat and women ought to use this medicinal herb before and after giving birth to a baby. It is effective to relieve shaoyang headache which can not be relieved by other herbs. It is used to treat the fullness and pain below the heart as the well as pain in the chest and diaphragm. It is used in the clinical practice with its root removed.

Xin [《用药心法》, *Gist for the Use of Medicinal Herbs*] says: Chaihu [柴胡, bupleurum, Radix Bupleuri] enters the meridian of shaoyang. It raises the stomach qi and eliminates the heat in exterior with its bitter and cold property.

Zhen [《珍珠囊》, *Pouch of Pearls*] says: The alternating cold and heat and gallbladder impediment can not be treated without Chaihu [柴胡, bupleurum,

Radix Bupleuri].

Ben Cao says: It is mainly used to treat the diseases of stomach and intestines. It can treat the binding depression in the stomach and intestines, remove food accumulation, cold pathogen, heat pathogen, evolve the new from the old, remove the heat below the heart, treat the phlegm heat accumulation, the retention of pathogenic qi in the chest, the wandering qi in the five zang-organs, the detention and water accumulation in the large intestine, hypertonicity and spasm caused by dampness pathogen. Chaihu [柴胡, bupleurum, Radix Bupleuri] can be added to bath water. The long-term taking of it can relax the body, brighten the eyes and replenish the essential qi. Banxia [半夏, pinellia, Rhizoma Pinelliae] is its envoy herb. It is averse to Zaojia [皂荚, gleditsia, Radix Gleditsiae] and restrained by Ziwan [紫菀, aster, Radix Asteris] and Lilu [藜芦, root and rhizome of black falsehellebore, Radix et Rhizoma Veratri]. It enters the meridian of foot shaoyang. It governs the east in direction. It governs the qi aspect in the meridian and blood aspect in the viscera and alternates cold and heat. Chaihu [柴胡, bupleurum, Radix Bupleuri] is slightly cold in property. Its taste is slightly bitter and that is why it can promote the circulation of the meridians. If assissted with Sanleng [三棱, Common Burreed Rhizome, Rhizome of Common Burreed], Guangshu [广术, Rhioxma Curcumae Aeruginosae, Curcuma Zedoary] and Badou [巴豆, croton, Fructus Crotonis], it will remove the stasis bump and that is why it can treat blood syndromes like irregular menstruation. Cold damage and miscellaneous diseases can be treated by Minor Bupleurum Decoction according to Yilao [Zhang Yansu]. If used together with Four Agents Decoction, Qinjiao [秦艽, root of largeleaf gentian, Radix Gentianae Macrophyuae] and Mudanpi [牡丹皮, moutan, Moutan Cortex], it can regulate menstruation.

Yan Yi [《衍义》, *Extension of the Materia Medica*] says: There is no record of Chaihu [柴胡, bupleurum, Radix Bupleuri] curing the consumptive disease in *Ben Jing* [《神农本草经》, *Agriculture God's Canon of Materia Medica*]. Nowadays people usually use Chaihu [柴胡, bupleurum, Radix Bupleuri] to treat the consumptive disease. This is a common mistake. The visceral deficiency affected by heat pathogen can cause the consumptive disease and that is why it is called Lao in Chinese (meaning overstrain), which has similar meaning with another Lao in Chinese (meaning prison). Think over before use. *Jing Yan Fang* [《经验方》, *Experienced Prescription*] says: Qinghao Pill is suitable with Chaihu [柴胡, bupleurum, Radix Bupleuri] included to abate the consumptive fever effectively.

Ri Hua Zi [《日华子》, *Materia Medica of Ri Hua-Zi*] says: It is sweet in taste. It can tonify five kinds of consumptive diseases and seven damages, eliminate vexation, ease fright, benefit qi and strength.

Yao Xing Lun [《药性论》, *Treatise on Medicinal Properties*] says: It can treat vexation diseases and emaciation. If doctors use this herb to treat the disease without excess heat, the life of the patient may be at risk. The annotation of materia medica should be correct and accurate, otherwise they can cause misunderstandings in later generations. Excellent doctors can deal with problems on their own while those ordinary ones, lack of observation and research, may cause the death of patients. Zhang Zhongjing used Chaihu [柴胡, bupleurum, Radix Bupleuri] to treat alternate cold and heat such as malaria effectively.

Tu Jing [《图经》, *Illustrated Classics of Materia Medica*] says: Major Bupleurum and Minor Bupleurum Decoction, Bupleurum Decoction together with Dragon Bone and Oyster Shell, Bupleurum Decoction together with Marabilite can be used to treat cold damage. So people in later generation regard Chaihu [柴胡, bupleurum, Radix Bupleuri] as the most important herb to treat cold damage and fever.

Li Dongyuan said: Chaihu [柴胡, bupleurum, Radix Bupleuri] conducts clear qi and directs yang. It is necessary to add Chaihu [柴胡, bupleurum, Radix Bupleuri] if there is a fever and not necessary if there is no fever. Chaihu [柴胡, bupleurum, Radix Bupleuri] can conduct stomach qi to ascend and corresponds to spring. That is the reason why it is added like this.

Haizang [Wang Haogu] said: It relieves the internal and external fatigue in the viscera. It not only conducts clear qi to ascend featured with yang property, but also enters the meridian of foot shaoyang. The qi of shaoyang that ascends just above the surface of the earth is called tender yang. That is why it enters the meridian of Shaoyang.

葛 根

气平,味甘。无毒。

阳明经引经药,足阳明经行经的药。《象》云:治脾虚而渴,除胃热,解酒毒,通行足阳明经之药。去皮用。

《心》云:止渴升阳。

《珍》云:益阳生津,勿多用,恐伤胃气。虚渴者,非此不能除。

《本草》云:主消渴,身大热,呕吐,诸痹,起阴气,解诸毒,疗伤寒中风头痛,解肌发表出汗,开腠理,疗金疮,止痛,胁风痛。生根汁,寒,治消渴,伤寒壮热。花,主消酒。粉,味甘,大寒、主压丹石,去烦热,利大小便,止渴。小儿热痱,以葛根浸、捣汁饮之,良。

东垣云:葛根甘平,温,世人初病太阳证,便服葛根升麻汤,非也。

朱奉议云:头痛如欲破者,连须葱白汤饮之不已者,葛根葱白汤。

易老云:用此以断太阳入阳明之络,即非太阳药也。故仲景治太阳、阳明合病,桂枝汤内加麻黄、葛根也。又有葛根黄芩黄连解肌汤,是知葛根非太阳药,即阳明药。

《食疗》云:葛根蒸食之消毒,其粉亦甚妙。其粉以水调三合,能解鸩毒。

《衍义》云:治中热酒渴病,多食行小便,亦能使人利。病酒及渴者,得之甚良。

易老又云:太阳初病未入阳明,头痛者,不可便服葛根发之;若服之,是引贼破家也。若头颅痛者,可服之葛根汤,阳明自中风之仙药也。

《本草》又云:杀野葛、巴豆百药毒。

Gegen [葛根, pueraria, Radix Puerariae]

It is mild in property and sweet in taste. It is nontoxic.

It conducts the circulation of the meridian of yangming. It promotes the circulation of stomach meridian of foot yangming.

Xiang [《药类法象》, *Rules for the Use of Medicinal Herbs*] says: Gegen [葛根, pueraria, Radix Puerariae] can treat the spleen deficiency and thirst, clear the stomach heat and resolve the toxin of liquor. It is the herb which runs through the meridian of foot yangming. The peel should be removed before use.

Xin [《用药心法》, *Gist for the Use of Medicinal Herbs*] says: Gegen [葛根, pueraria, Radix Puerariae] quenches thirst and makes the yang qi ascend.

Zhen [《珍珠囊》, *Pouch of Pearls*] says: It boosts the yang qi and engenders liquid. It shouldn't be overused because it may damage the stomach qi. The deficiency thirst can not be treated without Gegen [葛根, pueraria, Radix Puerariae].

Ben Cao says: It is mainly used to treat consumptive thirst, high fever, vomiting and various impediments, ascend the yin qi, resolve various toxins, treat cold damage, wind attack and headache, resolve flesh, effuse the exterior and sweating, open interstice, treat incised wounds, and relieve pain and hypochondria pain due to wind. Its juice of raw root is cold in property, which can relieve thirst, and treat cold damage and vigorous heat. Its flowers are mainly used to dispel the effects of alcohol. Its powder is sweet in taste and cold in property. It can be used to relieve mineral intoxication and vexation heat, disinhibit stool and urine, relieve thirst. It is effective to treat child fever if drinking after soaking in Gegen [葛根, pueraria, Radix Puerariae] juice.

Li Dongyuan said: Gegen [葛根, pueraria, Radix Puerariae] is sweet in taste and mild and warm in property. It is wrong for people who just catch taiyang diseases to take Gegen Shengma Decoction.

Zhu Fengyi [Zhu Gong] said: To treat the serious headache, if Lianxu Congbai decoction does not work, Gegen Congbai Decoction may work.

Yilao [Zhang Yuansu] said: Gegen [葛根, pueraria, Radix Puerariae] is used to prevent taiyang from entering the meridian of yangming. So it is not the taiyang medicinal herbs. Therefore when Zhang Zhongjing treats taiyang and yangming diseases, he includes Mahuang [麻黄, ephedra, Herba Ephedrae] and Gegen [葛根, pueraria, Radix Puerariae] in Guizhi Decoction. There is Gegen Huangqin Huanglian Flesh Resolving Decoction, indicating that Gegen [葛根, pueraria, Radix Puerariae] is not the medicinal of taiyang but of yangming.

Shi Liao [《食疗本草》, *Materia Medica for Dietotherapy*] says: The steamed Gegen [葛根, pueraria, Radix Puerariae] can detoxicate. Its powder is also very effective. Mix it with 0.3 He of water and it will remove poison.

Yan Yi [《衍义》, *Extension of the Materia Medica*] says: Gegen [葛根, pueraria, Radix Puerariae] treats the heat in chest and the thirst due to liquor.

Taking too much of it may promote urine and help to smooth stool. It is good to take Gegen[葛根, pueraria, Radix Puerariae] to resolve liquor and thirst.

Yilao[Zhang Yuansu] also said: In the early stage of taiyang diseases when they do not enter the meridian of yangming, and are accompanied with headache, Gegen[葛根, pueraria, Radix Puerariae] should not be taken. If taken, the diseases would be worsened. People who have headache can take Gegen Decoction. It is an effective medicinal herb to treat yangming diseases with wind pathogen.

Ben Cao also says: It is antidote for Yege[野葛, yellow jessamine, Gelsemii Herba] and Badou[巴豆, Croton Fruit, Fructus Crotonis] and resolves various toxins.

威 灵 仙

气温,味苦、甘,纯阳。

《象》云:主诸风湿冷,通五脏,去腹内痃滞,腰膝冷痛,及治伤损。铁脚者佳。去芦用。

《心》云:去大肠之风。

《本草》云:忌茗。

Weilingxian [威灵仙, clematis, Clematidis Radix]

It is mild in property, and bitter and sweet in taste. It is of yang property.

Xiang[《药类法象》, Rules for the Use of Medicinal Herbs] says: It is mainly used to treat various diseases caused by wind, dampness and cold, free the five zang-organs, and relieve abdominal conglomeration, cold pain in the lumbus and knees and injury. Clematis sinensis osbeck is the best. It is used in clinical practice with its root removed.

Xin[《用药心法》, Gist for the Use of Medicinal Herbs] says: It removes the wind in the large intestine.

Ben Cao says: Do not drink tea when taking Weilingxian[威灵仙, clematis, Clematidis Radix].

细　辛

气温,味大辛,纯阳。性温,气厚于味,阳也。无毒。

少阴经药,手少阴引经之药。

《象》云:治少阴头痛如神,当少用之。独活为使,为主用。去芦头并叶。华州者佳。

《珍》云:主少阴经头痛。

《心》云:止诸项头痛,诸风通用之。味辛热,温阴经,散水寒以去内寒。

《本草》云:主咳逆头痛脑动,百节拘挛,风湿痹痛,死肌,温中下气,破痰,利水道,开胸中,除喉痹,齆鼻,风痫癫疾,下乳结,汗不出,血不行,安五脏,益肝胆,通精气。久服明目,利九窍。

东垣云:治邪在里之表,故仲景少阴证,用麻黄附子细辛汤也。

易老云:治少阴头痛。太阳则羌活,少阴则细辛,阳明则白芷,厥阴则川芎、吴茱萸,少阳则柴胡。用者随经不可差。细辛香味俱细而缓,故入少阴,与独活颇相类。

《本草》又云:曾青、枣根为之使,得当归、芍药、白芷、川芎、牡丹、藁本、甘草,共疗妇人。得决明、鲤鱼胆汁、青羊肝,共疗目痛。恶狼毒、山茱萸、黄芪,畏硝石、滑石,反藜芦。

《衍义》云:治头面风痛,不可缺也。

Xixin [细辛, as arum, Herba Asari]

It is mild in property, pungent in taste, and pertaining to pure yang. It is warm and its property is thicker than the taste. That is why it is pure yang. It is nontoxic.

It is a medicinal herb entering the meridian of shaoyin. It functions as a guiding herb of the meridian of hand-shaoyin.

Xiang [《药类法象》, *Rules for the Use of Medicinal Herbs*] says: It is effective to treat the headache due to the disorder of the meridian of shaoyin. The dosage should be kept moderate. Duhuo [独活, pubescent angelica, Radix Angelicae Pubescentis] is its envoy herb. It is used in the clinical practice with its root head and leaves removed. Those growing in Huazhou are the best.

Zhen [《珍珠囊》, *Pounch of Pearls*] says: It is mainly used to treat headache due to disorder of the meridian of shaoyin.

Xin [《用药心法》, *Gist for the Use of Medicinal Herbs*] says: It can relieve various headache and can be used to treat various wind diseases. Its taste is pungent. It warms the yin meridian and dissipates the water cold to remove the internal cold.

Ben Cao says: It is mainly used to treat the cough due to the counter-flow of qi, headache, hypertonicity of joints, the impediment due to wind dampness, muscle necrosis, warm the middle energizer, promote qi to descend, dispel phlegm, free the waterways, diffuse the stagnant qi in the chest, eliminate the throat impediment and wind epilepsy, and disperse the breast nodule. It can treat anhidrosis, blood stasis, tranquilize the five zang-organs, benefit the liver and gallbladder, free the essential qi. The long-term taking of it will improve vision and disinhibit the nine orifices.

Li Dongyuan said: It treats the internal pathogen. That is why Zhang Zhongjing used Mahuang Fuzi Xixin Decoction to treat the shaoyin disease.

Yilao [Zhang Yuansu] said: It treats the shaoyin headache. Qianghuo [羌活, notopterygium, Notopterygii Rhizoma et Radix] is effective to treat taiyang disease; Xixin [细辛, as arum, Herba Asari] is effective to treat shaoyin disease; Baizhi [白芷, root of dahurian angelica, Radix Angelicae Dahuricae] is effective to treat yangming disease; Chuanxiong [川芎, sichuan lovage rhizome, Rhizoma Ligustici Chuanxiong] and Wuzhuyu [吴茱萸, evodia, Fructus Evodiae] are effective to treat jueyin disease; Chaihu [柴胡, bupleurum, Radix Bupleuri] is effective to treat shaoyang disease. The medicinal herbs should be used according to the meridian precisely. The taste of Xixin [细辛, as arum, Herba Asari] is fine and it enters the meridian of shaoyin. It is similar to that of Duhuo [独活, pubescent angelica, Radix Angelicae Pubescentis].

Ben Cao also says: Cengqing [曾青, azurite ore, Azuritum] and Zaogen [枣根, Root of Common Jujube, Ziziphus jujuba Mill] are its assistance. If used together with Danggui [当归, Chinese angelica, Radix Angelicae Sinensis], Shaoyao [芍药, peony, Radix Paeoniae], Baizhi [白芷, root of dahurian angelica, Radix Angelicae Dahuricae], Chuanxiong [川芎, sichuan lovage rhizome, Rhizoma Ligustici Chuanxiong], Mudan [牡丹, moutan, Cortex Moutan Radicis], Gaoben [藁本, Chinese Lovage, Rhizoma Ligustici] and Gancao [甘草, licorice, Radix Glycyrrhea Praeparata], it can treat female diseases. If used together with Juemingzi [决明子, seed of sickle senna, Semen Cassiae], Liyudan [鲤鱼胆, carp gall, Fel Cyprinus Carpio] and Qingyanggan [青羊肝, gora's liver, Naemorhedus goral Hardwicke], it can relieve the pain of eyes. It is averse to Langdu [狼毒, wolfsbane, Euphorbiae Nematocyphae Radix], Shanzhuyu [山茱萸, cornus, Fructus Corni] and Huangqi [黄芪, milkvetch root, Radix Astragali]. It is in mutual restraint with Xiaoshi [硝石, niter, Sal Nitri], Huashi [滑石, talcum, Talcum], and incompatible with Lilu [藜芦, root and rhizome of black falsehellebore, Radix et Rhizoma Veratri].

Yan Yi [《衍义》, Extension of the Materia Medica] says: It treats the wind attack at the head and face.

白 芷

气温,味大辛,纯阳。无毒。气味俱轻,阳也。

阳明经引经药,手阳明经本经药。行足阳明经,于升麻汤四味内加之。

《象》云:治手阳明头痛,中风寒热,解利药也。以四味升麻汤加之。

《珍》云:长肌肉,散阳明之风。

《心》云:治风通用,去肺经风热。

《本草》云:主女子漏下赤白,血闭阴肿,寒热风,头侵目泪出,长肌肤润泽,可作面脂,疗风邪,久渴吐呕,两胁满,风痛头眩目痒。

《日华子》云:补胎漏滑落,破宿血,补新血。乳痈发背,一切疮疥,排脓止痛生肌,去面皯疵瘢,明目。其气芳香,治正阳阳明头痛。与辛夷、细辛同用,治鼻病。内托,用此长肌肉,则阳明可知矣。又云:当归为之使,恶旋覆花。

Baizhi [白芷, root of dahurian angelica, Radix Angelicae Dahuricae]

Baizhi [白芷, root of dahurian angelica, Radix Angelicae Dahuricae] is mild in property and pungent in taste, pure yang. It is nontoxic. Both of its property and taste are light. It is of yang property.

It serves as the guiding drug of the meridian of yangming. It is regarded as a medicinal herb of the meridian of hand yangming. It conducts the meridian of foot yangming, and can be used in the four ingredients of Shengma Decoction.

Xiang [《药类法象》, *Rules for the Use of Medicinal Herbs*] says: It relieves the meridian of hand yangming headache, wind attack and cold heat. It resolves summer heat and dampness. It can be used with Siwei Shengma Decoction.

Zhen [《珍珠囊》, *Pouch of Pearls*] says: It promotes the growth of muscles and dissipate the yangming wind.

Xin [《用药心法》, *Gist for the Use of Medicinal Herbs*] says: It can be universally used to treat wind diseases and dissipate wind heat of the lung meridian.

Ben Cao says: It is mainly used to treat red and white vaginal discharge, blood stasis and genital swelling, cold heat, tearing due to head wind, engender muscles and moisturize the skin. It can be used as facial cream. It treats wind pathogen, long term thirst, vomiting, fullness in hypochondrium, wind pain, dizziness and itching eyes.

Ri Hua Zi [《日华子》, *Materia Medica of Ri Hua-Zi*] says: It can tonify the fetal spotting and abortion, break the blood stasis, and supplement blood. It can treat acute mastitis, charbuncle on the back, scabs, expel pus, relieve pain and engender muscles, remove blemish and scar on the face, brighten the eyes. It smells fragrant and is used to treat yangming headache. If used with Xinyi [辛夷, flower of biond magnolia, Flos Magnoliae] and Xixin [细辛, as arum, Herba Asari], it can treat the diseases of nose. Baizhi [白芷, root of dahurian angelica, Radix Angelicae Dahuricae] is used to treat the internal collapse to promote the growth of muscles. It also says: Danggui [当归, Chinese angelica, Radix Angelicae Sinensis] is its assistance. It is averse to Xuanfuhua [旋覆花, inula flower, Inulae Flos].

川 芎

气温,味辛,纯阳。无毒。

入手足厥阴经,少阳经本经药。

《象》云:补血,治血虚头痛之圣药,妊妇胎不动数月,加当归,二味各二钱,水二盏,煎至一半,服。神效。

《珍》云：散肝经之风，贯芎治少阳经苦头痛。

《心》云：治少阳头痛及治风通用。

《本草》云：主中风人脑头痛，寒痹筋挛缓急，金疮，妇人血闭无子，除脑中冷动，面上游风去来，目泪出，多涕唾，忽忽如醉，诸寒冷气，心腹坚痛，中恶，卒急肿痛，胁风痛，温中除内寒。

《日华子》云：能除鼻洪、吐血及溺血，破症结宿血，养新血。

易老云：上行头目，下行血海，故清神、四物汤所皆用也。入手足厥阴经。

《衍义》云：头面风不可缺也，然须以他药佐之，若单服久服，则走散真气，即使他药佐之，亦不可久服，中病即便已。

东垣云：头痛甚者，加蔓荆子；顶与脑痛，加川芎；若头痛者，加藁本；诸经若头痛，加细辛。若有热者，不能治。别有青空之剂，为缘诸经头痛，须用四味。

《本草》又云：白芷为之使，畏黄连。

Chuanxiong [川芎, Sichuan lovage rhizome, Rhizoma Ligustici Chuanxiong]

Chuanxiong [川芎, Sichuan lovage rhizome, Rhizoma Ligustici Chuanxiong] is mild in property and pungent in taste, pure yang. It is nontoxic.

It enters the meridian of hand and foot yueyin. It is regarded as a medicinal herb of the meridian of shaoyang.

Xiang [《药类法象》, *Rules for the Use of Medicinal Herbs*] says: It supplements the blood, very effective to treat the headache due to the blood deficiency, pregnancy without stirring fetus, and can be used with Danggui [当归, Chinese angelica, Radix Angelicae Sinensis]. The dosage of each medicinal herb is 10g. Put them in two cups of water, decoct to half of the water and take the decoction. It will be very effective.

Zhen [《珍珠囊》, *Pounch of Pearls*] says: It dissipates the wind in liver meridian. Chuanxiong [川芎, Sichuan lovage rhizome, Rhizoma Ligustici Chuanxiong] is effective to treat shaoyang headache.

Xin [《用药心法》, *Gist for the Use of Medicinal Herbs*] says: It can be used to treat shaoyang headache and wind diseases.

Ben Cao says: It is mainly used to treat wind attack, headache, spasm due to cold impediment, incised wound, blood block infertility. It treats the cold in the head, the wind on the face, tearing, frequent nasal mucus and saliva, unconsciousness like being drunk, cold qi, the pain in the heart and abdomen, malignity stroke, acute swelling and pain, rib-side pain. It warms the middle energizer and eliminates the internal cold.

Ri Hua Zi [《日华子》, *Materia Medica of Ri Hua-Zi*] says: It can stop nose blood, blood ejection, bloody urine, resolve the seriously stagnated blood, and nourish the blood.

Yilao [Zhang Yuansu] said: It promotes qi to flow upward to the head and eyes. It promotes qi to flow downward to the sea of blood and that is the reason why it is used to arouse the spirit and used in Four Herbs Decoction. It enters the meridian of hand-jueyin and foot-jueyin.

Yan Yi [《衍义》, *Extension of the Materia Medica*] says: The head and face wind disease can not be treated without it. However, it needs the assistance of other herbs. Long-time taking of it will dissipate the original qi. Even with the assistance of other herbs, it can not be taken for a long time.

Li Dongyuan said: If used together with Manjingzi [蔓荆子, fruit of shrub chastetree, Fructus Viticis], it can relieve serious headache; if used together with Chuanxiong [川芎, Sichuan lovage rhizome, Rhizoma Ligustici Chuanxiong], it can treat vertex headache and brain pain; if used together with Gaoben [藁本, Chinese Lovage, Rhizoma Ligustici], it can relieve headache; if used together with Xixin [细辛, as arum, Herba Asari], it can treat the meridian headache. It can not be used to treat fever. It is also used in Qing Kong Decoction because four ingredients should be used to treat the headache of various meridians.

Ben Cao also says: Baizhi [白芷, root of dahurian angelica, Radix Angelicae Dahuricae] is its assistance. It is restrained by Huanglian [黄连, coptis, Rhizoma Coptidis].

麻 黄

气温,味苦,甘而苦,气味俱薄,阳也,升也。甘热,纯阳无毒。

手太阴之剂,入足太阳经,走手少阴经,阳明经药。

《象》云:发太阳、少阴经汗。去节,煮三二沸,去上沫。否则,令人心烦闷。

《心》云:阳明经药,去表上之寒邪。甘热,去节,解少阴寒,散表寒、发浮热也。

《珍》云：去荣中寒。

《本草》云：主中风、伤寒头痛、温症，发表出汗，去邪热气。止厥逆上气，除寒热，破症坚积聚。

《液》云：入足太阳、手少阴，能泄卫实发汗，及伤寒无汗，咳嗽。根、节能止汗。夫麻黄，治卫实之药，桂枝，治卫虚之药，桂枝、麻黄虽为太阳经药，其实荣卫药也。以其在太阳地分，故曰太阳也。本病者即荣卫，肺主卫，心主荣为血，乃肺、心所主，故麻黄为手太阴之剂，桂枝为手少阴之剂。故伤寒、伤风而嗽者，用麻黄、桂枝，即汤液之源也。

《药性论》云：君。味甘平，治瘟疫。

《本草》又云：厚朴为之使，恶辛夷、石韦。

Mahuang [麻黄, ephedra, Herba Ephedrae]

Mahuang [麻黄, hedra, Herba Ephedrae] is warm in property, bitter in taste, sweet and bitter, thin in property and flavor, yang in property and ascending in functional tendency. It is sweet and hot, pure yang and nontoxic. The hand-taiyin formula enters the meridian of foot-taiyang, and goes along the meridian of hand-shaoyin, the medicinal herb of the meridian of yangming.

Xiang [《药类法象》, Rules for the Use of Medicinal Herbs] says: It promotes the sweating in the meridian of taiyang and shaoyin. When decocting, remove the nodes, boil twice or third times, and skim off the scum. If you do not follow the instruction, it may cause vexation and oppression.

Xin [《用药心法》, Gist for the Use of Medicinal Herbs] says: It is the medicinal herb of the meridian of yangming. It eliminates the external cold pathogen. It is sweet and heat. Remove the nodes before decoction. It can eliminate the shaoyin cold, dissipate the external cold, and effuse floating heat.

Zhen [《珍珠囊》, Pounch of Pearls] says: It eliminates the cold in luxuriance.

Ben Cao says: It is mainly used to treat wind attack, cold damage headache, warm pattern, relieve exterior syndrome, promote sweating, eliminate pathogenic heat, cough and the counter-flow of qi, eliminate cold heat, and resolve the hard lump and the accumulation.

Ye [《汤液本草》, Materia Medica for Decoctions] says: It enters the meridian of foot-taiyang, the meridian of hand-shaoyin, discharges defense excess, promotes sweating, and treats cold damage without sweat and cough. The root and knob of it can stop sweating. Mahuang [麻黄, ephedra, Herba Ephedrae] can treat the defense excess. Guizhi [桂枝, Cinnamon bark, Cortex Cinnamomum Cassia] is the medicinal herb to treat the defense deficiency. Guizhi [桂枝, Cinnamon bark, Cortex Cinnamomum Cassia] and Mahuang [麻黄, ephedra, Herba Ephedrae] are the medicinal herbs of the meridian of taiyang. The fact is that they are autually medicinal herbs to nourish the defense. They are in taiyang earthly branches and that is why they are called the medicinal herbs of taiyang. To treat the root disease, people need to nourish the defease. The lung governs the defense qi. The heart governs the nutrient qi and transforms into blood. So Mahuang [麻黄, ephedra, Herba Ephedrae] is a medicinal herb of the meridian of hand-taiyin. Guizhi [桂枝, Cinnamon bark, Cortex Cinnamomum Cassia] is a medicinal herb of the meridian of hand-shaoyin. This is the reason why Mahuang [麻黄, ephedra, Herba Ephedrae] and Guizhi [桂枝, Cinnamon bark, Cortex Cinnamomum Cassia] is used to treat cough due to cold damage and wind damage. It is regarded as the origin of decoction.

Yao Xing Lun [《药性论》, *Treatise on Medicinal Properties*] says: It is the monarch medicine. The taste is sweet and neutral. It can be used to treat the pestilence.

Ben Cao says: Houpu [厚朴, magnolia bark, Cortex Magnoliae Officinalis] is its assistance. It is averse to Xinyi [辛夷, flower of biond magnolia, Flos Magnoliae] and Shiwei [石韦, shearer's pyrrosia leaf, Folium Pyrrosiae].

藁 本

气温,味大辛。苦、微温,气厚味薄,阳也,升也,纯阳。无毒。

太阳经本经药。

《象》云:太阳经风药,治寒邪结郁于本经。治头痛、脑痛;大寒犯脑,令人脑痛,齿亦痛。

《心》云:专治太阳头痛,其气雄壮。

《珍》云:治巅顶痛。

《本草》云：主妇人疝瘕，阴中寒肿痛，腹中急。除风头痛，长肌肤，悦颜色，辟雾露，润泽，疗风邪辨曳，金疮。可作沐药、面脂。实，主流风四肢。恶䕡茹。此与木香，同治雾露之气；与白芷，同作面脂药治疗。

仲景云：清明已前，立秋已后，凡中雾露之气，皆为伤寒。又云清邪中于上焦，皆雾露之气，神术白术汤内加木香、藁本，择其可而用之。此既治风，又治湿，亦各从其类也。

Gaoben [藁本, Chinese Lovage, Rhizoma Ligustici]

Gaoben [藁本, Chinese Lovage, Rhizoma Ligustici] is mild in property and strongly pungent in taste. It is bitter and slightly warm. It is strong in property and thin in flavor. It is of yang property, ascending, and pure yang. It is nontoxic.

It is regarded as a medicinal herb of the meridian of taiyang.

Xiang [《药类法象》, *Rules for the Use of Medicinal Herbs*] says: As the wind medicine of the meridian of taiyang, it can be used to treat the cold damage in the meridian. It can be used to treat the headache and the painfal brain caused by great cold invading the brain accompanied with toothache.

Xin [《用药心法》, *Gist for the Use of Medicinal Herbs*] says: It specializes in curing taiyang headache and it is strong in property.

Zhen [《珍珠囊》, *Pounch of Pearls*] says: It can be used to treat the pain in the vertex of the head.

Ben Cao says: It is mainly used to treat the hernia and abdominal mass in women, genital coldness, swelling and pain, abdominal contracture and spasm. It is used to treat the headache caused by the invasion of wind into the head, promote the growth of muscles and luster the facial expression, eliminate dist, moisten the skin, and treat the wind pathogenic factors and incised wounds. It can be used in the bath water or face cream. Its fruit is mainly used to treat the wind damage in limbs. It is averse to Lüru [䕡茹, Lanru herb, Herba Lanru]. Both Gaoben [藁本, Chinese Lovage, Rhizoma Ligustici] and Muxiang [木香, root of common aucklandia, Radix Aucklandiae] can treat the cold damage caused by mist and dew; if used together with Baizhi [白芷, root of dahurian angelica, Radix Angelicae Dahuricae], it can be taken as grease to luster the face.

Zhang Zhongjing said: Before the Tomb-sweeping Day and after autumn begins, all the diseases caused by the mist and dew are cold damage. He also said that the clear pathogen in the upper energizer due to the mist and dew can be treated by Shenzhu Baizhu Decoction supplemented with Muxiang [木香, root of common aucklandia, Radix Aucklandiae] and Gaoben [藁本, Chinese Lovage, Rhizoma Ligustici]. It can treat wind pathogen and dampness according to various kinds of it.

桔　梗

气微温,味辛、苦,阳中之阳。味厚,气轻,阳中之阴也。有小毒。

入足少阴经,入手太阴脉经药。

《象》云:治咽喉痛,利肺气。去芦,米泔浸一宿,焙干用。

《珍》云:阳中之阴,谓之"舟楫",诸药有此一味,不能下沉。治鼻塞。

《心》云:利咽嗌胸膈之气。以其色白,故属肺。辛、甘、微温,治寒呕,若咽中痛,桔梗能散之也。

《本草》云:主胸胁痛如刀刺,腹满,肠鸣幽幽,惊恐悸气。利五脏肠胃,补血气,除寒热风痹,温中消谷,疗咽喉痛,下蛊毒。

易老云:与国老并行,同为舟楫之剂。如将军苦泄峻下之药,欲引至胸中至高之分成功,非此辛甘不居,譬如铁石入江,非舟楫不载,故用辛甘之剂以升之也。

《衍义》云:治肺热气奔促,咳逆,肺痈排脓。

《本草》又云:节皮为之使。得牡蛎、远志疗恚怒;得硝石、石膏疗伤寒。畏白及、龙眼、龙胆。

Jiegeng [桔梗, platycodon grandiflorum, Radix Platycodi]

Jiegeng [桔梗, platycodon grandiflorum, Radix Platycodi] is slightly warm in property and pungent and bitter in taste, pertaining to yin within yang. It is strong in taste and weak in property. It is yin within yang. It is slightly toxic.

It enters the meridian of foot-shaoyin and the meridian of hand-taiyin.

Xiang [《药类法象》, *Rules for the Use of Medicinal Herbs*] says: It treats the sore throat and disinhibits the lung qi. For processing purpose, remove the root, soak it in the washing water of rice for a night and dry it.

Zhen［《珍珠囊》, *Pounch of Pearls*］says: It is yin within yang, so it is called Zhouji (means ship in Chinese). Jiegeng［桔梗, platycodon grandiflorum, Radix Platycodi］can prevent the other herbs in a formula from sinkng. It is effective to treat the nasal congestion.

Xin［《用药心法》, *Gist for the Use of Medicinal Herbs*］says: It relieves the distention in the chest and diaphragm. It is white, so it belongs to the lung. It is pungent, sweet and slightly warm. It can be used to treat the cold vomiting. Jiegeng［桔梗, platycodon grandiflorum, Radix Platycodi］can treat the sore throat.

Ben Cao says: It is mainly used to treat the pain of the chest and rib-side like being stabbed by a knife, abdominal fullness, borborygum like deer crying, terror and palpitation. It smooths the intestines and stomach, tonifies qi and the blood, eliminates the wandering arthritis due to cold and heat, and warms the middle internal organs and swift digestion. It treats sore throat and removes poison produced by venomous insects.

Yilao［Zhang Yuansu］said: It is effective when used with Guolao［国老, licorice, Glycyrrhizae Radix］. Both of them are the medicinal herbs like boats (one that acts as a conductor to the upper energizer). The function of Jiegeng［桔梗, platycodon grandiflorum, Radix Platycodi］is like that of Jiangjun［将军, rhubarb, Radix et Rhizoma Rhei］which can be used to discharge with bitterness and purge drastically. Jiangjun［将军, rhubarb, Radix et Rhizoma Rhei］can not be conducted to the chest without the assistance of Jiegeng［桔梗, platycodon grandiflorum, Radix Platycodi］. It is like the iron stone in the river which needs the boat to bear and support. So sweet and pungent medicinal herbs should be used to conduct.

Yan Yi［《衍义》, *Extension of the Materia Medica*］says: It treats the lung heat, panting, cough and counterflow, and expels the pus and the carbuncle of the lung.

Ben Cao also says: Jiepi［节皮, Jiepi medicinal, Materia medica Jiepi］is its assistance. If used together with Muli［牡蛎, oyster shell, Concha Ostreae］and Yuanzhi［远志, polygala root, Radix Polygalae］, it can treat the resentment and anger; if used together with Xiaoshi［硝石, niter, Sal Nitri］and Shigao［石膏,

gypsum, Gypsum Fibrosum], it can treat the cold damage. It is restrained by Baiji [白芨, tuber of common bletilla, Rhizoma Bletillae], Longyan [龙眼, longan aril, Arillus Longan] and Longdan [龙胆, root of rough gentian, Radix Gentianae].

鼠黏子

气平,味辛,辛温。

《象》云:主风毒肿,利咽膈。吞一枚,可出痈疽疮头。

《珍》云:润肺散气。

Shunianzi [鼠黏子, arctium, Arctium Lappa L.]

Shunianzi [鼠黏子, arctium, Arctium Lappa L.] is mild in property, pungent in taste and warm in nature.

Xiang [《药类法象》, *Rules for the Use of Medicinal Herbs*] says: It is mainly used to treat the wind toxin swelling and disinhibit the throat. To take one can cure sore ulcer.

Zhen [《珍珠囊》, *Pouch of Pearls*] says: It moistens the lung and disperses qi.

秦艽

气微温,味苦、辛,阴中微阳。

手阳明经药。

《象》云:主寒热邪气,风湿痹,下水,利小便。治黄病骨蒸。治口噤及肠风泻血。去芦用。

《珍》云:去手阳明经下牙痛,口疮毒,去本经风湿。

《本草》云:菖蒲为之使。

Qinjiao [秦艽, largeleaf gentian root, Radix Gentianae Macrophyllae]

It is slightly warm in property, bitter and pungent in taste, and slightly yang within yin.

It is a medicinal herb of the meridian of hand-yangming.

Xiang [《药类法象》, *Rules for the Use of Medicinal Herbs*] says: It is mainly used to treat the cold heat pathogenic qi and the arthralgia due to wind dampness, discharge water and promote urination. It can be used to treat jaundice and hectic fever due to yin deficiency. It treats the lock jaw, intestine wind and bloody stool. It is used in the clinical practice with its root removed.

Zhen [《珍珠囊》, *Pounch of Pearls*] says: It relieves the toothache of the meridian of hand-yangming and resolves the toxin of mouth sore. It eliminates the wind dampness of the meridian.

Ben Cao says: Changpu [菖蒲, acorus, Acorus Calamus] is its assistance.

天 麻

气平,味苦。无毒。

《象》石:治头风。

《本草》云:主诸风湿痹,四肢拘挛,小儿风痫惊气,利腰膝,强筋力。其苗名定风草。

Tianma [天麻, gastrodia, Gastrodiae Rhizoma]

It is mild in property and bitter in taste. It is nontoxic.

Xiang [《药类法象》, *Rules for the Use of Medicinal Herbs*] says: It treats the head wind.

Ben Cao says: It is mainly used to treat the arthralgia due to wind dampness, the hypertonicity of limbs, the wind epilepsy and the fright of children, and strengthen the lumbus and knees, sinews and bones. Its plant is named Dingfengcao in Chinese.

黑 附 子

气热,味大辛,纯阳。辛、甘、温,大热。有大毒。通行诸经引用药。入手少阳经三焦、命门之剂。

《象》云:性走而不守。亦能除肾中寒甚,白术为佐,名术附汤,除寒湿之圣药也,湿药中少加之,通行诸经引用药也。治经闭。慢火炮。

《珍》云：治脾湿肾寒。

《本草》云：主风寒咳逆邪气，温中，金疮，破症坚积聚，血瘕，寒湿痿躄拘挛，膝痛脚疼，冷弱不能行步，腰脊风寒，心腹冷痛，霍乱转筋，下利赤白，坚肌骨，强阴，堕胎，为百药之长。

《液》云：入手少阳三焦、命门之剂，浮中沉无所不至。附子味辛大热，为阳中之阳，故行而不止，非若干姜 止而不行也。非身表凉而四肢厥者，不可僭用。如用之者，以其治四逆也。

《本草》又云：地胆为之使，恶蜈蚣，畏防风、黑豆、甘草、黄芪、人参。冬月采为附子，春月采为乌头。

Heifuzi［黑附子, aconite, Radix Aconiti Praeparata］

It is heat in property, pungent in taste, and pure yang. It is pungent, sweet, and warm, with great heat. It is toxic. It conducts herbs to all the meridians. It enters the triple energizer of the meridian of hand-shaoyang and it treats the disease concerning Mingmen acupoint.

Xiang［《药类法象》, *Rules for the Use of Medicinal Herbs*］says：It works in a wandering tendency. It also eliminates the cold in kidney. Baizhu［白术, rhizome of largehead atractyloes, Rhizoma Atractylodis Macrocephalae］is its assistance. Zhufu Decoction is very effective to eliminate the cold dampness. It can treat the menstrual block. It needs processing with slow flame.

Zhen［《珍珠囊》, *Pounch of Pearls*］says：It treats spleen dampness and kidney cold.

Ben Cao says：It is mainly used to treat wind cold cough, counter-flow and pathogenic qi, warm the middle internal organs, treat incised wounds, and disperse the accumulation of abdominal mass. It can treat blood conglomeration, cold dampness, atrophy and flaccidity, hypertonicity, knees and feet pain, inability to walk due to cold and weakness, cold damage in lumbus and spine, cold pain in the heart and abdomen, cholera cramps, dysenteric diarrhea. It can strengthen muscles, bones and yin, and induce abortion. It is the chief of medicinal herbs.

Ye［《汤液本草》, *Materia Medica for Decoctions*］says：It enters the triple energizer of the meridian of hand-shaoyang and it is the life gate formula. It works through the whole body. Fuzi［附子, aconite, Radix Aconiti Praeparata］is pungent in taste and extremely hot in property, yang within yang. It moves ceaselessly and differs with Ganjiang [干姜, dried ginger, Rhizoma Zingiberis], which is likely to cease instead of moving. It should only be used to treat the reversal cold limbs due to exterior cold. It is mainly applied to treat the reversal cold of limbs.

Ben Cao also says: Didan [地胆, all-grass of canton sonerila, Meloe coarctatus] is its assistance. It is averse to Wugong [蜈蚣, centipede, Scolopendra]. It is restrained by Fangfeng [防风, divaricate saposhnikovia root, Radix Saposhnikoviae], Heidou [黑豆, black soybean, Sojae Semen Atrum], Gancao [甘草, liquorice root, Glycyrrhiza uralensis Fisch.], Huangqi [黄芪, milkvetch root, Radix Astragali seu Hedysari] and Renshen [人参, ginseng, Radix Ginseng]. When collected in winter, it is called Fuzi [附子, aconite, Radix Aconiti Praeparata]; when collected in spring, it is called Wutou [乌头, root of Szechwan aconita, Radix Aconiti].

乌 头

气热,味大辛、辛、甘,大热。有大毒。

行诸经。

《象》云:治风痹血痹,半身不遂,行经药也。慢火炮坼,去皮用。

《本草》云:主中风恶风,洗洗出汗,除寒湿痹,咳逆上气,破积聚寒热,消胸上痰,冷食不下,心腹冷疾,胳间痛,肩胛痛,不可俯仰,目中痛,不可久视,堕胎。其汁煎之,名射罔,杀禽兽。

《液》云:乌、附,天雄侧子之属,皆水浸炮裂,去皮脐用之。多有外黄里白,劣性尚在,莫若乘热切作片子,再炒,令表里皆黄,内外一色,劣性皆去,却为良也。世人罕如此制之。

Wutou [乌头, common monkshood, Aconitum carmichaeli Debx.]

Wutou [乌头, common monkshood, Aconitum carmichaeli Debx.] is heat in property, extremely pungent in flavor, pungent and sweet in taste, and with great heat. It is severely toxic.

It conducts all the meridians.

Xiang [《药类法象》, *Rules for the Use of Medicinal Herbs*] says: It treats wind impediment, blood impediment and paralysis. It promotes the circulation of meridians. Prepare it with slow flame and the peel should be removed before use.

Ben Cao says: It is mainly used to treat the wind stroke marked by aversion to cold with chilliness, shivering and sweating, eliminate the cold-dampness impediment and cough with dyspnea and the counter-flow of qi, break accumulation and conglomeration, treat the cold-heat disease, transform phlegm, treat inability to get cold food down, cold pain in the heart region and abdomen, umbilical pain, shoulder blade pain, inability to raise head and bend forward, eye pain, and induce abortion. Its decoction is called Shewang and can be used to kill birds and beasts.

Ye [《汤液本草》, *Materia Medica for Decoctions*] says: Wutou [乌头, common monkshood, Aconitum carmichaeli Debx.], Fuzi [附子, aconite, Radix Aconiti Praeparata], Tianxiong [天雄, tianxiong conite, Aconiti Radix Lateralis Tianxiong] and Cezi [侧子, Branch Monkshood Daughter, Aconitum carmichaeli Debx.] need to be soaked in water and blast-fried, and remove the peel. Most of them are yellow outside and white inside. Slice them into pieces when they are hot, stir-fry again and make them yellow both outside and inside. It becomes effective medicinal with its toxin removed. People seldom process this medicinal herb in this way.

缩 砂

气温,味辛。无毒。

入手足太阴经、阳明经、太阳经、足少阴经。

《象》云:治脾胃气结滞不散,主劳虚冷泻,心腹痛,下气,消食。

《本草》云:治虚劳冷泻,宿食不消,赤白泄利,腹中虚痛,下气。

《液》云:与白檀、豆蔻为使,则入肺;与人参、益智为使,则入脾;与黄柏、茯苓为使,则入肾;与赤、白石脂为使,则入大小肠。

Suosha [缩砂, Fructus Amomi Xanthioidis, Amomum villosum Lour. Var. xanthioides T. L. Wu et Senjen]

It is warm and mild in property, and pungent in taste. It is nontoxic.

It enters the meridian of hand and foot taiyin, the meridian of yangming, the meridian of taiyang and the meridian of foot shaoyin.

Xiang [《药类法象》, *Rules for the Use of Medicinal Herbs*] says: It treats qi stagnation in the spleen and stomach and it is mainly used to treat the deficiency due to overstrain and cold diarrhea, pain in the heart and abdomen, promote qi to descend, and digest food.

Ben Cao [《神农本草经》, *Shennong's Classic of Materia Medica*] says: It treats the deficiency due to overstrain and cold diarrhea, abiding food accumulation, dysenteric diarrhea, deficiency pain in the abdomen, and descends qi.

Ye [《汤液本草》, *Materia Medica for Decoctions*] says: Baitan [白檀, sapphire-berry sweetleaf, Symplocoris Paniculatae Radix] and Doukou [豆蔻, Katsumada's galangal seed, Alpiniae Katsumadai Semen] work as its assistance, and it enters the lung. Renshen [人参, ginseng, Radix Ginseng] and Yizhi [益智, alpinia, Alpiniae Oxyphyllae Fructus] work as its assistance, and it enters the spleen. Huangbo [黄柏, bark of amur corktree, Cortex Phellodendri] and Fuling [茯苓, Indian bread, Poria] work as its assistance, and it enters the kidney. Chishizhi [赤石脂, halloysite, Halloysitum Rubrum] and Baishizhi [白石脂, kaolin, Kaolin] work as its assistance, and it enters the large and small intestines.

荜澄茄

气温，味辛。无毒。
本草云：主下气消食，皮肤风，心腹间气胀，令人能食。

Bichengqie [荜澄茄, cubeb, Litseae Fructus]

It is warm and mild in property and pungent in taste. It is nontoxic.

Ben Cao says: It is mainly used to descend qi, digest food, treat the wind of skin and the qi distention between the heart and the abdomen, and improve the appetite.

荜茇

气温,味辛。无毒。

《本草》云:主温中下气,补腰脚,杀腥气,消食,除胃冷、阴疝、痃癖。

《衍义》云:走肠胃中冷气,呕吐,心腹满痛。多服走泄真气,令人肠虚下重。

Biba [荜茇, long pepper, Piper Longum L.]

It is warm and mild in property, and pungent in taste. It is nontoxic.

Ben Cao says: It is mainly used to warm the middle internal organs and promote qi to descend. It can tonify the waist and feet, remove the fishy flavor, digest food, and eliminate cold in the stomach, yin hernia, hypochondroiun abdominal mass.

Yan Yi [《衍义》, *Extension of the Materia Medica*] says: It eliminates the cold qi in the intestines and stomach. It treats vomiting, fullness and the pain in the heart and abdomen. Taking too much of it may damage the genuine qi, cause the deficiency of the intestines and tenesmus.

香附子

气微寒,味甘,阳中之阴。无毒。

《本草》云:除胸中热,充皮毛,久服利人益气、长须眉。后世人用治崩漏,本草不言治崩漏。

《图经》云:膀胱、两胁气妨,常日忧愁不乐,饮食不多,皮肤瘙痒瘾疹,日渐瘦损,心忪少气。以是知益血中之气药也。方中用治崩漏,是益气而止血也。又能去凝血,是推陈也。与巴豆同治泄泻不止,又能治大便不通。

《珍》云:快气。

Xiangfuzi [香附子, cyperus, Cyperi Rhizoma]

Xiangfuzi [香附子, cyperus, Cyperi Rhizoma] is slightly cold in property and sweet in taste, pertaining to yin within yang. It is nontoxic.

Ben Cao says: It eliminates the heat in the chest, and fortifies the skin and hair. Long-term taking of it can benefit people's health, replenish qi and promote eyebrows. The people of later generations use it to treat the uterine bleeding but it is not mentioned in *Ben Cao*.

Tu Jing [《图经》, *Illustrated Classics of Materia Medica*] says: It can treat the qi stagnation in the bladder and rib-sides, anxiousness and unhappiness, poor appetite, itchy skin and measles, emaciation, palpitation and asthenic breathing, so it can replenish qi and blood. It is used to treat the uterine bleeding for its function of replenishing qi and stanching bleeding. It also can be used to coagulate blood and promote the discharge of waste. If used together with Badou [巴豆, croton, Fructus Crotonis], it can treat diarrhea and constipation.

Zhen [《珍珠囊》, *Pounch of Pearls*] says: It can disinhibit qi.

草豆蔻

气热,味大辛,阳也。辛温。无毒。

入足太阴经、阳明经。

《象》云:治风寒客邪在胃口之上,善去脾胃客寒,心与胃痛。面包煨熟,去面用。

《珍》云:益脾胃,去寒。

《本草》云:主温中,心腹痛,呕吐,去口臭气,下气,胀满短气,消酒进食,止霍乱,治一切冷气,调中补胃健脾,亦能消食。

《衍义》云:性温,而调散冷气力甚速。虚弱不能饮食,宜此与木瓜、乌梅、缩砂、益智、曲、糵、盐、草、姜也。

Caodoukou [草豆蔻, katsumada galangal seed, Semen Alpiniae Katsumadai]

Caodoukou [草豆蔻, katsumada galangal seed, Semen Alpiniae Katsumadai] is hot in property, strongly pungent in taste, and of yang propenty. It is pungent and warm in nature. It is nontoxic.

It enters the meridian of foot-taiyin and the meridian of yangming.

Xiang [《药类法象》, *Rules for the Use of Medicinal Herbs*] says: It is used to treat the pathogenic wind cold syndrome in stomach. It is effective to eliminate the cold in the spleen and stomach, heart pain and stomachache. Cover it with flour and bake, and then remove the flour.

Zhen〔《珍珠囊》, *Pouch of Pearls*〕says: It is beneficial for the spleen and stomach. It can eliminate cold.

Ben Cao says: It is mainly used to warm the middle internal organs, relieve the pain in the heart and the abdomen, treat vomiting and halitosis, descend qi, treat fullness and shortness of breath, resolve liquor and digest food, treat cholera and cold qi, regulate the middle energizer, strengthen the spleen and stomach, and digest food.

Yan Yi〔《衍义》, *Extension of the Materia Medica*〕says: It is warm in nature, and it can dissipate cold qi at a fast speed. It can treat weakness and poor appetite when used together with Mugua〔木瓜, common floweringqince fruit, Fructus Chaenomelis〕, Wumei〔乌梅, smoked plum, Fructus Mume〕, Suosha〔缩砂, Fructus Amomi Xanthioidis, Amomum villosum Lour. Var. xanthioides T. L. Wu et Senjen〕, Yizhi〔益智, sharp-leaf glangal fruit, Fructus Alpiniae oxyphyllae〕, leaven, tiller, salt, grass and ginger.

白豆蔻

气热,味大辛,味薄气厚,阳也。辛,大温。无毒。

入手太阴经。

《珍》云:主积冷气,散肺中滞气,宽膈,止吐逆,治反胃,消谷下气进食,去皮用。

《心》云:专入肺经,去白睛翳膜。红者,不宜多用。

《本草》云:主积聚冷气,止吐逆反胃,消谷下气。

《液》云:入手太阴,别有清高之气,上焦元气不足,以此补之。

Baidoukou〔白豆蔻, cardamom, Amomi Fructus Rotundus〕

It is hot in property and extremely pungent in taste. It is light in taste, and strong in smell, pertaining to yang. It is pungent and warm. It is nontoxic.

It enters the meridian of hand-taiyin.

Zhen〔《珍珠囊》, *Pouch of Pearls*〕says: It is mainly used to treat cold qi accumulation, dissipate qi stagnation in the lung, disinhibit the chest and diaphragm, treat vomiting, regurgitation, accelerate digestion, promote qi to descend, and promote appetite. Its peel should be removed before use.

Xin [《用药心法》, *Gist for the Use of Medicinal Herbs*] says: It enters the meridian of lung to remove the slight corneal opacity. Do not use too much when it is red.

Ben Cao says: It is mainly used to treat the accumulation of cold, vomiting, regurgitation, accelerate digestion, and descend qi.

Ye [《汤液本草》, *Materia Medica for Decoctions*] says: It enters the meridian of hand-taiyin. It can tonify the original qi in the upper energizer.

延 胡 索

气温,味辛。苦、辛,温。无毒。

入手足太阴经。

《象》云:破血治气,月水不调,小腹痛,暖腰膝,破症瘕。碎用。

《液》云:治心气痛、小腹痛,有神。主破血,产后诸疾,因血为病者。妇人月水不调,腹中结块,崩漏淋露,暴血上行,因损下血。

Yanhusuo [延胡索, yanhusuo, Rhizoma Corydalis]

It is warm in property and pungent in taste. It is bitter, pungent and warm. It is nontoxic.

It enters the meridian of hand and foot taiyin.

Xiang [《药类法象》, *Rules for the Use of Medicinal Herbs*] says: It breaks bloody conglomeration, regulates qi, and treats menstrual disorder and lower abdomen pain. It warms the waist and knees and breaks the lump. Break it into pieces when using it.

Ye [《汤液本草》, *Materia Medica for Decoctions*] says: It treats the pain in the heart and the lower abdomen, and brings the presence of spirit. It is mainly used to break bloody conglomeration, postpartum diseases and diseases related to blood. It treats menstrual disorder, abdominal lump, uterine bleeding, prolonged bleeding, the counter-flow of blood which damages the blood in the lower part.

茴 香

气平,味辛。无毒。

入手足少阴经,太阳经药。

《象》云:破一切臭气,调中止呕下食。炒黄色,碎用。

《本草》云:主诸瘘、霍乱及蛇伤。又能治肾劳,癫疝气,开胃下食。又治膀胱阴痛,脚气,少腹痛不可忍。

《液》云:茴香本治膀胱药,以其先丙,故云小肠也,能润丙燥。以其先戊,故从丙至壬。又手足少阴二药,以开上下经之通道,所以壬与丙交也。

Huixiang [茴香, fennel, Foeniculum Vulgare]

It is mild in property and pungent in taste. It is nontoxic.

It enters the meridian of hand and foot shaoyin. It is the medicinal herb of the meridian of taiyang.

Xiang [《药类法象》, *Rules for the Use of Medicinal Herbs*] says: It removes the foul smell, harmonizes the spleen and the stomach, stops vomiting and promotes digestion. Fry until it turns to yellow and break it into pieces before use.

Ben Cao says: It is mainly used to treat scrofula, cholera and snake bite. It can also be used to treat kidney overstain and hernia. It promotes appetite and digestion. It also treats bladder genital pain, beriberi, and intolerable lower abdomen pain.

Ye [《汤液本草》, *Materia Medica for Decoctions*] says: Huixiang [茴香, fennel, Foeniculum vulgare] is a medicinal herb to treat bladder diseases, and moisten dryness in the small intestine, corresponding to the third heavenly stem, then the fifth heavenly stem, and then the ninth heavenly stem. As the medicinal herb of the meridian of hand and foot shaoyin, it can free the passage of the meridians. The ninth heavenly stem is associated with the third heavenly stem.

红 蓝 花

气温,味辛。辛而甘、温、苦,阴中之阳。无毒。

《象》云：治产后口噤血晕，腹内恶血不尽，绞痛。破留血，神效。搓碎用。

《心》云：和血，与当归同用。

《珍》云：入心养血。谓苦为阴中之阳，故入心。

《本草》云：主产后血晕，胎死腹中，并酒煮服。亦主蛊毒下血。其苗，生捣傅游肿。其子，吞数粒，主天行疮子不出。其胭脂，主小儿聤耳，滴耳中。仲景治六十二种风，兼腹中血气刺痛，用红花一大两，分为四分，酒一大升，煎强半，顿服之。

Honglanhua ［红蓝花, Tulipa, Carthamus Tinctorius L.］

It is warm and mild in property, and pungent in taste. It is pungent and sweet, warm, bitter, pertaining to yang within yin. It is nontoxic.

Xiang ［《药类法象》, *Rules for the Use of Medicinal Herbs*］ says: It treats the postpartum lockjaw and blood dizziness, persistent malign blood in abdomen and colic pain. It is very effective in treating blood retention. Rub it into pieces before use.

Xin ［《用药心法》, *Gist for the Use of Medicinal Herbs*］ says: It harmonizes the blood, and can be used with Danggui ［当归, Chinese angelica, Radix Angelicae Sinensis］.

Zhen ［《珍珠囊》, *Pounch of Pearls*］ says: It enters the heart and nourishes the blood. It is bitter, and of yang within yin. That is why it enters the heart.

Ben Cao says: It is mainly used to treat the postpartum hemorrhagic syncope, and the death in utero. Boil it with liquor before use. It also resolves toxin and descends blood. Pound its plant for the wandering swelling. Take several seeds and it will treat the epidemic non-eruption of sores. Its rouge can treat the purulent ear of children. Zhang Zhongjing used it to treat 62 kinds of wind pathogens, the abdominal pain due to blood stasis and qi stagnation. Divide 1 Liang of Honglanhua ［红蓝花, Tulipa, Carthamus tinctorius L.］ into four portions, and boil it with 1 Sheng of liquor until fifty percent of liquor left and take at a draught.

良 姜

气热，味辛，纯阳。

《本草》云：治胃中冷逆，霍乱腹痛，反胃呕食，转筋泻痢。下气，消宿食。

《心》云：健脾胃。

Liangjiang［良姜，lesser galangal rhizome, Rhizoma Alpiniae Officinarum］

It is heat in property and pungent in taste. It is of pure yang.

Ben Cao says：It treats the coldness and qi counter-flow in the stomach, cholera, abdominal pain, regurgitation, vomiting, cramp and diarrhea. It promotes qi to descend, and digests retained food.

Xin［《用药心法》，*Gist for the Use of Medicinal Herbs*］says：It fortifies the spleen and the stomach.

黄 芪

气温，味甘，纯阳。甘，微温，性平。无毒。

入手少阳经、足太阴经，足少阴、命门之剂。

《象》云：治虚劳自汗，补肺气，入皮毛，泻肺中火。如脉弦自汗，脾胃虚弱，疮疡血脉不行，内托，阴证疮疡必用之。去芦用。

《珍》云：益胃气，去肌热，诸痛必用之。

《心》云：补五脏诸虚不足，而泻阴火，去虚热，无汗则发之，有汗则止之。

《本草》云：主痈疽久败疮，排脓止痛，大风癞疾，五痔鼠瘘，补虚；小儿百病，妇人子脏风邪气，逐五脏间恶血，补丈夫虚损，五劳羸瘦，腹痛泄痢。益气，利阴气。

有白水芪、赤水芪、木芪，功用皆同。惟木芪茎短而理横，折之如绵，皮黄褐色，肉中白色，谓之绵黄芪。其坚脆而味苦者，乃苜蓿根也。又云，破症癖，肠风血崩，带下，赤白痢，及产前、后一切病，月候不调，消渴痰嗽。又治头风热毒，目赤，骨蒸。生蜀郡山谷、白水、汉中，今河东陕西州郡多有之。芪与桂同功，特味稍异，比桂但甘平，不辛热耳。世人以苜蓿根代之，呼为土黄芪，但味苦，能令人瘦，特味甘者能令人肥也。颇能乱真，用者宜审。治气虚盗汗并自汗，即皮表之药；又治肤痛，则表药可知；又治咯血，柔脾胃，是为中州药也；又治伤寒尺脉不至，又补肾脏元气，为里药。是上中下内外三焦之药。

今《本草图经》只言河东者，沁州绵上是也，故谓之绵芪。味甘如蜜，兼体骨柔软如绵，世以为如绵，非也。《别说》云，黄芪本出绵上为良，故《图经》所绘者，宪水者也，与绵上相邻，盖以地产为"绵"。若以柔韧为"绵"，则伪者亦柔，但以干脆甘苦为别耳。

东垣云：黄芪、人参、甘草三味，退热之圣药也。《灵枢》曰：卫气者，所以温分肉而充皮肤，肥腠理而司开阖。黄芪既补三焦、实卫气，与桂同，特益气异耳。亦在佐使。桂则通血也，能破血而实卫气，通内而实外者欤。桂以血言，一作色求，则芪为实气也。恶鳖甲。

Huangqi [黄芪, milkvetch root, Radix Astragali seu Hedysari]

It is mild in property and sweet in taste, and of pure yang. It is sweet, slightly warm and neutral in nature. It is nontoxic.

It enters the meridian of hand-shaoyang, the meridian of foot-taiyin, the meiridian of foot-shaoyin, and acts as the medicinal herb of lifegate.

Xiang [《药类法象》, *Rules for the Use of Medicinal Herbs*] says: It is used to treat the deficiency due to overstrain, spontaneous sweating, tonify the lung qi, hair and skin, and clear the lung heat. It is effective to treat wiry pulse, spontaneous sweating, spleen and stomach vacuity, inhibited blood and vessels in ulcerated sores, internal expulsion, and ulcerated sores due to yin damage pattern. The root and hair should be removed before use.

Zhen [《珍珠囊》, *Pounch of Pearls*] says: It boosts the stomach qi and the heat in flesh. It can be used to treat all kinds of pains.

Xin [《用药心法》, *Gist for the Use of Medicinal Herbs*] says: It can tonify the deficiency of the five zang-organs, clear the yin fire, and relieve the deficiency heat. If there is no sweat, it will promote sweat; and if there is sweating, it will check sweating.

Ben Cao says: It is mainly used to treat the injury caused by chronic carbuncle and ulcer, to resolve pus, to relieve pain, to treat severe leprosy, five kinds of hemorrhoids and scrofula, to improve deficiency and to treat various infantile diseases, uterine pathogenic qi, expel the malign blood in the five zang-organs, treat impotence, weakness due to five kinds of overstrain, abdominal pain and diarrhea. It replenishes qi and disinhibits yin qi.

Baishuiqi, Chishuiqi and Muqi have the same effect. The plant of Muqi is short and has lateral veins. It is as soft as cotton when it is folded. Its skin is yellowish-brown and its flesh is white. It is called Mianhuangqi. Those with hard and crispy part which tastes bitter are the root of Muxu [苜蓿, alfalfa, Medicago sativa L.]. It also says: It resolves stagnated blood, and treats intestine wind, flooding, vaginal discharge, red-white dysentery, antepartum and postpartum diseases, menstrual irregularities, consumptive thirst, phlegm and cough. It can also be used to treat head wind, heat toxin, red eyes and steaming bone. It grows in the valleys in Shujun, Baishui and Hanzhong. Presently it can be found in many counties in Hedong, Shanxi. Huangqi [黄芪, milkvetch root, Radix Astragali seu Hedysari] has the same effect as Guizhi [桂枝, Cinnamon bark, Cortex Cinnamomum Cassia]. They have unique smell. Comparing with Guizhi [桂枝, Cinnamon bark, Cortex Cinnamomum Cassia], Huangqi [黄芪, milkvetch root, Radix Astragali seu Hedysari] is sweeter and milder, but not so pungent and hot in property. People use the root of Muxu [苜蓿, alfalfa, Medicago sativa L.] to take its place and call it Tuhuangqi. However, it tastes bitter, and makes people lose weight. Those with unique smell and sweet taste will make people gain weight. It is easy to mix them up with each other. Check carefully before use. It can be used to treat the deficiency of qi, night sweating, spontaneous sweating. It is a medicinal herb of skin and exterior. It can also be used to treat skin pain. That is why it is a medicinal of exterior. It can also be used to treat the expectoration of blood, and fortify the spleen and the stomach. That is why it is a medicinal herb of the central region. It can also be used to treat the cold damage and the failure to feel chi pulse, and tonify the original qi of the kidney. So it is also an interior medicinal herb. It is the medicinal herb involving externally and internally the triple energizer.

Ben Cao Tu Jing [《本草图经》, *Illustrated Classic of the Materia Medica*] says: Huangqi [黄芪, milkvetch root, Radix Astragali seu Hedysari] in Jinshang, Qinzhou, southwest of Shanxi is called Mianqi. It is as sweet as honey in taste and the plant is as soft as cotton. It is wrong for people to call it "Mian" in Chinese.

Bie Shuo [《别说》, *Annotated Version of Agriculture God's Canon of Materia Medica*] says: Huangqi [黄芪, milkvetch root, Radix Astragali seu Hedysari] growing in Mianshang is good in quality. The picture in *Tu Jing* [《图经》,

Illustrated Classics of Materia Medica] is from Xianshui which is next to Mianshang. So the place of the origin is called Mian. Those which can not be taken as Mianqi are crispy, sweet and bitter.

Li Dongyuan said: Huangqi [黄芪, milkvetch root, Radix Astragali seu Hedysari], Renshen [人参, ginseng, Radix Ginseng] and Gancao [甘草, liquorice root, Glycyrrhiza uralensis Fisch.] are very effective to clear heat. *Lingshu* [《灵枢》, *Spiritual Pivot*] says: The defensive qi can engender mustcles and nourish the skin, benefit interstices and govern opening and closing. Huangqi [黄芪, milkvetch root, Radix Astragali seu Hedysari] can not only tonify the triple energizer but also replenish the defensive qi. The effect of Guizhi [桂枝, Cinnamon bark, Cortex Cinnamomum Cassia] is similar to that of Huangqi [黄芪, milkvetch root, Radix Astragali seu Hedysari] but the latter is used to replenish qi. The effect is also related to its assistance. Guizhi [桂枝, Cinnamon bark, Cortex Cinnamomum Cassia] promtes blood circulation, treats blood stasis, fortifies defense qi, dredges the interior and strengthens the exterior. It is related with blood aspect and color while Huangqi [黄芪, milkvetch root, Radix Astragali seu Hedysari] replenishes qi. It is averse to Biejia [鳖甲, turtle carapace, Carapax Trionycis].

苍 术

气温，味甘。

入足阳明、太阴经。

《象》云：主治同白术，若除上湿、发汗，功最大；若补中焦、除湿，力小，如白术也。

《衍义》云：其长如大拇指，肥实，皮色褐，气味辛烈，须米泔浸洗，再换泔浸二日，去上粗皮。

东垣云：入足阳明、太阴，能健胃安脾。

《本草》但言：术，不分苍、白。其苍术别有雄壮之气，以其经泔浸、火炒，故能出汗，与白术止汗特异，用者不可以此代彼。

海藏云：苍、白有止、发之异，其余主治，并见《图经》。

Cangzhu [苍术, atractylodes rhizome, Rhizoma Atractylodis]

It is warm in property and sweet in taste.

It enters the meridian of foot yangming and the meridian of taiyin.

Xiang [《药类法象》, *Rules for the Use of Medicinal Herbs*] says: It has the same effect as Baizhu [白术, argehead atractylodes rhizome, Rhizoma Atractylodis Macrocephalae]. It is very effective to eliminate the upper dampness and promote sweating. It is less effective to tonify the middle energizer and eliminate dampness. It is just like Baizhu [白术, argehead atractylodes rhizome, Rhizoma Atractylodis Macrocephalae].

Yan Yi [《衍义》, *Extension of the Materia Medica*] says: It is as long as the thumb, large, with brown peel and pungent smell. It needs to be soaked in the rice-washed water for two days, and in changed rice-washed water for another two days. Remove the rough peel before use.

Li Dongyuan said: It enters the meridian of foot-yangming and taiyin. It fortifies the stomach and calms the spleen.

Ben Cao says: There is no need to make a distinction between Cangzhu [苍术, atractylodes rhizome, Rhizoma Atractylodis] and Baizhu [白术, argehead atractylodes rhizome, Rhizoma Atractylodis Macrocephalae] but Cangzhu [苍术, atractylodes rhizome, Rhizoma Atractylodis] is strong in nature. After being soaked in the rice-washed water and being fryied on fire, it can promote sweating. It is different from the effect of Baizhu [白术, argehead atractylodes rhizome, Rhizoma Atractylodis Macrocephalae] which can be used to stop sweating. So they can not be used interchangeably.

Haizang [Wang Haogu] said: Cangzhu [苍术, atractylodes rhizome, Rhizoma Atractylodis] and Baizhu [白术, argehead atractylodes rhizome, Rhizoma Atractylodis Macrocephalae] are different. The former can promote sweating and the latter can stop sweating. One can refer to *Tu Jing* [《图经》, *Illustrated Classic of Materia Medica*] to know other effects of the medicinal herb.

白　术

气温，味甘。苦而甘、温，味厚气薄，阴中阳也。无毒。

入手太阳、少阴经，足阳明、太阴、少阴、厥阴四经。

《象》云：除湿益燥，和中益气，利腰脐间血，除胃中热，去诸经之湿，理胃。

洁古云：温中去湿，除热，降胃气，苍术亦同，但味颇厚耳。下行则用之，甘温补阳，健脾逐水，寒淫所胜，缓脾生津去湿，渴者用之。

《本草》在本条下，无苍、白之名。近多用白术治皮间风，止汗消痞，补胃和中，利腰脐间血。通水道，上而皮毛，中而心胃，下而腰脐。在气主气，在血主血。

洁古又云：非白术，不能去湿；非枳实，不能消痞。除湿利水道，如何是益津液。

Baizhu [白术, argehead atractylodes rhizome, Rhizoma Atractylodis Macrocephalae]

It is warm in property, and sweet and bitter in taste, with the former being strong and the later being weak, so it is regarded as yang within yin. It is nontoxic.

It enters the meridian of hand taiyang and shaoyin, and the meridian of foot yangming, taiyin, shaoyin and yueyin.

Xiang [《药类法象》, *Rules for the Use of Medicinal Herbs*] says: It can eliminate dampness and moisten dryness, harmonize the middle energizer and replenish qi, dredge blood retention in the waist and navel, clear the heat in the stomach, dispel the dampness in the channels, and regulate the stomach.

Jiegu [Zhang Yuansu] said: It can warm the middle internal organs and expel dampness, eliminate heat, and make the stomach qi descend. Cangzhu [苍术, atractylodes rhizome, Rhizoma Atractylodis] has the same effect, but its taste is rather stronger. It can be used to descend, tonify yang with its sweet and warm property, fortify the spleen, expel water, restrict cold pathogen, smooth the spleen, engender liquid, expel dampness and disperse thirst.

Ben Cao says: Baizhu [白术, argehead atractylodes rhizome, Rhizoma

Atractylodis Macrocephalae] is mostly used to treat the wind in skin, check sweating, disperse glomus, tonify the stomach, and harmonize the middle energizer. It is good for the blood between the waist and the umbilicus. It frees the waterways, going upward to the skin and hair, middle to the heart and stomach, downward to the waist and navel. It governs qi when it is in qi and governs the blood when it is in the blood.

Jiegu [Zhang Yuansu] also said: One can not eliminate dampness without Baizhu [白术, argehead atractylodesrhizome, Rhizoma Atractylodis Macrocephalae] and disperse glomus without Zhishi [枳实, immature orange fruit, Fructus Aurantii Immaturus]. It can eliminate dampness, regulate the waterways and nourish the fluids.

当 归

气温,味辛甘而大温,气味俱轻,阳也。甘辛,阳中微阴。无毒。

入手少阴经,足太阴经、厥阴经。

《象》云:和血补血,尾破血,身和血。先水洗去土,酒制过,或火干、日干入药,血病须用。去芦用。

《心》云:治血通用。能除血刺痛,以甘故能和血,辛温以润内寒,当归之苦以助心散寒。

《珍》云:头,止血;身,和血;梢,破血。治上,酒浸;治外,酒洗。糖色,嚼之大辛,可能溃坚。与菖蒲、海藻相反。

《本草》云:主咳逆上气,温疟,寒热洗在皮肤中,妇人漏下绝子,诸恶疮疡金疮,煮汁饮之。温中止痛及腰痛,除客血内塞,中风痉,汗不出,湿痹中恶,客气虚冷。补五脏,生肌肉。气血昏乱,服之即定。有各归气血之功,故名当归。

雷公云:得酒浸过,良。若要破血,即使头节硬实处;若要止痛止血,即用尾。若一时用,不如不使。

易老云:用头,则破血;用尾,则止血;若全用,则一破一止,则和血也。入手少阴,以其心主血也;入足太阴,以其脾裹血也;入足厥阴,以其肝藏血也。头能破血,身能养血,尾能行血。用者不分,不如不使。若全用,在参、芪皆能补血;在牵牛、大黄皆能破血,佐使定分,用者当知。从桂、附、茱萸则热;从大黄、芒硝则寒。诸经头痛,俱在细辛条下。惟酒蒸当归,又治头痛,以其诸头痛皆属木,故以血药主之。

《药性论》云：臣。畏生姜，恶湿面。

《经》云：当归主咳逆上气。当归血药，如何治胸中气。

《药性论》云：补女子诸不足。此说尽当归之用矣。

Danggui [当归, Chinese angelica, Radix Angelicae Sinensis]

It is mild in property, and pungent and sweet in taste. Both of its property and taste are light. It is of yang property. For being sweet and pungent in taste, it is also slightly yin within yang. It is nontoxic.

It enters the meridian of hand-shaoyin, the meridian of foot-taiyin, and the meridian of yueyin.

Xiang [《药类法象》, *Rules for the Use of Medicinal Herbs*] says: It can be used to harmonize and supplement the blood. The end part of it can break the bloody conglomeration, and the main part of it can harmonize the blood. Wash off the mud in water firstly, process it with liquor, and then dry and fry it with fire or sunlight. It can be used to treat blood diseases. The root and hair should be removed before use.

Xin [《用药心法》, *Gist for the Use of Medicinal Herbs*] says: Generally, it can be used to treat all kinds of blood diseases. It can be used to eliminate blood heat and stabbing pain. It harmonizes the blood because it is sweet, and moistens the internal cold because it is pungent and mild. Its bitterness can disperse the cold of the heart.

Zhen [《珍珠囊》, *Pouch of Pearls*] says: Its top can stanch bleeding; the main part can harmonize the blood; the end part can break the bloody conglomeration. It can treat the diseases in the upper body after liquor soaking, and the external diseases after liquor washing. Those in caramel colour are greatly pungent in taste when chewing and they can break hardness. It is averse to Changpu [菖蒲, acorus, Acorus Calamus] and Haizao [海藻, seaweed, sargassum].

Ben Cao says: It is mainly used to treat the cough with dyspnea and the upward counterflow of qi, the warm malaria with cold and the heat in the skin, the infertility with vaginal bleeding, various severe sores, ulcers and the injuries caused by metal. Decoct it and drink the juice. It can warm the middle internal organs, relieve pain and waist pain, eliminate blood cold, wind stroke, the absence of sweating, the impediment due to dampness and the unconsciousness caused by severe wind, and eliminate guest qi and deficiency cold. It can be used to tonify the five zang-organs and engender muscles. It can calm the confused qi and blood. The reason why it is called Danggui〔当归, Chinese angelica, Radix Angelicae Sinensis〕is that it can make qi and blood back to the place where they are supposed to be.

Leigong〔Lei Xiao〕said: It is good in quality after soaking in liquor. The top part of it can break the bloody conglomeration; the end part of it can relieve pain and stanch bleeding. People would rather not use it if it is used only for a short period of time.

Yilao〔Zhang Yuansu〕said: The top part can break the bloody conglomeration; the end part can stanch bleeding. It can harmonize the blood when the whole plant is used. It enters the meridian of hand-shaoyin because the heart governs the blood; it enters the meridian of foot-taiyin because the spleen commands the blood; it enters the meridian of foot-yueyin, because the liver stores the blood. The top part can break the bloody conglomeration; the body part can nourish the blood; the end part can conduct the blood. Different parts have different effects. They should be used separately. Quandanggui〔全当归, whole tangkuei, Angelicae Sinensis Radix Integra〕, Renshen〔人参, ginseng, Radix Ginseng〕and Huangqi〔黄芪, root of milkvetch, Radix Astragali seu Hedysari〕can supplement the blood. With the assistance of Qianniu〔牵牛, morning glory, Pharbitidis Semen〕and Dahuang〔大黄, rhubarb root and rhizome, Radix et Rhizoma Rhei〕, it can break the bloody conglomeration. Doctors should make a clear distinction between its assistant and guiding drugs. With Guizhi〔桂枝, Cinnamon bark, Cortex Cinnamomum Cassia〕, Fuzi〔附子, aconite, Radix Aconiti Praeparata〕and Zhuyu〔茱萸, evodia, Evodiae Fructus〕, it is hot in property; with Dahuang〔大黄, rhubarb root and rhizome, Radix et Rhizoma Rhei〕and Mangxiao〔芒硝, crystallized sodium sulfate, Natrii Sulfas〕, it is cold in property. The treatment of the headache of various meridians is listed in the item of Xixin〔细辛, asarum, Asarum sieboldii Miq.〕. Steamed Danggui〔当归, Chinese angelica, Radix Angelicae Sinensis〕with liquor can treat headache. Various headaches belong to wood, so the medicinal herb to treat blood diseases is needed.

Yao Xing Lun [《药性论》, *Treatise on Medicinal Properties*] says: It is a minister medicinal herb. It is restrained by Shengjiang [生姜, fresh ginger, Rhizoma Zingiberis Recens]. It is averse to the unleavened dough.

Jing says: Danggui [当归, Chinese angelica, Radix Angelicae Sinensis] is used to treat cough with dyspnea and is a medicinal herb to treat blood diseases. How can it treat the qi in the chest?

Yao Xing Lun [《药性论》, *Treatise on Medicinal Properties*] says: It can tonify the insufficiency of women. This is all about the effect of Danggui [当归, Chinese angelica, Radix Angelicae Sinensis].

芍 药

气微寒,味酸而苦。气薄味厚,阴也,降也。阴中之阳。有小毒。

入手、足太阴经。

《象》云:补中焦之药,得炙甘草为佐,治腹中痛。夏月腹痛少加黄芩,如恶寒腹痛,加肉桂一钱,白芍药三钱,炙甘草一钱半,此仲景神方也。如冬月大寒腹痛,加桂二钱半,水二盏,煎一半。去皮用。

《心》云:脾经之药,收阴气,能除腹痛,酸以收之,扶阳而收阴气,泄邪气,扶阴。与生姜同用,温经散湿,通塞,利腹中痛,胃气不通,肺燥气热。酸收甘缓,下利必用之药。

《珍》云:白补、赤散,泻肝、补脾胃。酒浸,行经,止中部腹痛。

《本草》云:主邪气腹痛,除血痹,破坚积,寒热疝瘕,止痛,利小便,益气,通顺血脉,缓中,散恶血,逐贼血,去水气,利膀胱。

《衍义》云:芍药,全用根,其品亦多。须用花红而单叶者,山中者佳,花叶多则根虚。然其根多赤色,其味涩。有色白粗肥者,亦好,余如《经》。然血虚寒人禁此一物,古人有言:减芍药以避中寒。诚不可忽。今见花赤者,为赤芍药;花白者,为白芍药。俗云白补而赤泻。

东垣云:但涩者为上。或问:古今方论中多以涩为收,今《本经》有利小便一句者,何也? 东垣云:芍药能停诸湿而益津液,使小便自行,本非通行之药,所当知之。又问:有缓中一句,何谓缓中? 东垣云:损其肝者缓其中。又问:当用何药以治之? 东垣云:当用四物汤,以其内有芍药故也。赤者,利小便、下气,白者,止痛、散气血。入手、足太阴经。大抵酸涩者为上,为收敛停湿之剂,故主手、足太阴经。收降之体,故又能至血海而入于九地之下,后至厥阴经也。后人用赤泻白补者,以其色在西方故补,色在南方故泄也。

《本草》云:能利小便。非能利之也,以其肾主大小二便,既用此以益阴滋湿,故小便得通也。

《难经》云:损其肝者缓其中。即调血也。没药、乌药、雷丸为之使。

《本草》又云:恶石斛、芒硝。畏硝石、鳖甲、小蓟。反藜芦。

《液》云:腹中虚痛,脾经也,非芍药不除。补津液停湿之剂。

Shaoyao [芍药, Chinese herbaceous peony, Paeonia Lactiflora Pall]

It is slightly cold in nature, and sour and bitter in taste. It is weak in property and strong in flavor, pertaining to yin with descending tendency. It is of the property of yang within yin. It is slightly toxic.

It enters the meridian of hand-taiyin and the meridian of foot-taiyin.

Xiang [《药类法象》, *Rules for the Use of Medicinal Herbs*] says: It is the medicinal herb to tonify the middle energizer. It can relive the abdominal pain with the assistance of Zhigancao [炙甘草, mix-fried licorice, Glycyrrhizae Radix cum Liquido Fricta]. In summer, it can be used together with Huangqin [黄芩, baical skullcap root, Radix Scutellariae] to relieve the abdominal pain. If there is adversion to cold as well as the abdominal pain, add 1 Qian of Rougui [肉桂, cassia bark, Cortex Cinnamomi], 3 Qian of Baishaoyao [白芍药, white peony root, Radix Paeoniae Alba] and one and a half Qian of Zhigancao [炙甘草, mix-fried licorice, Glycyrrhizae Radix cum Liquido Fricta]. This is a formula from Zhang Zhongjing. To treat the great cold abdomen pain, add two and a half Qian of it, boil it in 2 cups of water till only one cup of water left. The peel should be removed before use.

Xin [《用药心法》, *Gist for the use of Medicinal Herbs*] says: It is the medicinal herb of the spleen meridian and it astringes the yin qi. It can relieve abdomen pain. Being sour and astringent, it can support yang and contract yin, clear pathogenic qi, and support yin. Taken with Shengjiang [生姜, fresh ginger, Rhizoma Zingiberis Recens], it can warm the meridians and dissipate dampness, open congestion, and relieve abdomen pain. Sourness can contract and sweetness can moderate. One can not treat diarrhea without it.

Zhen [《珍珠囊》, *Pounch of Pearls*] says: Baishaoyao [白芍药, white peony root, Radix Paeoniae Alba] can nourish and Chishaoyao [赤芍药, red peony, Paeoniae Radix Rubra] can drain. It can drain the liver and tonify the spleen and the stomach. Soak it in liquor, and it will treat the abdominal pain during menstruation.

Ben Cao says: It is mainly used to treat the pathogenic qi and abdominal pain, eliminate the blood impediment, dispel the hard accumulation of cold and heat, cease pain, promote urination, replenish qi, free the blood vessels, harmonize the middle energizer, dissipate the malign blood, dispel stasis, and disinhibit the bladder.

Yan Yi [《衍义》, *Extension of the Materia Medica*] says: The root of Shaoyao [芍药, Chinese herbaceous peony, Paeonia lactiflora Pall.] should be used. It has many varieties. Those with red flowers and single leaves should be used. Shaoyao [芍药, Chinese herbaceous peony, Paeonia lactiflora Pall.] which grows in the mountain is better in quality. Those with more flowers and leaves have less roots. Most of its roots are red and astringent in taste. The white and strong ones are also good in quality and the other properties are the same with what was addressed in *Jing*. The patients with the cold and blood deficiency syndrome can not take this medicinal herb. The ancients said: take less Shaoyao [芍药, Chinese herbaceous peony, Paeonia lactiflora Pall] so as to treat the center cold. This can not be ignored. Those with red flowers are Chishaoyao [赤芍药, red peony, Paeoniae Radix Rubra]. Those with white flowers are Baishaoyao [白芍药, white peony root, Radix Paeoniae Alba]. Baishaoyao [白芍药, white peony root, Radix Paeoniae Alba] can nourish and Chishaoyao [赤芍药, red peony, Paeoniae Radix Rubra] can drain.

Li Dongyuan said: Those which are astringent are good in quality. One may ask: In the ancient and modern prescriptions, it is said that astringency is contraction. *Ben Cao* says it can promote urination. Why? Li Dongyuan said: Shaoyao [芍药, Chinese herbaceous peony, Paeonia lactiflora Pall] can eliminate various dampness, benefit fluids and promote urination. It is not a medicinal herb to free. One may ask: What is the meaning to harmonize the middle energizer? Li

Dongyuan said: It can emolliate the liver and relax tension. One may ask: What medicinal herbs should be used to treat it? Li Dongyuan said: Four Agents Decoction can treat it because there is Shaoyao [芍药, Chinese herbaceous peony, Paeonia lactiflora Pall] in it. Chishaoyao [赤芍药, red peony, Paeoniae Radix Rubra] can promote urination, promote qi to descend; Baishaoyao [白芍药, white peony root, Radix Paeoniae Alba] can relieve pain, and dissipate qi and blood. It enters the meridian of hand-taiyin and the meridian of foot-taiyin. Baishaoyao [白芍药, white peony root, Radix Paeoniae Alba], sour and astringent, is an atriction-promoting and dampness-eliminating medicinal herb. It governs the meridian of hand and foot taiyin. It has the functional tendency of descending, so it can reach the sea of blood, the lower body part, and then the jueyin meridian. In later generations, Baishaoyao [白芍药, white peony root, Radix Paeoniae Alba] is used to tonify for its color is connected with the direction of west and Chishaoyao [赤芍药, red peony, Paeoniae Radix Rubra] is used to dredge for its color is related with the direction of south.

Ben Cao says: It can promote urination in an indirect way. The reason is that the kidney governs stool and urine. It can nourish yin, moisten dampness and promote urination.

Nan Jing [《难经》, *Canon of Difficult Issues*] says: It can emolliate the liver and harmonize the middle energizer. This is blood-harmonizing. Moyao [没药, myrrh, Myrrha], Wuyao [乌药, lindera, Linderae Radix] and Leiwan [雷丸, stone-like omphalia, Omphalia Lapidescens] are its assistance.

Ben Cao also says: It is averse to Shihu [石斛, dendrobe, Herba Dendrobii] and Mangxiao [芒硝, crystallized sodium sulfate, Natrii Sulfas]. It is restrained by Xiaoshi [硝石, niter, Sal Nitri], Biejia [鳖甲, turtle carapace, Carapax Trionycis] and Xiaoji [小蓟, field thistle, Cirsii Herba]. It is averse to Lilu [藜芦, black false hellebore, Veratrum nigrum L.].

Ye [《汤液本草》, *Materia Medica for Decoctions*] says: The abdominal pain is the problem of the spleen meridian. It can not be treated without Shaoyao [芍药, Chinese herbaceous peony, Paeonia lactiflora Pall.]. It is the medicinal herb to nourish the fluids and eliminate dampness.

熟 地 黄

气寒,味苦,阴中之阳。甘,微苦,味厚气薄,阴中阳也。无毒。

入手、足少阴经,厥阴经。

《象》云:酒洒,蒸如乌金,假酒力则微温,大补,血衰者须用之。善黑须发。忌萝卜。

《珍》云:若治外、治上,酒制。

《心》云:生则性大寒而凉血,熟则性寒而补肾。

《本草》云:主折跌、绝筋、伤中,逐血痹,填骨髓,长肌肉。作汤,除寒热积聚,除痹;主男子五劳七伤,女子伤中、胞漏下血;破恶血,溺血。利大小肠,去胃中宿食,饱力断绝,补五脏内伤不足;通血脉,益气力,利耳目。生者,尤良。得清酒、麦门冬,尤良。恶贝母,畏芜夷。

东垣云:生地黄,治手足心热及心热。入手足少阴、手足厥阴,能益肾水而治血,脉洪实者,宜此,若脉虚,则宜熟地黄。地黄假火力蒸九数,故能补肾中元气。仲景制八味丸,以熟地黄为诸药之首,天一所生之源也。汤液四物以治藏血之脏,亦以干熟地黄为君者,癸乙同归一治也。蒸捣不可犯铁,若犯铁,令人肾消。

陈藏器云:蒸干即温补,生干即平宣。

《机要》云:熟地黄,脐下发痛者,肾经也,非地黄不能除。补肾益阴之剂,二宜丸加当归为补髓。

Shudihuang [熟地黄, prepared rehmannia root, Radix Rehmanniae Preparata]

It is cold in property and bitter in taste, pertaining to yang within yin. It is sweet and slightly bitter. It is strong in taste, and thin in property. It is yang within yin. It is nontoxic.

It enters the meridian of hand and foot shaoyin, and the jueyin meridian.

Xiang [《药类法象》, *Rules for the Use of Medicinal Herbs*] says: Add some liquor and steam until it turns to jet-black. It is slightly warm with liquor and supplements the blood greatly and can be used to treat the blood depletion. It is effective to blacken the hair and beard. Do not eat radish in the period of taking the medicinal herb.

Zhen [《珍珠囊》, *Pounch of Pearls*] says: To treat the diseases located in the external and upper parts of the body, process it with liquor.

Xin [《用药心法》, *Gist for the use of Medicinal Herbs*] says: Shengdihuang [生地黄, unprocessed rehmannia root, Radix Rehmanniae Recens] is greatly cold in property and can cool the blood; Shudihuang [熟地黄, prepared rehmannia root, Radix Rehmanniae Preparata] is cold in nature and can tonify the kidney.

Ben Cao says: It is mainly used to treat the fracture of bones and sinews due to falling and visceral injury, middle damage, expel blood impediment, enrich marrow, and promote the growth of muscles. When made into decoction, it can eliminate the accumulation of cold, heat and impediment. It is mainly used to treat the five consumptive diseases and seven damages of men, the middle damage, the uterine bleeding of women, and dispel the malign blood and the bloody urine. It can disinhibit the large intestine and small intestine, disperse the abiding food, tonify the internal injury and the insufficiency of the five zang-organs, regulate the blood and vessels, replenish qi and strength, sharpen hearing and brighten eyes. The therapeutic effect of raw Dihuang [地黄, rehmannia, Radix Rehmanniae] is better than the processed one. It is especially effective with the assistance of liquor and Maimendong [麦门冬, radix ophiopogonis, Ophiopogon japonicus Ker-Gawl]. It is averse to Beimu [贝母, fritillaria, Bulbus Fritillaria]. It is restrained by Wuyi [芜荑, great elm seed, Semen Ulmus Macrocarpa].

Li Dongyuan said: Shengdihuang [生地黄, unprocessed rehmannia root, Radix Rehmanniae Recens] can treat the heat in the heart of palms and soles, and the heart heat. It enters the meridian of hand and foot shaoyin, and the meridian of hand and foot jueyin. It can boost the kidney water and treat blood diseases. The patients who have surging pulse should take it. The patients who have vacuous pulse should take Shudihuang [熟地黄, prepared rehmannia root, Radix Rehmanniae Preparata]. Steam Dihuang [地黄, unprocessed rehmannia root, Rehmannia glutinosa Libosch. ex Fisch. et Mey.] with fire for nine times, and it can tonify the primordial qi in the kidney. Zhang Zhongjing processed Bawei Pill and took Shudihuang [熟地黄, prepared rehmannia root, Radix Rehmanniae Preparata] as the primary medicinal herb. It is the origin of Tianyi Decoction.

Four Agent Decoction can treat the viscera which store the blood. Take dry Shudihuang [熟地黄, prepared rehmannia root, Radix Rehmanniae Preparata] as the sovereign drug. It is a combined treatment of the liver and the kidney. Iron can not be used when it is steamed or pounded. If iron is involved, it will damage the kidney.

Chen Zangqi said: Steam-dried Shudihuang [熟地黄, prepared rehmannia root, Radix Rehmanniae Preparata] can warm and supplement, and the sun-dried can calm and disperse.

Ji Yao [《活法机要》, *Prescriptions and Therapies for Keeping Alive*] says: The pain below the navel and the kidney meridian can not be treated without Shudihuang [熟地黄, prepared rehmannia root, Radix Rehmanniae Preparata]. It is the medicinal herb to tonify the kidney and nourish yin. Er'yi Pill and Danggui [当归, Chinese angelica, Radix Angelicae Sinensis] can nourish the marrow.

生 地 黄

气寒,味苦,阴中之阳。甘、苦,大寒。无毒。

入手太阳经、少阴经之剂。

《象》云:凉血补血,补肾水真阴不足。此药大寒,宜斟酌用之,恐损胃气。

《珍》云:生血凉血。

《本草》云:主妇人崩中血不止,及产后血上薄心闷绝,伤身胎动下血,胎不落,堕坠腕折,瘀血留血,衄鼻吐血,皆捣饮之。

《液》云:手少阴,又为手太阳之剂,故钱氏泻丙与木通同用,以导赤也。诸经之血热与他药相随,亦能治之,溺血便血亦治之,入四散例。

《心》云:苦甘,阴中微阳,酒浸上行、外行。生血,凉血去热。恶贝母,畏芜荑。

Shengdihuang [生地黄, unprocessed rehmannia root, Radix Rehmanniae Recens]

It is cold in property and bitter in taste, pertaining to yang within yin. It is sweet, bitter and greatly cold. It is nontoxic.

It enters the meridian of hand-taiyang and shaoyin.

Xiang [《药类法象》, *Rules for the Use of Medicinal Herbs*] says: It can be used to cool the blood, nourish the blood, and tonify the kidney water and the insufficiency of genuine yin. It is greatly cold in property, so one needs to think over before use. It probably damages the stomach qi.

Zhen [《珍珠囊》, *Pounch of Pearls*] says: It engenders the blood and cool the blood.

Ben Cao says: It is mainly used to treat the blood flooding of women, the oppression due to the reverse flowing of blood in the heart after delivery, vaginal bleeding with fetal movement, difficult delivery, bone fractures and dislocation, blood stasis, epistaxis, and blood spitting. Pound it before use.

Ye [《汤液本草》, *Materia Medica for Decoctions*] says: It enters the meridian of hand-shaoyin, and the meridian of hand-taiyang. Qian used it with Mutong [木通, akebia stem, *Caulis Akebiae*] to drain the small intestine in order to conduct blood. It, together with other medicinals, can treat the blood heat in all the meridians, as well as the bloody urine and the bloody stool. The Four Ingredients Decoction is a good example.

Xin [《用药心法》, *Gist for the Use of Medicinal Herbs*] says: It is bitter and sweet, slightly yang within yin, with functional tendency of ascending and dispersing if soaked in liquor. It can engender the blood and can eliminate the heat by cooling the blood. It is averse to Beimu [贝母, fritillaria bulb, *Bulbus Fritillaria*]. It is restrained by Wuyi [芜荑, great elm seed, *Semen Ulmus Macrocarpa*].

山 药

气温，味甘平。无毒。

手太阴经药。

《本草》云：主补中益气，除热强阴。主头面游风，风头眼眩。下气，充五脏，长肌肉，久服耳目聪明，轻身耐老，延年不饥。手太阴药，润皮毛燥，凉而能补，与二门冬、紫芝为之使，恶甘遂。

东垣云：仲景八味丸用干山药，以其凉而能补也。亦治皮肤干燥，以此物润之。

Shanyao [山药, common yam rhizome, Dioscorea Opposita Thunb.]

It is warm in property, and sweet and mild in taste. It is nontoxic.

It enters the meridian of hand-taiyin.

Ben Cao says: It is mainly used to tonify the middle internal organs and replenish qi, eliminate heat and strengthen yin. It is mainly used to treat facial alopecia and dizzy vision. It is used to promote qi to descend, tonify the five zang-organs, and engender muscles. The long-term taking of it will improve vision and hearing, relax the body and prolong life, make people free from hunger. It is a medicinal herb of the meridian of hand-taiyin. It moistens the dry skin and the body hair. It is cold and can be used to tonify. Ermendong Decoction and Zizhi [紫芝, purple fragrant herb] are its assistance. It is averse to Gansui [甘遂, gansui root, Radix Euphorbiae Kansui].

Li Dongyuan said: The dried one is used in Zhang Zhongjing's Bawei Pill because it is cold in property and can also tonify. It also treats the skin dryness by moistening the skin.

麻 仁

味甘、平。无毒。

入足太阴经,手阳明经。

本草云:主补中益气,中风汗出,逐水,利小便,破积血,复血脉,乳妇产后余疾。长发,可为沐药。久服,肥泽不老。

《液》云:入足太阴、手阳明。汗多、胃热、便难,三者皆燥湿而亡津液,故曰脾约。约者,约束之义,《内经》谓:燥者润之,故仲景以麻仁润足太阴之燥及通肠也。

Maren [麻仁, cannabis fruit, Cannabis Fructus]

It is sweet in taste and mild in property. It is nontoxic.

It enters the meridian of foot-taiyin, and the meridian of hand-yangming.

Ben Cao says: It is mainly used to tonify the middle internal organs, replenish qi, treat wind stroke, sweating, expel water, promote urination, expel blood stasis, and restore the blood, vessels and treat postpartum diseases. It can be used to promote hair growth or can be used in bath water. The long-term taking of it will promote the growth of muscles and prevent aging.

Ye [《汤液本草》, *Materia Medica for Decoctions*] says: It enters the meridian of foot-taiyin and the meridian of hand-yangming. Copious sweat, stomach heat and difficult defecation will dry dampness and cause fluid collapse. It is called the constrained spleen. "Constrain" means to set a limit. *Nei Jing* [《黄帝内经》, *Yellow Emperor's Canon of Medicine*] says: To moisten dryness, Zhang Zhongjing used Maren[麻仁, cannabis fruit, Cannabis Fructus] to moisten dryness in the meridian of foot-taiyin and free the stool.

薏苡仁

气微寒,味甘。无毒。

《本草》云:主筋急拘挛,不可屈伸,风湿痹,下气。除筋骨邪气不仁,利肠胃,消水肿,令人能食,久服,轻身益气。其根能下三虫。仲景治风湿燥痛,日晡所剧者,与麻黄杏子薏苡仁汤。

Yiyiren [薏苡仁, coix, Semen Coicis]

It is slightly cold in property and sweet in taste. It is nontoxic.

Ben Cao says: It is mainly used to treat the tension of the sinews and hypertonicity, inhibited bending and stretching, wind-dampness impediment, and promote qi to descend. It is used to relieve the numbness of limbs due to the pathogenic qi, harmonize the stomach and intestines, disperse the water swelling, and promote appetite. The long-term taking of it can relax the body and replenish qi. Its root can kill three kinds of worms. Zhang Zhongjing treated the pain and restlessness due to wind-dampness, especially those worsened in later afternoon [3 p.m. – 5 p.m.] with Mahuang Xingzi Yiyiren Decoction.

甘 草

气平,味甘,阳也。无毒。

入足厥阴经、太阴经、少阴经。

《象》云：生用大泻热火，炙之则温，能补上焦、中焦、下焦元气。和诸药，相协而不争，性缓，善解诸急，故名国老。去皮用。甘草梢子生用为君，去茎中痛，或加苦楝、酒煮玄胡索为主，尤妙。

《心》云：热药用之缓其热，寒药用之缓其寒。《经》曰：甘以缓之。阳不足，补之以甘，中满禁用。寒热皆用，调和药性，使不相悖，炙之散表寒，除邪热，去咽痛，除热，缓正气，缓阴血，润肺。

《珍》云：养血补胃，梢子去肾中之痛。胸中积热，非梢子不能除。

《本草》云：主五脏六腑寒热邪气，坚筋骨，长肌肉，倍力。金疮𪘏，解毒。温中下气，烦满短气，伤脏咳嗽，止渴，通经脉，利血气，解百药毒。为九土之精，安和七十二种石，一千二百种草，故名国老。

《药性论》云：君。忌猪肉。

《内经》曰：脾欲缓，急食甘以缓之。甘以补脾，能缓之也，故《汤液》用此以建中。又曰：甘者令人中满。又曰：中满者勿食甘。即知非中满药也。甘入脾，归其所喜攻也。

或问：附子理中、调胃承气皆用甘草者，如何是调和之意？答曰：附子理中用甘草，恐其僭上也；调胃承气用甘草，恐其速下也。二药用之非和也，皆缓也。小柴胡有柴胡、黄芩之寒，人参、半夏之温，其中用甘草者，则有调和之意。中不满而用甘，为之补，中满者用甘，为之泄，此升降浮沉也，凤髓丹之甘，缓肾温而生元气，亦甘补之意也。《经》云：以甘补之，以甘泻之，以甘缓之。《本草》谓：安和七十二种石、一千二百种草，名为国老，虽非君而为君所宗，所以能安和草、石而解诸毒也。于此可见调和之意。夫五味之用，苦直行而泄，辛横行而散，酸束而收敛，咸止而软坚，甘上行而发，如何《本草》言下气？盖甘之味，有升降浮沉，可上可下，可内可外，有和有缓，有补有泻，居中之道尽矣。入足厥阴、太阴、少阴，能治肺痿之脓血而作吐剂，能消五发之疮疽。每用水三碗，慢火熬至半碗，去渣服之。消疮与黄芪同功，黄芪亦能消肿毒痈疽。修治之法与甘草同。

《本草》又云：术、干漆、苦参为之使。恶远志，反大戟、芫花、甘遂、海藻四物。

Gancao [甘草, liquorice root, Glycyrrhiza uralensis Fisch.]

It is mild in property and sweet in taste, pertaining to yang. It is nontoxic. It enters the meridian of foot-yueyin, taiyin, shaoyin.

Xiang [《药类法象》, *Rules for the Use of Medicinal Herbs*] says: It can be used to clear heat and fire when taken raw. It turns to warm property after frying and can tonify the original qi in the triple energizers. It can harmonize various medicinal herbs, assist other medicinal herbs rather than oppose the effect of them. It is mild and good at relaxing tension so it is called Guolao. The peel should be removed before use. Rootlet of Gancao [甘草, liquorice root, Glycyrrhiza uralensis Fisch.] is a sovereign medicinal herb when used raw and can relieve the pain in the penis. If used together with Kulian [苦楝, chinaberry bark, Meliae Cortex] and Xuanhusuo [玄胡索, corydalis, Corydalis Rhizoma] and boiled in liquor, it may be very effective.

Xin [《用药心法》, *Gist for the Use of Medicinal Herbs*] says that *Jing* [《黄帝内经》, *Yellow Emperor's Internal Canon of Medicine*] says: Sweetness can relieve. It can treat yang deficiency, and promote yang with sweetness. Do not use it when there is abdominal distention. It can be used to treat cold and heat, and harmonize medicinal herbs. Fried Gancao [甘草, liquorice root, Glycyrrhiza uralensis Fisch.] can dissipate exterior cold, eliminate heat pathogen, relieve soar throat, eliminate heat, harmonize the healthy qi, yin blood, and moisten the lung.

Zhen [《珍珠囊》, *Pounch of Pearls*] says: It can nourish blood and tonify the stomach. Its rootlet can relieve the pain in the kidney. Its rootlet is very effective to treat the accumulation of heat in the chest.

Ben Cao says: It is mainly used to treat the diseases caused by the pathogenic cold and heat in the five zang-organs and six fu-organs, strengthen sinews and bones, promote muscles and increase strength. It can be used to treat traumatic injury and swollen foot, and resolve toxin. It can warm the middle internal organs and promote qi to descend, treat vexation and fullness, shortness of breath, damage of the viscera, cough, relieve thirst, free the meridians, promote the circulation of blood and the flow of qi, and resolve various toxins. It is the essence of the earth, and harmonizes 72 kinds of stones and 1,200 kinds of plants. That is why it is called Guolao.

Yao Xing Lun [《药性论》, *Treatise on Medicinal Properties*] says: It is a sovereign medicinal herb. Patients should avoid pork in the period of taking it.

Nei Jing [《黄帝内经》, *Yellow Emperor's Internal Canon of Medicine*] says:

Sweet food can relieve the spleen. Sweetness can tonify and relieve the spleen. So it can be used to fortify the middle energizer according to *Tang Ye Ben Cao* [《汤液本草》, *Materia Medica for Decoctions*]. It also says: Sweetness may lead to abdominal fullness. It also says: The patients with abdominal fullness should not eat sweet food. It is not a medicinal herb to treat abdominal fullness. Sweetness enters the spleen and pertains to the organ that it takes effect.

One may ask that Fuzi [附子, aconite, Radix Aconiti Praeparata] can regulate the middle and Gancao [甘草, liquorice root, Glycyrrhiza uralensis Fisch.] can regulate the stomach and coordinate qi. What is the meaning of regulation? The answer is that Fuzi [附子, aconite, Radix Aconiti Praeparata] can rectify the middle and Gancao [甘草, liquorice root, Glycyrrhiza uralensis Fisch.] can harmonize and avoid great heat. Fuzi [附子, aconite, Radix Aconiti Praeparata] can regulate the stomach and coordinate qi. Gancao [甘草, liquorice root, Glycyrrhiza uralensis Fisch.] can harmonize and avoid the accelerated draining precipitation. Gancao [甘草, liquorice root, Glycyrrhiza uralensis Fisch.] is used to slow down the effect of Fuzi [附子, aconite, Radix Aconiti Praeparata]. Xiaochaihu [小柴胡, Common Goldenrop, Common Goldenrop] is as cold as Chaihu [柴胡, Chinese thorowax root, Radix Bupleuri] and Huangqin [黄芩, baical skullcap root, Radix Scutellariae]. It is as warm as Renshen [人参, ginseng, Radix Ginseng] and Banxia [半夏, pinellia, Rhizoma Pinelliae]. Gancao [甘草, liquorice root, Glycyrrhiza uralensis Fisch.] is used to harmonize. Sweetness can be used to tonify the middle energizer without fullness, and discharge the middle energizer with fullness. This is called the ascending, descending, dispersing and sinking properties of medicinal herbs. The sweetness of Fengsui pill can relieve the warmth of the kidney and promote the original qi. This is also an example to illustrate the tonifying function of sweetness. *Jing* says: Sweetness can be used to tonify, discharge or relieve.

Ben Cao says: It harmonizes all medicinal herbs, so it is called Guolao. Although it is not a sovereign drug, it is the clan relative of sovereign drugs. So it can harmonize all medicinal herbs and resolve all the toxins. This is the meaning of harmonization. Here is the effectiveness of the five flavors: bitterness goes straight and discharges; acridity goes laterally and dissipates; sourness restricts and astringes; saltiness relieves and softens hardness; sweetness goes upward and disperses. Why does it precipitate qi according to *Ben Cao*? It is because the medicinal herbs with sweetness can ascend, descend, float, and sink medicinal bearings. The sweetness may conduct the medicinal herbs upward or downward, internal or external, being harmonious and moderate, acting as supplementation and drainage. It plays a good role of mediator. It enters the meridian of foot-Jueyin, Taiyin, Shaoyin. It can treat purulent blood due to lung atrophy as emetic formula, the severe sore of the five organs. Add three bowls of water and boil it with slow fire until half a bowl of water left. Remove the dregs and then take it. It has the same effect as Huangqi [黄芪, milkvetch root, Radix Astragali seu Hedysari] to heal the sore. Huangqi [黄芪, milkvetch root, Radix Astragali seu Hedysari] can relieve swelling, toxin and carbuncle-abscesses. Its processing is the same as that of Gancao [甘草, liquorice root, Glycyrrhiza uralensis Fisch.].

Ben Cao also says: Cangzhu [苍术, atractylodes rhizome, Rhizoma Atractylodis], Ganqi [干漆, dried lacquer of true lacquertree, Resina Toxicodendri] and Kushen [苦参, flavescent sophora, Radix Sophorae Flavescentis] are its assistance. It is averse to Yuanzhi [远志, polygala root, Radix Polygalae]. It is restrained by Daji [大戟, root of Peking euphorbia, Radix Euphorbiae Pekinensis], Yuanhua [芫花, immature flower of lilac daphne, Flos Genkwa], Gansui [甘遂, gansui root, Radix Euphorbiae Kansui] and Haizao [海藻, seaweed, Sargassum].

白 前

气微温, 味甘, 微寒。无毒。

《本草》云: 主胸胁逆气, 咳嗽上气。状似白薇、牛膝辈。

《衍义》云: 白前保定肺气, 治嗽多用, 白而长于细辛, 但粗而脆, 不似细辛之柔。若以温药相佐使则尤佳。仲景用。

Baiqian [白前, willowleaf rhizome, Rhizoma Cynanchi Stauntonii]

It is slightly warm in property, sweet in taste, and slightly cold. It is nontoxic.

Ben Cao says: It is mainly used to treat the counter-flow of qi in chest and hypochondrium, the panting and cough with qi ascent. Its shape is like that of Baiwei〔白薇, blackend swallowwort root, Radix Cynanchi Atrati〕and Niuxi〔牛膝, root of twotooth achyranthes, Radix Achyranthis Bidentatae〕.

Yan Yi〔《衍义》, *Extension of the Materia Medica*〕says：Baiqian〔白前, willowleaf rhizome, Rhizoma Cynanchi Stauntonii〕secures the lung qi. It is chiefly used to treat cough. It is whiter and longer than Xixin〔细辛, asarum, Asarum sieboldii Miq.〕, thick and crispy. It is not as tender as Xixin〔细辛, asarum, Asarum sieboldii Miq.〕. It will be more effective with the assistance of warm medicinal herbs. Zhang Zhongjing used it.

白　薇

气大寒，味苦、咸，平。无毒。

《本草》云：主暴中风身热，肢满，忽忽不知人，狂惑邪气，寒热酸疼，温疟洗洗发作有时。疗伤中淋露，下水气，利阴气，益精。近道处处有之，状似牛膝、白前而短小。疗惊邪风狂痓病。

《液》云：《局方》中多有用之治妇人，以《本经》疗伤中、下淋露故也。

《本草》又云：恶黄芪、大黄、大戟、干姜、干漆、山茱萸、大枣。

Baiwei〔白薇, blackend swallowwort root, Radix Cynanchi Atrati〕

It is greatly cold in property, bitter and salty in taste, and mild in property. It is nontoxic.

Ben Cao says：It is mainly used to treat the severe wind stroke, fever, the distension of limbs, unconsciousness, manic confusion, the cold-heat disease caused by pathogenic qi, aching muscles and the warm malaria with shivering and regular onset. It can be used to treat stranguria due to damage of the triple energizer, relieve edema, and disinhibit yinqi and boost essence. It is easily found near roads. Its shape is like that of Niuxi〔牛膝, twotoothed achyranthes root, Radix Achyranthis Bidentatae〕and Baiqian〔白前, willowleaf rhizome, Rhizoma Cynanchi Stauntonii〕. It is short and small. It treats fright, wind pathogen, manic disease and tetany.

Ye〔《汤液本草》, *Materia Medica for Decoctions*〕says：According to *Ju*

Fang [《局方》, *Welfare Pharmacy*], it is mainly used to treat women diseases. According to *Ben Cao*, it is used to treat stranguria due to damage of the triple energizer.

Ben Cao says: It is averse to Huangqi [黄芪, milkvetch root, Radix Astragali seu Hedysari], Dahuang [大黄, rhubarb root and rhizome, Radix et Rhizoma Rhei], Ganjiang [干姜, dried ginger, Rhizoma Zingiberis], Shanzhuyu [山茱萸, cornus, Fructus Corni] and Dazao [大枣, Chinese date, Fructus Jujubae].

前 胡

气微寒,味苦。无毒。

《本草》云:主痰满,胸胁中痞,心腹结气,风头痛。去痰实,下气,治伤寒寒热,推陈致新,明目益精。半夏为使。恶皂荚,畏藜芦。

Qianhu [前胡, hogfennel root, Radix Peucedani]

It is slightly cold in property, bitter in taste and nontoxic.

Ben Cao says: It is mainly used to treat the fullness due to phlegm, the hard lump in the chest and rib-sides, the stagnation of qi in the heart and abdomen, and the wind headache. It is used to remove phlegm and descend qi, treat cold damage and the diseases due to cold and heat, get rid of the stale to bring forth the fresh, improve vision and replenish essence. In compatibility, Banxia [半夏, pinellia Tuber, Rhizoma Pinelliae] is its assistance. It is averse to Zaojia [皂荚, soap pod, Gleditsia sinensis Lam.] and restrained by Lilu [藜芦, veratrum, Veratri Nigri Radix et Rhizoma].

木 香

气热,味辛、苦,纯阳。味厚于气,阴中阳也。无毒。

《象》云:除肺中滞气,若治中、下焦气结滞,须用槟榔为使。

《珍》云:治腹中气不转运,和胃气。

《心》云:散滞气,调诸气。

《本草》云：治邪风，辟毒疫瘟鬼，强志，主淋露，疗气劣，肌中偏寒，主气不足，消毒，瘟疟蛊毒，行药之精。

《本经》云：主气劣、气不足，补也；通壅气、导一切气，破也。安胎、健脾胃，补也；除癖块，破也。与本条补破不同，何也？易老以为破气之剂，不言补也。

Muxiang [木香, root of common aucklandia, Radix Aucklandiae]

It is hot in property, pungent and bitter in taste, and of yang property. Its flavor is thicker than its property, which pertains to yang within yin. It is nontoxic.

Xiang [《药类法象》, *Rules for the Use of Medicinal Herbs*] says: It removes the qi stagnation in the lung. If the qi stagnation in the middle and lower energizer is treated, Binglang [槟榔, areca seed, Semen Arecae] should be its assistance.

Zhen [《珍珠囊》, *Pouch of Pearls*] says: It treats the syndrome of qi stagnation in the abdomen and harmonizes the stomach qi.

Xin [《用药心法》, *Gist for the Use of Medicinal Herbs*] says: It disperses the qi stagnation and regulates all kinds of qi.

Ben Cao says: It is mainly used to eliminate the evil qi, prevent the invasion of toxin and pestilence, strengthen memory, and treat the severe heat disease and the disease caused by metrostaxis. In addition, it cures the qi disorder and the cold in muscles. It is also used to treat the insufficiency of qi, eliminate the toxin and pestilence due to malaria. It is the herb with guiding function.

Ben Jing [《神农本草经》, *Agriculture God's Canon of Materia Medica*] says: It is mainly used to treat the qi disorder and the insufficiency of qi, which exemplifies supplement function. It can be used for removing the stagnation qi and conducting all kinds of qi, which exemplifies to its breaking function. Its supplement method can be used for preventing abortion and replenishing the spleen and stomach, whereas its breaking function is used for removing the abdominal mass. Why do people treat diseases with different methods other than the supplement and breaking methods mentioned here? Yi Lao [Zhang Yuansu] regarded it as the medicinal herb with breaking effect but did not address its supplement effect.

知 母

气寒,味大辛。苦寒,味厚,阴也,降也。苦,阴中微阳。无毒。

入足阳明经,手太阴、肾经本药。

《象》云:泻足阳明经火热,补益肾水膀胱之寒。去皮用。

《心》云:泻肾中火,苦寒,凉心去热。

《珍》云:凉肾,肾经本药,上颈行经,皆须用酒炒。

《本草》云:主消渴热中,除邪气,肢体浮肿,下水,补不足,益气,疗伤寒,久疟烦热,胁下邪气,膈中恶,及风汗内疸。多服,令人泄。

东垣云:入足阳明、手太阴,味苦,寒润。治有汗骨蒸,肾经气劳,泻心。仲景用此为白虎汤,治不得眠者,烦躁也。烦者,肺也;躁者,肾也。以石膏为君主,佐以知母之苦寒,以清肾之源。缓以甘草、粳米之甘,而使不速下也。《经》云:胸中有寒者,瓜蒂散吐之。又云:表热里寒者,白虎汤主之。瓜蒂、知母味皆苦寒,而治胸中寒及里寒,何也?答曰:成无己注云:即伤寒寒邪之毒为热病也。读者要逆识之,如《论语》言:乱臣十人,书言唯以乱民,其能而乱四方。乱,皆治也,乃治乱者也,故云乱民,乱四方也。仲景所言"寒"之一字,举其初而言之,热病在其中矣。若以"寒"为寒冷之寒,无复用苦寒之剂。兼言白虎证"脉尺寸俱长",则热可知矣。

Zhimu [知母, rhizome of common anemarrhena, Rhizoma Anemarrhenae]

It is cold in property and extremely pungent in taste. It is bitter and cold with thick flavor, which pertains to yin and descent in functional tendency. Its bitterness pertains to mild yang within yin. It is nontoxic.

It enters the meridian of foot-yangming and hand-taiyin, and is regarded as the medicinal herb of the kidney meridian.

Xiang [《药类法象》, *Rules for the Use of Medicinal Herbs*] says: It clears away the fire and heat through the meridian of foot-yangming, and supplements the cold caused by the kidney fluid in the bladder. It can be used after peeling.

Xin [《用药心法》, *Gist for the Use of Medicinal Herbs*] says: It clears away the kidney fire, cold and bitterness, and it has the function of clearing away the heart fire.

  Zhen [《珍珠囊》, *Pouch of Pearls*] says: It has the function of clearing away the kidney fire, being the medicinal herb of kidney meridian and menstruating, but it should be used after being fried by liquor.

  Ben Cao says: It is mainly used to treat diabetes and heat attack, eliminate the evil qi, relieve the dropsy of limbs, promote urination, improve insufficiency and replenish qi. It cures cold damage, chronic malaria vexing fever and pathogenic qi in rib-sides. It treats pathogen in diaphragm, wind sweat and interior jaundice. The long-term taking of it will lead to diarrhea.

  Li Dongyuan said: It enters the meridian of foot-yangming and hand-taiyin. It is bitter in flavor and moist in nature. It is used to treat the syndrome of abnormal sweating due to the deficiency of yin and bone steaming, as well as the consumptive diseases in the kidney meridian and clears away the heart fire. Zhang Zhongjing used it to make White Tiger Decoction to treat dysphoria and insomnia. Dysphoria often bothers the lung, and agitation often attacks the kidney. Shigao [石膏, gypsum, Gypsum Fibrosum] is used as the sovereign medicinal herb, and Zhimu [知母, rhizome of common anemarrhena, Rhizoma Anemarrhenae] is used as the assistant medicinal herb to clear away the kidney fire with its cold and bitter property. The sweet flavor of Gancao [甘草, liquorice root, Glycyrrhiza uralensis Fisch.] and Jingmi [粳米, Rice, Oryza sativa L.] can be used to moderate and purge gradually instead of abruptly. *Jing* says: If the patient has cold syndrome in his chest, Guadi Powder can be used to eliminate cold. It also says that if one has the interior cold syndrome with exterior heat, White Tiger Decoction can be used to treat it. Both Guadi [瓜蒂, fruit pedicel of muskmelon, Pedicellus Melo Fructus] and Zhimu [知母, rhizome of common anemarrhena, Rhizoma Anemarrhenae] are cold and bitter in flavor, but they are used to treat the cold syndrome in the chest and interior. Why? The answer lies in the annotation of Cheng Wuji: The cold pathogen caused by cold damage pertains to the heat syndrome. Readers should know about it from the oppostite perspective, as what was said in *Lun Yu* [《论语》, *The Analects of Confucius*], "As stated in the book, if ten rebels who unleash chaos, they would bring about the disturbance in the whole country. Therefore, what they did must be stopped and controlled by the governor, for those rebels may make the whole country in chaos. " When it comes to the "cold", Zhang Zhongjing took its original meaning as an example, indicating the heat disease in the internal body. If the "cold" is caused by cold weather, there is no need to take medicines with bitter and cold property. It is also said that White Tiger Decoction can be used to treat the heat syndrome with long pulse.

贝　母

气平，微寒，味辛、苦。无毒。

《本草》云：主伤寒烦热，淋沥、邪气，疝瘕、喉痹，乳难，金疮，风痉。疗腹中结实，心下满，洗洗恶风寒，目眩项直，咳嗽上气。止烦渴，出汗，安五脏，利骨髓。

仲景：寒实结胸，外无热证者，三物小陷胸汤主之，白散亦可。以其内有贝母也。别说，贝母能散胸中郁结之气，殊有功。

《本草》又云：厚朴、白薇为之使，恶桃花，畏秦艽、矾石、莽草，反乌头。

海藏祖方，下乳三母散：牡蛎、知母、贝母三物为细末，猪蹄汤调下。

Beimu [贝母, fritillaria, Bulbus Fritillariae Thunbergii]

It is mild and slightly cold in property, as well as pungent and bitter in taste. It is nontoxic.

Ben Cao says: It is mainly used to treat the cold damage with vexing fever, the dribbling urination due to the evil qi, hernia, abdominal mass, throat impediment, dystocia, and the injury caused by metal and tetanus. It can be used to treat the cold pathogen caused by cold damage, cease dizziness and the stiffness of the neck, ascend qi due to cough. It removes polydipsia, promote perspiration, tranquilizes the five zang-organs and promotes the function of bone marrow.

Zhang Zhongjing said: For those suffering from the chest binding syndrome due to cold excess without exterior heat, Sanwu Xiaoxianxiong Decoction can be adopted, so is true with the white powder for it contains Beimu [贝母, fritillaria, Bulbus Fritillariae Thunbergii]. It is also said that Beimu [贝母, fritillaria the, Bulbus Fritillariae Thunbergii] has the special function of dispersing the qi stagnation in the thorax.

Ben Cao also says: In compatibility, Houpu [厚朴, magnolia bark, Cortex Magnoliae Officinalis] and Baiwei [白薇, blackend swallowwort root, Radix Cynanchi Atrati] are its assistant herbs. It is averse to Taohua [桃花, peach blossom, Prunus persica [L.] Batsch.], restrainted by Qinjiao [秦艽, root of largeleaf gentian, Radix Gentianae Macrophyllae], Fanshi [矾石, aluminite, Alumen] and Mangcao [莽草, Illicium aniaatum, Magnoliaceae], and anatagonizes Wutou [乌头, common monkshood, Aconitum carmichaeli Debx.].

According to the prescription of Hai Zang's [Wang Haogu] ancestor, there were three kinds of powder to promote lactation, including Muli [牡蛎, oyster shell, Concha Ostreae], Zhimu [知母, common anemarrhena rhizome, Rhizoma Anemarrhenae] and Beimu [贝母, fritillaria, Bulbus Fritillariae Thunbergii]. Grind them into powder and take them together with the stewed pig's trotter soup.

黄 芩

气寒,味微苦,苦而甘。微寒,味薄气厚,阳中阴也。阴中微阳,大寒。无毒。

入手太阴经之剂。

《象》云:治肺中湿热,疗上热,目中赤肿,瘀肉壅盛,必用之药。泄肺受火邪上逆于膈上。补膀胱之寒不足,乃滋其化源也。

《心》云:泻肺中之火。

洁古云:利胸中气,消膈上痰。性苦寒,下痢脓血稠粘,腹疼后重,身热,久不可者。与芍药、甘草同用。

《珍》云:除阳有余,凉心去热,通寒格。阴中微阳,酒炒上行,主上部积血,非此不能除。肺苦气上逆,急食苦以泄之。

《本草》云:主诸热黄胆,肠澼泄痢,逐水,下血闭,恶疮疽蚀,火伤,疗痰热,胃中热,小腹绞痛。消谷,利小肠,女子血闭,淋露下血,小儿腹痛。

东垣云:味苦而薄,中枯而飘,故能泻肺火而解肌热,手太阴剂也。细实而中不空者,治下部妙。

陶隐居云:色深坚实者好。又治奔豚、脐下热痛。飘与实,高下之分,与枳实、枳壳同例。黄芩,其子主肠澼脓血。

《本草》又云：得厚朴、黄连，治腹痛；得五味子、牡蒙、牡蛎，令人有子；得黄芪、白蔹、赤小豆，疗鼠瘘。山茱萸、龙骨为之使。恶葱实。畏丹砂、牡丹、藜芦芦。

张仲景治伤寒心下痞满，泻心汤四方皆用黄芩，以其去诸热、利小肠故也。又，太阳病下之，利不止，有葛根黄芩黄连汤。亦主妊娠，安胎散内多用黄芩，今医家常用有效者，因著之。《千金方》：巴郡太守奏加减三黄丸，疗男子五劳七伤、消渴、不生肌肉，妇人带下、手足寒热者。久服之，得行及奔马。甚验。

陶隐居云：黄芩，圆者名子芩，仲景治杂病方多用之。

Huangqin [黄芩, baical skullcap root, Radix Scutellariae]

It is cold in property, and slightly bitter and sweet in taste. For its cold property, its flavor is thin and property is thick, which pertains to yin within yang. It pertains to mild yang within yin, and it is extremely cold. It is nontoxic.

It is the medicinal herb entering the heart meridian of hand-taiyin.

Xiang [《药类法象》, *Rules for the Use of Medicinal Herbs*] says: It is used for treating the dampness and heat of the lung and curing the heat-syndrome in the upper part. It is effective to treat red swollen eyes and pterygium. It clears away the lung fire counter-flowing above the diaphragm and supplements the cold-insufficiency in bladder so as to nourish its source.

Xin [《用药心法》, *Gist for the Use of Medicinal Herbs*] says: It clears away the lung fire.

Jie Gu [Zhang Yuansu] said: It is used to promote the middle qi of the chest and remove the phlegm of the diaphragm. It is bitter and cold in nature and can be used to purge the thick purulent blood due to dysentery and diarrhea, and it can treat abdominal pain and persistent fever. It is also used together with Shaoyao [芍药, Chinese herbaceous peony, Paeonia lactiflora Pall.] and Gancao [甘草, liquorice root, Glycyrrhiza uralensis Fisch.].

Zhen [《珍珠囊》, *Pounch of Pearls*] says: It removes the excessive yang, cools the heart by clearing away the heat, and eliminates the repelling of cold and heat. It pertains to the slight yang within yin and guides the medicinal herb to go upward after frying with liquor. It is mainly used to treat the hematocele in the upper body, which can not be eliminated otherwise. The counter-flow of the lung qi can be discharged rapidly with the medicinal bitter in taste.

Ben Cao says: It is mainly used to treat various heat syndromes or patterns, jaundice and bloody stool, expel water, relieve amenorrhea, and cure severe sore, ulcer and scald. It removes the phlegm heat, the cardiothoracic fever in the stomach, and the colic in the lower abdomen. It digests food, promotes the function of small intestines, treats the amenorrhea, menorrhagia and the infantile abdominal pain.

Li Dongyuan said: Bitter but thin in flavor, hollow and light, it can clear away the lung fire and expel the heat in the muscle, so it is a medicinal herb to enter the meridian of hand-taiyin. The herb which is slim and solid in the middle can be used in the treatment of syndromes in the lower body.

Tao Yinju said: The dark colored and solid one is of good quality. It can also be used in the treatment of Bentun① and the heat pain below the umbilicus. The difference between the hollow and the solid is just like the difference between Zhishi [枳实, immature orange fruit, Fructus Aurantii Immaturus] and Zhiqiao [枳壳, orange fruit, Fructus Aurantii]. The seeds of Huangqin [黄芩, baical skullcap root, Radix Scutellariae] are mainly used to treat dysentery and purulent blood.

Ben Cao also says: It can be used in the treatment of the abdominal pain with Houpu [厚朴, magnolia bark, Cortex Magnoliae Officinalis] and Huanglian [黄连, golden thread, Rhizoma Coptidis]. Besides, it helps woman conceive if used together with Wuweizi [五味子, Chinese magnoliavine fruit, Fructus Schisandrae Chinensis], Mumeng [牡蒙, Chinese Sage Herb, Herba Salviae Chinesnsis] and Muli [牡蛎, oyster shell, Concha Ostreae]. It also cures the rat fistula if used together with Huangqi [黄芪, milkvetch root, Radix Astragali seu Hedysari], Bailian [白蔹, ampelopsis, Radix Ampelopsis] and Chixiaodou [赤小豆, rice bean, Semen Phaseoli]. In compatibility, Shanzhuyu [山茱萸, cornus, Fructus Corni] and Longgu [龙骨, bone fossil of big mammals, Os Draconis] are its assistance. It is averse to Congshi [葱实, Fistular Onion Seed, Allium fistulosum L.], and restrained by Dansha [丹砂, cinnabar, Cinnabaris], Mudan [牡丹,

---

① It refers to the palpitation underneath the navel similar to a running pig.

moutan, Cortex Moutan Radicis] and Lilu [藜芦, veratrum, Veratri Nigri Radix et Rhizoma].

Zhang Zhongjing used Huangqin [黄芩, baical skullcap root, Radix Scutellariae] to form Xiexin Decoction to treat cold damage as well as abdominal distention and fullness because it is responsible for removing all kinds of heat pathogen and promoting the function of the small intestines. In addition, Gegen Huangqi Huanglian Decoction can be used to treat taiyang diseases as well as dysentery and diarrhea. It is also used in Antai Powder to prevent abortion. It is recorded here because presently it is still widely used by doctors and proved effective. *Qian Jin Fang* [《千金方》, *Prescriptions Worth a Thousand Gold For Emergencies*] recorded: Prefecture chief of Bajun in feudal China found that modified Jiajian Sanhuang Pill can be used to cure five kinds of consumptive diseases and seven damages of men, consumptive thirst, the syndrome of failing to generate muscles, leukorrhea as well as cold and the heat of hands and feet. The long-term taking of it will make people strong and walk fast like a running horse. It proves to be effective in clinic.

Tao Yinju said: The round kind of Huangqin [黄芩, baical skullcap root, Radix Scutellariae] is called Ziqin, which is used by Zhang Zhongjing to treat miscellaneous diseases.

黄 连

气寒,味苦。味厚气薄,阴中阳也,升也。无毒。

入手少阴经。

《象》云:泻心火,除脾胃中湿热,治烦躁恶心,郁热在中焦,兀兀欲吐,心下痞满必用药也。仲景治九种心下痞,五等泻心汤皆用之。去须用。

《心》云:泻心经之火,眼暴赤肿,及诸疮,须用之。苦寒者主阳有余,苦以除之。安蛔,通寒格,疗下焦虚,坚肾。

《珍》云:酒炒上行,酒浸行上头。

《本草》云:主热气,目痛眦伤泣出,明目。肠澼腹痛下痢,妇人阴中肿痛。五脏冷热,久下泄澼脓血,止消渴大惊,除水利骨,调胃厚肠,益胆,疗口疮。久服令人不忘。

《液》云：入手少阴，苦燥，故入心，火就燥也。然泻心其实泻脾也，为子能令母实，实则泻其子。治血，防风为上使，黄连为中使，地榆为下使。

海藏祖方，令终身不发斑疮，煎黄连一口，儿生未出声时，灌之，大应。已出声灌之，斑虽发，亦轻。古方以黄连为治痢之最。

《衍义》云：治痢有微血，不可执以黄连。为苦燥剂，虚者多致危困，实者宜用之。

《本草》又云：龙骨、理石、黄芩为之使，恶菊花、芫花、玄参、白藓皮。畏款冬花。胜乌头，解巴豆毒。

Huanglian ［黄连，golden thread，Rhizoma Coptidis］

It is cold in property and bitter in taste. Its taste is thick, its property is thin, and it pertains to yang within yin with the ascending functional tendency. It is nontoxic.

It enters the meridian of hand-shaoyin.

Xiang ［《药类法象》，*Rules for the Use of Medicinal Herbs*］ says：It clears away the heart fire, removes the dampness-heat of the spleen and the stomach, and cures dysphoria and nausea. It is regarded as an indispensable medicinal herb for the intense nausea and the epigastric fullness due to stagnated heat in the middle energizer. Zhang Zhongjing used it to treat nine kinds of epigastric stuffiness and five kinds of Xiexin Decoction. It is used after the tassel is removed.

Xin ［《用药心法》，*Gist for the Use of Medicinal Herbs*］ says：It can be used to clear away the fire in the heart meridian, and treat epidemic red eyes as well as sorts of sores. Being bitter and cold in property, the excessive yang can be removed with medicinal bitter in taste. It can prevent ascaris from moving, regulate the repelling of cold and heat, cure the deficiency in the lower energizer, and replenish the kidney.

Zhen ［《珍珠囊》，*Pounch of Pearls*］ says：It is used to guide the medicinal herb to go upward after its being fried with liquor and guide the medicinal herb to go upward to head after soaking with liquor.

Ben Cao says：It is mainly used to to relieve the pain in eyes due to heat qi and the epiphora due to eyelid injury, improve vision, treat diarrhea, abdominal pain, dysentery, vulval swelling and pain, cold, and the heat in the five zang-organs.

It can persistently discharge purulent blood, cease diabetes and terror, remove water to promote the function of bones, regulate the stomach and thicken the intestine, replenish gallbladder, and cure oral aphthae. The long-term taking of it will invigorate memory.

Ye [《汤液本草》, *Materia Medica for Decoctions*] says: It enters the meridian of hand-shaoyin because of its bitterness and dryness. It enters the heart, and the fire pertains to dryness. However, it clears away the heart fire, which is equivalent to clearing away the spleen-fire. The spleen that pertains to the child-organ of the heart make the mother-organ fulfilled, that is why it equals to purging the child-organ. It is used to treat the deficiency with tonification function and the excess syndromes with purging function. It is mainly used to treat blood diseases, for Fangfeng [防风, divaricate saposhnikovia root, Radix Saposhnikoviae] is used as its upper assistance, Huanglian [黄连, golden thread, Rhizoma Coptidis] is its middle assistance, and Diyu [地榆, garden burnet root, Radix Sanguisorbae] is its lower assistance.

According to the prescription by Haizang's [Wang Haogu] ancestor, people may never suffer from dermatirtis for lifelong. That is, feed a newly-born baby a spoon of the decoction of Huanglian [黄连, golden thread, Rhizoma Coptidis] before he utters, he will have a loud response. But if he utters before feeding, and has dermatitis, the syndrome will be mitigated. The ancient prescription shows that Huanglian [黄连, golden thread, Rhizoma Coptidis] has the best curative effect in the treatment of diarrhea.

Yan Yi [《衍义》, *Extension of the Materia Medica*] says: Huanglian [黄连, golden thread, Rhizoma Coptidis] can not be used to treat the diarrhea with slight bleeding. It is used as the bitter and drying agent, and the deficiency may be worsened after taking it, whereas the excess may be relieved.

Ben Cao also says: In compatibility, Longgu [龙骨, loong bone, Os Draconis], Lishi [理石, fibrous gypsum, Gypsum et Anhydritum] and Huangqin [黄芩, baical skullcap root, Radix Scutellariae] are its assistance. It is averse to Juhua [菊花, chrysanthemums, Dendranthema morifolium Tzvel.], Yuanhua [芫花, immature flower of lilac daphne, Flos Genkwa], Xuanshen [玄参, figwort root, Radix Scrophulariae] and Baixianpi [白藓皮, densefruit pittany root-bark,

Cortex Dictamni], and restrained by Kuandonghua [款冬花, common coltsfoot flower, Flos Farfarae]. In property, it is more excessive than Wuton [乌头, common monkshood, Aconitum carmichaeli Debx.] in toxicity and detoxifies the toxicity of Badou [巴豆, Croton Fruit, Fructus Crotonis].

大 黄

气寒。味苦,大寒。味极厚,阴也,降也。无毒。

入手足阳明经。酒浸,入太阳经;酒洗,入阳明经。余经不用酒。

《象》云:性走而不守,泻诸实热不通,下大便,涤荡肠胃间热,专治不大便。

《心》云:涤荡实热。

《珍》云:热淫于内,以苦泄之。酒浸入太阳经,酒洗入阳明经,余经不用酒。

《本草》云:主下瘀血,血闭寒热,破症瘕积聚,留饮宿食,荡涤肠胃,推陈致新,通利水谷,调中化食,安和五脏。平胃下气,除痰实,肠间结热,心腹胀满,女子寒血闭胀,小腹痛,诸老血留结。

《液》云:味苦、寒,阴中之阴药。泄漏,推陈致新,去陈垢而安五脏,谓如戡定祸乱以致太平无异,所以有将军之名。入手足阳明,以酒引之,上至高巅;以舟楫载之,胸中可浮;以苦泄之,性峻至于下。以酒将之,可行至高之分,若物在巅,人迹不及,必射以取之也。故太阳阳明、正阳阳明承气汤中俱用酒浸,惟少阳阳明为下经,故小承气汤中不用酒浸也。杂方有生用者,有面裹蒸熟者,其制不等。

《衍义》云:损益前书已具。仲景治心气不足,吐血衄血,泻心汤用大黄、黄芩、黄连。或曰:心气既不足矣,而不用补心汤,更用泻心汤,何也?答曰:若心气独不足,则须当不吐衄也,此乃邪热因心气不足而客之,故令吐衄。以苦泄其热,就以苦补其心,盖一举而两得之。有是证者,用之无不效,惟在量其虚实而已。

《本草》又云:恶干漆。

Dahuang [大黄, rhubarb, Radix et Rhizoma Rhei]

It is cold in property, bitter in taste, and extremely cold in property. Its flavor is extremely thick, which pertains to yin with the descending functional tendency. It is nontoxic.

It enters the meridian of hand and foot yangming. If soaked in liquor, it can enter the meridian of taiyang. If washed in liquor, it can enter the meridian of yangming. To treat diseases on other meridians, it needs no processing with liquor.

Xiang [《药类法象》, *Rules for the Use of Medicinal Herbs*] says: It can go through each part in the body according to its property, purge the excessive heat due to obstruction, discharge the excrement, and clear away the heat of the intestines and stomach. It specializes in treating constipation.

Xin [《用药心法》, *Gist for the Use of Medicinal Herbs*] says: It is used to purge the excessive heat.

Zhen [《珍珠囊》, *Pouch of Pearls*] says: It is used to purge the internal heat pathogen by its bitter property. When soaked in liquor, it enters the meridian of taiyang; when washed in liquor, it enters the meridian of yangming. The herbs that are not processed by liquor can enter other meridians.

Ben Cao says: It is mainly used to treat blood stasis, amenorrhea and cold-heat disease, purge abdominal mass, conglomeration and accumulation, fluid retention and indigestion, activate the intestines and stomach, bring forth the new by reducing the old, unobstruct and disinhibit water and food, regulate the middle energizer, digest food, harmonize the five zang-organs, pacify the stomach and promote qi to flow downwards, remove the fullness due to phlegm, clear away the heat accumulation in the intestines, and remove the fullness in the chest and hypochondrium, amenorrhea due to the cold syndrome as well as the pain in the lower abdomen and any other accumulation in the stale blood.

Ye [《汤液本草》, *Materia Medica for Decoctions*] says: It is bitter in taste and cold in nature, pertaining to yin within yin. It has the function of purging and discharging to bring forth the new by reducing the old and take the old filthy so as to harmonize the five zang-organs. It says that its function is just like a man who can conquer the disturbance and pacify the world therefore he is also called the General. It enters the meridians of hand and foot yangming. It is guided by liquor, as if up to the summit and being carried by boat. It can float in the chest and purge by its bitterness because of its thick property, being used as the purgative method. It is possible to use liquor to make it as high as possible. If something is in it, it will not be traced. Therefore, both taiyang-yangming and zhengyang-yangming Chengqi Decoction are soaked in liquor, and only the meridians of shaoyang-yangming pertain to the lower meridians, so it is not necessarily soaked in liquor in Xiaochengqi Decoction. According to other prescriptions, the raw one can be used, or the steamed one wrapped with flour can be used, the processing methods of which are different.

Yan Yi [《衍义》, *Extension of the Materia Medica*] says: Both its damage and tonifying function are recorded in previous books. Zhang Zhongjing treated the deficiency of heart-qi, hematemesis and bleeding by Xiexin Decoction which contains the herbs of Dahuang [大黄, rhubarb, Radix et Rhizoma Rhei], Huangqin [黄芩, baical skullcap root, Radix Scutellariae] and Huanglian [黄连, golden thread, Rhizoma Coptidis]. The question is why the deficiency of heart-qi is treated by Xiexin Decoction rather than Buxin Decoction. The answer is if only the heart-qi is deficient, the patient would not have hematemesis or bleeding from the five sense organs. This syndrome is caused by the insufficieny of heart qi due to heat pathogen. The heat is purged with bitter medicinal herbs, equaling to replenishing the heart with bitterness, just as the saying goes "killing two birds with one stone". It is proved effective if correct decision is made about whether the syndrome is deficient or excessive.

Ben Cao also says: It is averse to effective Ganqi [干漆, Dried Lacquer, Resina Toxicodendri].

连 翘

气平,味苦。苦,微寒,气味俱轻,阴中阳也,无毒。

手足少阳经、阳明经药。

《象》云:治寒热瘰疬,诸恶疮肿,除心中客热,去胃虫,通五淋。

《心》云:泻心经客热,诸家须用,疮家圣药也。

《珍》云:诸经客热,非此不能除。

《本草》云:主寒热鼠瘘,瘰疬,痈肿瘿瘤,结热蛊毒,去寸白虫。

《液》云:入手、足少阳。治疮、疡、瘤、气瘿起、结核有神。与柴胡同功,但分气血之异耳。与鼠粘子同用,治疮疡别有神功。

Lianqiao [连翘, fruit of weeping forsythia, Fructus Forsythiae]

It is mild in property, bitter in taste and slightly cold in nature. Both its property and flavor are thin, pertaining to yang within yin. It is nontoxic.

It enters the meridian of hand and foot shaoyang and yangming.

Xiang [《药类法象》, *Rules for the Use of Medicinal Herbs*] says: It is mainly used to treat the diseases due to cold and heat, cervical scrofula, as well as all kinds of obstinate sore and abscessus. It clears away the guest heat caused by the terror in the heart and maw worm, and dredges five types of stranguria.

Xin [《用药心法》, *Gist for the Use of Medicinal Herbs*] says: It clears away the guest heat in the heart channel, and especially it is regarded as a kind of effective medicine for the patient who suffers from sore and ulcer.

Zhen [《珍珠囊》, *Pounch of Pearls*] says: The guest heat in the meridian can not be eliminated without it.

Ben Cao says: It is mainly used to treat cold-heat disease, tuberculosis, scrofula, abscess, severe sore, goiter, tumor, heat stagnation and worm toxin, and remove taeniasis.

Ye [《汤液本草》, *Materia Medica for Decoctions*] says: It enters the meridians of hand-shaoyang and foot-shaoyang. It is used to treat the diseases such as sore, ulcer, lump, hyperthyreosis of qi, especially tuberculosis. It is similar to Chaihu [柴胡, Chinese thorowax root, Radix Bupleuri] in function, but different in the treatment of qi and blood. It has good therapeutic effect on sore and ulcer when used with Niubangzi [牛蒡子, great burdock achene, Fructus Arctii].

连轺

气寒,味苦。

《本经》不见所注,但仲景古方所注云,即连翘之根也。方言熬者,即今之炒也。

Lianyao [连轺, the root of weeping forsythia capsule, Forsythia Suspensa (Thunb.) Vahl]

It is cold in property and bitter in taste.

There is no related record in Ben Jing [《本经》, Agriculture God's Canon of Materia Medica], but according to Zhang Zhongjing's ancient prescription, it was the root of Lianqiao [连翘, weeping forsythia capsule, Fructus Forsythiae]. The boiling method recorded in a local dialect, actually means stir frying now.

人 参

气温，味甘。甘而微苦，微寒，气味俱轻，阳也。阳中微阴，无毒。

《象》云：治脾肺阳气不足，及能补肺。气促，短气、少气。补而缓中，泻脾肺胃中火邪，善治短气。非升麻为引用，不能补上升之气，升麻一分、人参三分，为相得也。若补下焦元气，泻肾中火邪，茯苓为之使。

《心》云：补气不足而泻肺火，甘温而补阳利气。脉不足者，是亡血也，人参补之。益脾，与干姜同用补气，里虚则腹痛，此药补之，是补不足也。

《珍》云：补胃，喘嗽勿用，短气用之。

《本草》云：主补五脏，安精神，定魂魄，止惊悸，除邪气，明目，开心益智。疗肠胃中冷，心腹鼓痛，胸胁逆满，霍乱吐逆，调中，止消渴，通血脉，破坚积，令人不忘。

《液》云：味既甘温，调中益气，即补肺之阳、泻肺之阴也。若便言补肺，而不论阴阳寒热何气不足，则误矣。若肺受寒邪，宜此补之；肺受火邪，不宜用也。肺为天之地，即手太阴也，为清肃之脏，贵凉而不贵热，其象可知。若伤热则宜沙参。沙参味苦、甘微寒，无毒，主血积惊气，除寒热，补中益肺气，疗胃痹心腹痛，结热邪气，头痛，皮间邪热。安五脏，补中。人参补五脏之阳也，沙参苦，微寒，补五脏之阴也。安得不异。

易老云：用沙参代人参，取其味甘可也。

葛洪云：沙参，主卒得诸疝，小腹及阴中相引，痛如绞，自汗出，欲死。细末。酒调服方寸匕，立瘥。

《日华子》云：治恶疮疥癣及身痒，排脓，消肿毒。

海藏云：今易老取沙参代人参，取其甘也。若微苦则补阴，甘者则补阳，经虽云补五脏，亦须各用本脏药相佐使，随所引而相辅一脏也，不可不知。

Renshen [人参, ginseng, Radix Ginseng]

It is warm in property, sweet and slightly bitter in taste. It is slightly cold and is light in property and flavor, pertaining to yang. It pertains to slight yin within yang, and it is nontoxic.

Xiang [《药类法象》, *Rules for the Use of Medicinal Herbs*] says: It can treat the insufficiency of yang qi in the spleen and the lung so as to supplement the lung. It can also be used to treat panting, shortness of breath and so on. It tonifies and moderates the middle qi, discharges the fire pathogen in the spleen, lung and stomach, and is especially effective in treating shortness of breath. If Shengma [升麻, largetrifoliolious bugbane rhizome, Rhizoma Cimicifugae] is not used as the guiding medicinal herb, it will not tonify the ascending qi. Therefore, it would be effective to combine 1 Fen of Shengma [升麻, largetrifoliolious bugbane rhizome, Rhizoma Cimicifugae] and 3 Fen of Renshen [人参, ginseng, Radix Ginseng]. If there is the need of supplementing the primordial qi in the lower energizer and purging the fire pathogen of the kidney, Fuling [茯苓, Indian bread, Poria] serves as its assistance.

Xin [《用药心法》, *Gist for the Use of Medicinal Herbs*] says: It can supplement the insufficiency of qi so as to purge the lung fire, strengthen yang and benefit qi by its property of being warm and sweet. The asthenia of vessels pertains to hemorrhage bleeding, so Renshen [人参, ginseng, Radix Ginseng] can be used to tonify it. It can strengthen the spleen. If used together with Ganjiang [干姜, dry ginger, Rhizoma Zingiberis], it can supplement qi. The abdominal pain due to the interior deficiency can be treated by this herb, which is used to supplement the deficiency.

Zhen [《珍珠囊》, *Pouch of Pearls*] says: It can be used to replenish the stomach and treat shortness of breath. Do not use it to treat dyspnea and cough.

Ben Cao says: It is mainly used to supplement the five zang-organs, calm the spirit, tranquilize the ethereal soul and corporeal soul, cease fright and palpitation, eliminate the pathogenic qi, improve vision, soothe the heart, and promote intelligence. It is used to remove the cold in the stomach, abdominal distention on and pain, the qi counter-flow due to the fullness in the chest and hypochondrium, vomiting due to cholera, and regulate the middle energizer, cease thirst, smoothen vessels and break hard accumulation. It has the function of preventing amnesia.

Ye [《汤液本草》, *Materia Medica for Decoctions*] says: It is sweet in flavor and warm in nature, and it regulates the spleen and the stomach and replenishes qi, i. e., it supplements the lung yang and purges lung yin. As to its function to supplement the lung, it may be mistaken to neglect the differentiation of yin, yang, cold and heat that lead to qi deficieny. If the lung is attacked by the pathogenic factor due to cold, it is better to supplement with the herb; if the lung is attacked by the fire pathogen, the herb can not be used. The lung pertains to the meridian of hand-taiyin, which governs purification and descending, prefering cold to heat, which can be seen from its manifestation. Shashen [沙参, fourleaf ladybell root, Radix Adenophorae] is advisable to be used in the treatment of syndromes caused by the heat pathogen. Shashen [沙参, fourleaf ladybell root, Radix Adenophorae] is bitter, sweet in flavor and slightly cold in property, being nontoxic. It is mainly used to treat the accumulation of the extravasated blood and the qi turbulence due to fright, remove cold and heat, supplement the middle energizer and replenish the lung qi. Besides, it is used to treat the stomach impediment, the pain in the heart and the abdomen, heat pathogen, headache, and the heat pathogen in the skin. It calms the five zang-organs and supplements the middle energizer. Renshen [人参, ginseng, Radix Ginseng] can supplement the yang of the five zang-organs, but Shashen [沙参, fourleaf ladybell root, Radix Adenophorae] is bitter, slightly cold and supplements yin in the five zang-organs. How can we not distinguish them?

Yi Lao [Zhang Yuansu] said: Renshen [人参, ginseng, Radix Ginseng] can be substituted by Shashen [沙参, fourleaf ladybell root, Radix Adenophorae], for it is sweet in flavor.

Ge Hong said: Shashen [沙参, fourleaf ladybell root, Radix Adenophorae] is mainly used to treat all kinds of acute hernias, coupling between lower abdomen and pudendum, angina, spontaneous perspiration, and moribund syndrome. Grind it into fine powder, take it after mixing with liquor by square-inch-spoon, one can recover immediately.

Ri Hua Zi [《日华子》, *Materia Medica of Ri Hua-Zi*] says: It can be used to treat obstinate sores, scabies as well as pruritus. Besides, it can expel pus and relieve pyogenic infections.

Hai Zang [Wang Haogu] said: Presently, Yi Lao [Zhang Yuansu] replaced

Renshen［人参, ginseng, Radix Ginseng］with Shashen［沙参, fourleaf ladybell root, Radix Adenophorae］because of its sweet flavor. If it is slightly bitter, it will supplement yin and yang if it is sweet. Though *Jing* said that it is used to supplement the five zang-organs, one should be clear that it ought to be assisted with each organ's own drugs and be guided to benefit one specific organ.

沙 参

味苦、甘，微寒。无毒。

治证附前人参条下。

Shashen［沙参, fourleaf ladybell root, Radix Adenophorae］

It is bitter and sweet in flavor, and slightly cold in nature. It is nontoxic.

See its diagnosis and treatment in the clause of Renshen［人参, ginseng, Radix Ginseng］.

半 夏

气微寒，味辛、平。苦而辛，辛厚苦轻，阳中阴也。生微寒，熟温。有毒。

入足阳明经、太阴经、少阳经。

《象》云：治寒痰，及形寒饮冷伤肺而咳。大和胃气，除胃寒，进食。治太阴痰厥头痛，非此不能除。

《心》云：能胜脾胃之湿，所以化痰。渴者禁用。

《珍》云：消胸中痞，去膈上痰。

《本草》云：主伤寒寒热，心下坚，下气，咽喉肿痛，头眩，胸胀，咳逆，肠鸣。止汗。消心腹、胸膈痰热满结，咳嗽上气，心下急痛坚痞，时气呕逆，消痈肿，堕胎，疗痿黄，悦泽面目。生，令人吐；熟，令人下。用之汤洗去滑令尽。用生姜等分制用，能消痰涎，开胃健脾。射干为之使。恶皂荚。畏雄黄、生姜、干姜、秦皮、龟甲。反乌头。

《药性论》云：半夏使。忌羊血、海藻、饴糖。柴胡为之使。俗用为肺药，非也。止吐，为足阳明；除痰，为足太阴。小柴胡中虽为止呕，亦助柴胡能止恶寒，是又为足少阳也；又助黄芩能去热，是又为足阳明也。往来寒热在表里之中，故用此有各半之意。本以治伤寒之寒热，所以名半夏。《经》云：肾主五液，化为五湿，自入为唾，入肝为泣，入心为汗，入脾为痰，入肺为涕。有涎曰嗽，无涎曰咳，痰者因咳而动脾之湿也。半夏能泄痰之标，不能泄痰之本，泄本者，泄肾也。咳无形，痰有形；无形则润，有形则燥，所以为流湿润燥也。

Banxia［半夏, pinellia Tuber, Rhizoma Pinelliae］

It is slightly cold in property, pungent in flavor and mild in nature. It is bitter and pungent, the former being light and the latter being heavy. It pertains to yin within yang. It is slightly cold in property when it is raw, but warm when cooked. It is toxic.

It enters the meridian of foot-yangming, taiyin and shaoyang.

Xiang［《药类法象》, *Rules for the Use of Medicinal Herbs*］says: It is used to treat the phlegm due to cold and the cough due to the lung deficiency by drinking something cold. It harmonizes the stomach qi and removes the stomach cold, which is helpful for appetite. The taiyin headache due to phlegm syncope can not be treated otherwise.

Xin［《用药心法》, *Gist for the Use of Medicinal Herbs*］says: It can treat the dampness in the spleen and the stomach, so it can eliminate phlegm. It can not be used for the people suffering from the consumptive thirst.

Zhen［《珍珠囊》, *Pounch of Pearls*］says: It can eliminate the distention and fullness in the chest and remove the phlegm in the diaphragm as well.

Ben Cao says: It is pungent in taste and mild in property. It is mainly used to treat cold damage, cold-heat disease and the lumps below the heart, promote qi to flow downwards, treat the swelling and pain of the throat, vertigo, chest distension, the cough with dyspnea and borborygmus, and stop sweating. It can eliminate the phlegm-heat and agglomeration in the abdomen, chest and diaphragm, cough and suffocating catarrh, sharp pain and distention and fullness below the heart, vomiting due to seasonal epidemic pathogens. Besides, it dispels abscess, induces abortion and cures chlorosis to make the complexion lustrous. The raw one can lead to vomit, and the cooked one can lead to diarrhea. Before using, wash it to get rid of the slithery substances on the surface for lessening its toxicity. Process it with Shengjiang［生姜, fresh ginger, Rhizoma Zingiberis

Recens] to dissolve phlegm and saliva, and improve the stomach qi and tonify the spleen. In compatibility, Shegan [射干, blackberry lily rhizome, Rhizoma Belamcandae] is its assistance. It is averse to Zaojia [皂荚, soap pod, Gleditsia sinensis Lam.], restrained with Xionghuang [雄黄, realgar, Realgar], Shengjiang [生姜, fresh ginger, Rhizoma Zingiberis Recens], Qinpi [秦皮, ash bark, Cortex Fraxini], Ganjiang [干姜, dry ginger, Rhizoma Zingiberis] and Guijia [龟甲, tortoise shell, Carapax et Plastrum Testudinis]. It antagonizes Wutou [乌头, common monkshood, Aconitum carmichaeli Debx.]

Yao Xing Lun [《药性论》, *Treatise on Medicinal Properties*] says: In compatibility, Banxia [半夏, pinellia Tuber, Rhizoma Pinelliae] is used as an assistant drug. It is prohibited to be used together with goat blood, Haizao [海藻, seaweed, Sargassum] and malt sugar. In compatibility, Chaihu [柴胡, Chinese thorowax root, Radix Bupleuri] is its assitance. It is commonly regarded as a herb for the treatment of lung diseases, but this is wrong. It can stop vomiting when entering the meridian of foot-yangming; it eliminates phlegm when entering the meridian of foot-taiyin. Although it can stop vomiting when used together with Xiaochaihu [小柴胡, Common Goldenrop, Bupleurum tenue], it also helps Chaihu [柴胡, Chinese thorowax root, Radix Bupleuri] remove the syndrome of aversion to cold, which indicates that it enters the meridian of foot-shaoyang. Besides, it can assist Huangqin [黄芩, baical skullcap root, Radix Scutellariae] to remove heat, which indicates that it enters the meridian of foot-yangming. The alternate cold and heat exists between the interior and the exterior; therefore, it is used in the treatment with corresponding effect. Originally, it is used in the treatment of cold and heat due to cold damage, so it is given the name Banxia. *Jing* says: The kidney governs the five humors, which are transformed into five kinds of dampness, associated with salivia when entering the kidney, tears when entering the liver, perspiration when entering the heart, phlegm when entering the spleen, and snot when entering the lung. The cough with saliva is called Sou in Chinese, the cough without saliva is called Ke in Chinese. The phlegm is caused by spleen dampness disturbed by coughing. Banxia [半夏, pinellia, Rhizoma Pinelliae] can have a temporary effect on discharging the phlegm, but not a permanent one. To treat the root cause, one needs to discharge the kidney. The cough is invisible, the phlegm is tangible. The invisible cough should be treated with moistening and the tangible phlegm should be treated with drying. Therefore, Banxia [半夏, pinellia, Rhizoma Pinelliae] is the medicinal herb for drying dampness and moistening dryness.

五味子

气温,味酸,阴中阳。酸而微苦,味厚气轻,阴中微阳。无毒。

入手太阴经,入足少阴经。

《象》云:大益五脏。

孙真人云:五月常服五味子,以补五脏气,遇夏月季夏之间,困乏无力,无气以动,与黄芪、人参、麦门冬,少加黄柏,煎汤服,使人精神顿加,两足筋力涌出。生用。

《珍》云:治咳嗽。

《心》云:收肺气,补气不足,升也。酸以收逆气,肺寒气逆,则以此药与干姜同用治之。

《本草》云:主咳逆上气,劳伤羸瘦,补不足,益气强阴益精,养五脏,除热。

《日华子》云:明目,暖水脏,治风,下气消食。霍乱转筋,痃癖,奔豚冷气。消水肿,反胃,心腹气胀。止渴,除烦热,解酒毒,壮筋骨。五味皮甘肉酸,核中辛苦,都有咸味,故名五味子。仲景八味丸用此为肾气丸,述类象形也。

孙真人云:六月常服五味子,以益肺金之气,在上则滋源,在下则补肾,故入手太阴、足少阴也。

Wuweizi [五味子, Chinese magnoliavine fruit, Fructus Schisandrae Chinensis]

It is warm in property and sour in taste, pertaining to yang within yin. It is slightly sour and bitter. Its flavor is thick and its property is light. It pertains to mild yang within yin and is nontoxic.

It enters the meridian of hand-taiyin and foot-shaoyin.

Yao Lei Fa Xiang [《药类法象》, *Rules for the Use of Medicinal Herbs*] says: It greatly tonifies the five zang-organs.

Sun Zhenren (Sun Simiao) said: If Wuweizi [五味子, Chinese magnoliavine fruit, Fructus Schisandrae Chinensis] is often taken in May, it can supplement the qi of the five zang-organs; if people feel sleepy, tired and feeble between months in summer, they can not become energetic without activating qi. Wuweizi [五味子, Chinese magnoliavine fruit, Fructus Schisandrae Chinensis] is used together with Huangqi [黄芪, milkvetch root, Radix Astragali seu Hedysari], Renshen [人参, ginseng, Radix Ginseng], Maimendong [麦门冬, radix ophiopogonis, Ophiopogon japonicus Ker-Gawl] and a bit of Huangbo [黄柏, bark of amur corktree, Cortex Phellodendri] to form the decoction, and people will feel invigorated and powerful after taking the decoction. It should be used when raw.

Zhen [《珍珠囊》, Pounch of Pearls] says: It treats cough.

Xin [《用药心法》, Gist for the Use of Medicinal Herbs] says: It astringes the lung qi and supplements the insufficiency of qi, which pertains to ascent function. Therefore, its sourness can treat the counter-flow of qi. Used together with Ganjiang [干姜, dried ginger, Rhizoma Zingiberis], it can treat the counter-flow of qi due to the lung cold.

Ben Cao says: It is mainly used to treat the cough with dyspnea and the upward counter-flow of qi, resolve the overexertion with emaciation, tonify insufficiency, benefit qi, strengthen yin, replenish the essence, nourish the five zang-organs and eliminate heat.

Ri Hua Zi [《日华子》, Materia Medica of Ri Hua-Zi] says: It is used to improve vision, warm the water organ, treat the wind syndrome, descend qi and promote digestion, treat cholera and cramp, hypochondrial mass, palpitation underneath the navel similar to a running pig and the diseases caused by cold qi. In addition, it removes edema, gastric disorder causing nausea, etiminates flatulence of the chest and abdomen, quenches thirst, dysphoria and heat, dispels the to xin of alcohol and strengthen the body. The coating of Wuweizi [五味子, Chinese magnoliavine fruit, Fructus Schisandrae Chinensis] is sweet and its flesh is sour. Its pit is pungent and bitter. It is also salty, so it is named Wuweizi, which means five flavors in Chinese. Zhang Zhongjing used it in Bawei Pills to change it into Shenqi Pills according to its description.

Sun Zhenren [Sun Simiao] said: Wuweizi [五味子, Chinese magnoliavine fruit, Fructus Schisandrae Chinensis] is often taken in lunar June to replenish the lung qi, providing the nourishment in the upper and supplementing the kidney in the lower; therefore, it enters the meridians of hand-taiyin and foot-shaoyin.

甘 遂

气大寒,味苦、甘。甘,纯阳。有毒。

《本草》云:主大腹疝瘕,腹满,面目浮肿,留饮宿食。破坚消积,利水谷道;下五水,散膀胱留热,皮中痞热,气肿满。瓜蒂为使。恶远志,反甘草。

《液》云:可以通水,而其气直透达所结处。

《衍义》云:此药专于行水,攻决为用,入药须斟酌用之。

《珍》云:若水结胸中,非此不能除。

Gansui [甘遂, kansui, Radix Euphorbiae Kansui]

It is extremely cold in property, bitter and sweet in flavor, and its sweetness pertains to yang property. It is toxic.

Ben Cao says: It is mainly used to treat the hernia and conglomeration in the abdomen, the abdominal fullness, the dropsy of the face and eyes, the retention of fluid and the retention of undigested food, break lump and accumulation, and promote urination and defecation. It is used to treat five kinds of edema, clear away the heat in the bladder and the skin, and remove emplysema and the abdominal fullness. In compatibility, it is assisted by Guadi [瓜蒂, muskmelon fruit pedicel, Pedicellus Melo], restrained by Yuanzhi [远志, polygala root, Radix Polygalae] and averse to Gancao [甘草, liquorice root, Glycyrrhiza Uralensis Fisch.]

Ye [《汤液本草》, *Materia Medica for Decoctions*] says: It can regulate the water passage, and can go straight to the affected area of the body.

Yan Yi [《衍义》, *Extension of the Materia Medica*] says: It can be used to regulate the water passage and purge in disease treatment, therefore it should be used appropriately.

Zhen [《珍珠囊》, *Pounch of Pearls*] says: The hydrothorax can not be eliminated without Gansui [甘遂, gansui root, Radix Euphorbiae Kansui].

大 戟

气大寒,味苦、甘,阴中微阳。有小毒。

《本草》云:治蛊毒,十二水,腹满急痛,积聚,中风,皮肤疼痛,吐逆,颈腋痈肿,头疼,发汗,利大小肠。此泽漆根也。

《液》云:与甘遂同为泄水之药,湿胜者苦燥除之。反甘草。与芫花、黄药子等分,水糊为丸,桐子大,每服十丸,伤风寒,葱白汤下;伤食,陈皮汤下。或十五丸,微加至止,亦可。芫花别有条,海藏十枣汤同用。

《珍》云:泻肺,损真气。

Daji [大戟, peking euphorbia root, Radix Euphorbiae Pekinensis]

It is extremely cold in property, bitter and sweet in taste, and it pertains to slight yang within yin. It is slightly toxic.

Ben Cao says: It is mainly used to treat the disease caused by worm toxin, various edema, abdominal fullness and sharp pain, accumulation, aggregation, wind stroke, cutaneous pain and vomiting, carbuncle swollen, headache, and sweating. It can promote large and small intestines. It is the root of Zeqi [泽漆, spurge, Herba Euphorbiae Helioscopiae].

Ye [《汤液本草》, *Materia Medica for Decoctions*] says: It is used similarly as Gansui [甘遂, kansui, Radix Euphorbiae Kansui] for discharging water. The excessive dampness in the body can be dried with its bitterness. It anagonizes Gancao [甘草, liquorice root, Glycyrrhizae Uralensis Fisch.]. It can be used together with Yuanhua [芫花, immature flower of lilac daphne, Flos Genkwa] and Huangyaozi [黄药子, air potato, Rhizoma Dioscoreae Bulbiferae] in the same amount to make pills as big as Tongzi [桐子, phoenix tree seed, Firmiana plantanifoliaa (L. f.) Marsili.]. Ten pills can be taken with Congbai Decoction each time to treat the cold pathogen due to wind; they can be taken with chenpi decoction to treat dyspepsia caused by excessive eating or improper diet. Or fifteen pills or a bit more can be taken each time. Haizang [Wang Haogu] once used it with Yuanhua [芫花, immature flower of lilac daphne, Flos Genkwa] which needs removing stripes to make Shizao Decoction.

Zhen [《珍珠囊》, *Pounch of Pearls*] says: It can purge the lung fire, but damage the genuine qi.

莞 花

气微寒,味苦、辛。有毒。

《本草》云:主伤寒温疟,下十二水,破积聚大坚症瘕,荡涤肠胃中留癖,饮食寒热邪气。利水道,疗痰饮咳嗽。

《衍义》云:仲景以莞花治利者,以其行水也,水去则利止,其意如此。用时斟酌,不可太过与不及也。仍察其须有是证,方可用之。仲景小青龙汤:若微利,去麻黄,加莞花,如鸡子,熬令赤色用之。盖利水也。

Raohua [莞花, flower of longflower stringbush, Wikstroemia Canescens (Wall.) Meisn.]

It is slightly cold in property, and bitter and pungent in flavor. It is toxic.

Ben Cao says: It is mainly used to treat cold damage, malaria and various edema, break accumulation, hard mass and conglomeration, remove the retention of undigested food, the cold-heat and evil-qi in the intestines and stomach, disinhibit the waterway in the body, treat the cough due to phlegm and fluid retention.

Yan Yi [《衍义》, *Extension of the Materia Medica*] says: Zhang Zhongjing used Raohua [莞花, flower of longflower stringbush, Wikstroemia canescens (Wall.) Meisn.] in the treatment of diarrhea to expel water. When the water is discharged, the diarrhea is cured to that effect. The dosage should be considered carefully to avoid excessive or inappropriate usage. It can only be used after careful synderome differentiation. According to Zhang Zhongjing's Xiaoqinglong Decoction, if the edema is mild, get rid of Muahuang [麻黄, ephedra, Herba Ephedrae] and add Raohua [莞花, flower of Long flower String bush, Wikstroemia canescens (Wall.) Meisn.] in the prescription, just like egg yolk, and then make it into red decoction to promote the water passage.

海 藻

气寒,味咸。

《本草》云:主瘿瘤气,颈下核,破散结气,痈肿症瘕坚气,腹中上下鸣,下十二水肿。疗皮间积聚,暴㿗,留气热结,利小便。

《珍》云:洗,去咸。泄水气。

Haizao [海藻, seaweed, Sargassum]

It is cold in property and salty in taste.

Ben Cao says: It is mainly used to treat goiter, tumor and the lump in the neck, remove qi stagnation, carbuncle, abdominal mass, the borborygum in the upper and the lower abdomen, and resolve twelve kinds of edema. It proves effective in treating the accumulative pathogen in the skin, acute swelling of heat accumulation, scrotum, qi stagnation, and promoting urination.

Zhen [《珍珠囊》, *Pouch of Pearls*] says: Wash it to remove its salt. It can treat water retention.

商 陆 根

气平,味辛、酸。有毒。

《本草》云:主水胀满,瘕痹,熨除痈肿,杀鬼精物。治胸中邪气、水肿、痿痹、腹满洪,直疏五脏,散水气。如人形者,有神。

《珍》云:辛酸同用,导肿气。

Shanglugen [商陆根, pokeberry root, Radix Phytolaccae]

It is mild in property, and pungent and sour in taste. It is toxic.

Ben Cao says: It is mainly used to treat the distension and fullness due to edema, conglomeration and impediment, eliminate abscess through external application and strange pathogenic factors like ghost and monster. It can be used to treat pathogenic qi in the chest, edema, flaccidity and impediment, abdomial distension, dredge the five zang-organs to purge water and resolve swelling. The one that is shaped like the human body may be more effective.

Zhen [《珍珠囊》, *Pounch of Pearls*] says: It can be used to guide and remove the water retention with its pungency and sourness.

旋 覆 花

气温,味咸、甘。冷利,有小毒。

《本草》云:主补中下气,消坚软痞,消胸中痰结,吐如胶漆。脐下膀胱留饮。利大肠,通血脉。发汗吐下后,心下痞,噫气不除者,宜此。

仲景治伤寒汗下后,心下痞坚,噫气不除,旋复代赭汤。

胡洽治痰饮,两胁胀满,旋覆花丸,用之尤佳。

Xuanfuhua [旋覆花, inula flower, Flos Inula Japonica]

It is warm in property, and salty and sweet in taste. It can cause cold diarrhea, and it is slightly toxic.

Ben Cao says: It is mainly used to tonify the middle qi and descend qi, soften distention and fullness, and remove the retention of phlegm in the chest with vomiting product like glue. It can treat the fluid retention in the bladder below the umbilicus. It promotes large intestines and circulates vessels. It is advisable to be used in the treatment of the distension and fullness below the rib-side as well as belching which are not cured after sweating, purging and vomitting.

Zhang Zhongjing used Xuanfu Daizhe Decoction to treat the hard epigastric stuffiness and belching uncured after diaphoresis in cold damage. Hu Qia used Xuanfuhua Pill to treat the phlegm-fluid retention, distention and the fullness of both sides of ribs, which has a better effect.

泽 泻

气平,味甘。甘、咸、寒,味厚,阴也,降也,阴中微阳。

入足太阳经、少阴经。

《象》云:除湿之圣药。治小便淋沥,去阴间汗。无此疾,服之令人目盲。

《心》云:去旧水,养新水。寒水气,须用。

《珍》云:渗泻止渴。

《本草》云:治风寒湿痹,乳难,消水,养五脏,益气力,肥健。补虚损五劳,除五脏痞满,起阴气,止泄精,消渴淋沥,逐膀胱三焦停水。

扁鹊云:多服病人眼。

《衍义》云:其功尤长于行水。

仲景云:水畜烦渴,小便不利,或吐或泻,五苓散主之。方用泽泻,故知其用长于行水。《本经》又引扁鹊云:多服病人眼。诚为行去其水故也。仲景八味丸用之者,亦不过接引桂、附等归就肾经,别无他意。凡服泽泻散人,未有不小便多者,小便既多,肾气焉得复实。今人止泄精,多不敢用。

《本经》云:久服明目;扁鹊谓:多服昏目,何也? 易老云:去胞中留垢,以其味咸能泄伏水,故去留垢,即胞中陈积物也。入足太阳、少阴,仲景治太阳中风入里,渴者,五苓散主之。

Zexie [泽泻, oriental waterplantain rhizome, Rhizoma Alismatis]

It is mild in property and sweet in taste. It is sweet and salty in taste, and cold in nature. The flavor is thick, which pertains to yin with descending funtional tendency and slight yang within yin as well.

It enters the meridian of foot-taiyang and shaoyin.

Xiang [《药类法象》, *Rules for the Use of Medicinal Herbs*] says: It is an effective medicinal herb for removing dampness. It has the function in the treatment of dribbling urine, and removing the perspiration at night. People may be blind after taking it without the symptoms mentioned above.

Xin [《用药心法》, *Gist for the Use of Medicinal Herbs*] says: It can discharge the stale water to raise the fresh water. It should be used to remove cold and water retention.

Zhen [《珍珠囊》, *Pounch of Pearls*] says: It can be used to treat diarrhea and relieve thirst.

Ben Cao says: It is mainly used to treat the disease due to wind, cold, the impediment due to dampness and agalactia, eliminate water, nourish the five zang-organs, increase energy and strengthen the body. It can also treat consumptive diseases, remove the distention and fullness in the five zang-organs, raise yin qi, stop seminal emission, treat diabetes and dribbling urination. Besides, it is used to expel the water retention in the bladder and the triple energizers.

Bian Que said: Patients may suffer from eye diseases if taking it too much.

Yan Yi [《衍义》, *Extension of the Materia Medica*] says: It is effective in regulating the water passge.

Zhang Zhongjing said: When the patient feels vexation and thirst and has the syndromes such as dysuria, vomiting, diarrhoea, Wuling Powder may be adopted to treat them. Zexie [泽泻, oriental waterplantain rhizome, Rhizoma Alismatis] is used in the prescription for its effect at the regulation of water passage. *Ben Jing* [《本经》, *Agriculture God's Canon of Materia Medica*] quoted Bian Que's words: The patient will suffer from eye diseases if taking it too much, which is the result of its function in the regulation of water passage. In Zhang Zhongjing's Bawei Pill, Zexie [泽泻, oriental waterplantain rhizome, Rhizoma Alismatis] is used to guide Gui [桂, cassia twig, Ramulus Cinnamomi], Fu [附, aconite, Aconiti Radix Lateralis Praeparata] and other herbs to enter the kidney meridian. People who take Zexie Powder will urinate more, which may damage the kidney qi. Presently, it is used to stop seminal emission but should not be used excessively.

Ben Jing [《神农本草经》, *Agriculture God's Canon of Materia Medica*] says: The long-term taking of it will improve vision. However, Bian Que said: It may cause blurred vision if taking too much. Why do they have different views about it? Yi Lao [Zhang Yuansu] said: It can remove the retention in the uterus because it can purge water retention with its saltiness. The retention in the uterus is actually substance accumulated in it. It enters the meridians of foot-taiyang and shaoyin. Zhang Zhongjing used Wuling Powder to treat the wind-stroke syndrome of taiyang meridian and diabetes.

红豆蔻

气温,味辛。无毒。

《本草》云:主肠虚水泻,心腹绞痛,霍乱,呕吐酸水。解酒毒。不宜多,令人舌粗不能饮食。

《液》云:是高良姜子,用红豆蔻复用良姜,如用官桂复用桂花同意。

Hongdoukou [红豆蔻, galanga galangal fruit, Fructus Alpiniae Galangae]

It is warm in property and pungent in taste. It is nontoxic.

Ben Cao says: It is mainly used to treat the intestinal asthenia and watery diarrhea, heart and abdominal colic, cholera, and acid regurgitation and vomiting. It can also be used to dispel the effects of alcohol. Excessive taking of it may cause bulky tongue hindering food intake, which ought to be avoided.

Ye [《汤液本草》, *Materia Medica for Decoctions*] says: It is the seed of Gaoliangjiang [高良姜, lesser galangal rhizome, Rhizoma Alpiniae Officinarum]. That Hongdoukou [红豆蔻, galanga galangal fruit, Fructus Alpiniae Galangae] is used repeatedly together with Liangjiang [良姜, lesser galangal rhizome, Rhizoma Alpiniae Officinarum] is the same as the Guangui [官桂, Cassia Cortex Cinnamomi] is used repeatedly with Guihua [桂花, murraya jasminorage, Folium et Cacumen Murrayae].

肉豆蔻

气温,味辛。无毒。

入手阳明经。

《本草》云:主鬼气,温中,治积冷心腹胀痛,霍乱中恶,冷痃呕沫,冷气,消食止泄,小儿伤乳霍乱。

Roudoukou [肉豆蔻, nutmeg, Semen Myristicae]

It is warm in property, pungent in taste and nontoxic.

It enters the meridian of hand-yangming.

Ben Cao says: It is mainly used to treat pathogenic factors, warm the middle internal organs, and treat the distending pain due to the accumulated cold in the heart and the abdomen, as well as cholera, noxious pathogen attack, chronic infectious disease caused by cold, vomiting, and diseases caused by cold pathogen, improve digestion, stop diarrhea, and cure the dyspepsia due to improper feeding as well as cholera of infants.

甘　松

气平，味甘温。无毒。

《本草》云：主恶气，卒心腹痛满。治黑皮䵟䵳，风疳齿䘌。

Gansong［甘松，nardostachys root，Radix et Rhizoma Nardostachyos］

It is mild in property, sweet in taste and warm in nature. It is nontoxic.

Ben Cao says: It is mainly used to treat evil qi, heart stroke and abdominal fullness abruptly. It is also used to treat dark skin, black mole, haggard complexion, dental deseases, and ulcerative gingivitis.

蜀　漆

气微温，味辛，纯阳。辛平，有毒。

《珍》云：破血。

《心》云：洗去腥，与苦酸同用，导胆。

《本草》云：主疟及咳逆寒热，腹中症坚痞结，积聚邪气，蛊毒鬼疰，疗胸中邪结气，能吐出之。

成无己注云：火邪错逆，加蜀漆之辛以散之。

Shuqi［蜀漆，dichroa，Ramulus et Folium Dichroae］

It is slightly warm in property and pungent in taste, pertaining to pure yang. It is pungent and mild in nature, but toxic.

Zhen［《珍珠囊》，*Pounch of Pearls*］says: It breaks blood stasis.

Xin［《用药心法》，*Gist for the Use of Medicinal Herbs*］says: Its fishy flavor can be deodorized after washing. It is used to guide the gallbladder when prescribed together with herbs bitter and sour in flavor.

Ben Cao says: It is mainly used to treat malaria, cough with dyspnea, cold-heat disease, abdominal lump, conglomeration and accumulation due to evil-qi, the disease caused by worm toxin and strange pathogenic factors like ghost, and cure the qi stagnation in the chest by expiration and vomitting.

According to Cheng Wuji's annotation, Shuqi [蜀漆, dichroa, Ramulus et Folium Dichroae] can be used to disperse the reverse flow of fire pathogen with its pungency.

蒲 黄

气平，味甘。无毒。

《本草》云：主心腹膀胱寒热，利小便，止血，消瘀血。又云：治一切吐、衄、唾、溺、崩、泻、扑、症、带下等血，并皆治之。并疮疖，通月候，堕胎，儿枕急痛，风肿鼻洪，下乳，止泄精血利。如破血消肿则生用，补血止血则炒用。

Puhuang [蒲黄, cattail pollen, Pollen Typhae]

It is mild in property, sweet in taste and nontoxic.

Ben Cao says: It is mainly used to treat the cold-heat in the heart, abdomen and bladder, promote urination, cease bleeding and resolve blood stasis. It is also said to be used to treat the bleeding caused by vomiting, epistaxis, spitting, drowning, flooding, purging, diving, blood stasis and leukorrhea, treat sore and furuncle, regulate menstruation, induce abortion, treat abdominal pain after the delivery of baby, swelling and epistaxis, promote lactation, and cease seminal emission and bleeding. The raw kind can be used to break blood stasis and reduce swelling, The stir-fried kind can be used to replenish blood and cease bleeding.

天门冬

气寒，味微苦。苦而辛，气薄味厚，阴也。甘平，大寒。无毒，阳中之阴。入手太阴经，足少阴经。

《象》云：保肺气，治血热侵肺，上喘气促。加人参、黄芪为主，用之，神效。

《心》云：苦以泄滞血，甘以助元气，及治血妄行，此天门冬之功也。

《本草》云：主诸暴风湿偏痹，强骨髓，杀三虫，去伏尸。保定肺气，去寒热，养肌肤，益气力，利小便，冷而能补。久服延年，多子孙，能行步，益气。入手太阴、足少阴经，荣卫枯涸，湿剂所以润之，二门冬、人参、北五味子、枸杞子，同为生脉之剂。此上焦独取寸口之意。

《日华子》云：贝母为使。镇心，润五脏，益皮肤，悦颜色。补五劳七伤，治肺气并嗽，消痰，及风痹热毒，游风烦闷，吐血。去心用。

Tianmendong [天门冬, asparagus, Radix Asparagi]

It is cold in property and slightly bitter in taste. Being bitter and pungent, with thick property and thin flavor, it pertains to yin. It is sweet, mild and great cold in property. It is nontoxic, pertaining to yin within yang.

It enters the meridian of hand-taiyin and foot-shaoyin.

Xiang [《药类法象》, *Rules for the Use of Medicinal Herbs*] says: It assists the lung qi and treats the invasion of blood heat into the lung, asthma and polypnea. In compatibility, it has a good effect when combined with Renshen [人参, ginseng, Radix Ginseng] and Huangqi [黄芪, milkvetch root, Radix Astragali seu Hedysari].

Xin [《用药心法》, *Gist for the Use of Medicinal Herbs*] says: It can be used to disperse the stagnated blood according to its property of being bitter, and its sweetness assists the original qi and treats hematemesis during menstruation, which is the function of Tianmendong [天门冬, asparagus, Radix Asparagi] for medical purpose.

Ben Cao says: It is mainly used to treat the wind-dampness that causes paralysis, strengthen bones and marrows, kill three kinds of worms and eliminate Fushi, a serious disease caused by overstrain. It can be used to protect and calm the lung qi, remove cold and heat, tonify the skin, replenish qi and energy, and promote urination. It can be used to tonify with its cold. The long-term taking of it will prolong life, help women conceive, benefit walking and replenish qi. It enters the meridian of hand-taiyin, foot-shaoyin and nourishes the nutrient and defensive qi because it is the medicinal herb for moistening. Tianmendong [天门冬, asparagus, Radix Asparagi], Maimendong [麦门冬, radix ophiopogonis, Ophiopogon Japonicus Ker-Gawl], Renshen [人参, ginseng, Radix Ginseng], Bei Wuweizi [北五味子, Chinese Magnolcavine FruitSchizandra sinensis Baill., Schisandra Chinensis] and Gouqizi [枸杞子, lycium, Lycii Fructus] are of similar herbs with the function of activating pulse. This means to take the Cunkou pulse to treat the diseases in the upper energizer.

Ri Hua Zi [《日华子》, *Materia Medica of Ri Hua-Zi*] says: In compatibility, Beimu [贝母, fritillaria (bulb), Bulbus Fritillaria) is its assistance. It is used to calm the heart, moisten the five zang-organs, tonify the skin and make face lustrous. It supplements five consumptions and seven damages, treats the cough caused by lung qi, dissolves phlegm, removes wandering arthritis, heat-pathogen, urticaria, depression and hematemesis. It is used after removing the plumule.

麦门冬

气寒,味微苦甘。微寒,阳中微阴也。无毒。

入手太阴经。

《象》云:治肺中伏火,脉气欲绝。加五味子、人参。三味为生脉之剂,补肺中元气不足。

《珍》云:行经,酒浸、汤浸。去心,治经枯。

《心》云:补心气不足,及治血妄行,补心不足。

《本草》云:主心腹结气,伤中伤饱,胃络脉绝,羸瘦短气。身重目黄,心下支满,虚劳客热,口干燥渴,止呕吐,愈痿蹶,强阴益精,消谷调中,保神,定肺气,安五脏,令人肥健,美颜色,有子。地黄、车前子为之使,恶款冬花、苦瓠。畏苦参、青蘘。入手太阴。

《衍义》云:治肺热之功为多,其味苦,但专泄而不专收,寒多人禁服。治心肺虚热及虚劳。麦门冬、地黄、麻仁、阿胶,润经益血,复脉通心。二门冬、五味子、枸杞子,同为生脉之剂。

Maimendong [麦门冬, radix ophiopogonis, Ophiopogon Japonicus Ker-Gawl]

It is cold in property, slightly bitter and sweet in taste. Its light coldness pertains to slight yin within yang and it is nontoxic.

It enters the meridian of hand-taiyin.

Xiang [《药类法象》, *Rules for the Use of Medicinal Herbs*] says: It is used to treat the latent fire in the lung, and the weak pulse in extremis. When used together with Wuweizi [五味子, Chinese magnoliavine fruit, Fructus Schisandrae Chinensis] and Renshen [人参, ginseng, Radix Ginseng] to make a prescription, it can supplement the insufficiency of the original qi in the lung. The reason is that the three herbs can activate pulse.

Zhen [《珍珠囊》, *Pounch of Pearls*] says: It can be used to guide herbs to circulate in the meridians after its being soaked in liquor and decoction, and can be used for treating amenorrhea after removing the plumule.

Xin [《用药心法》, *Gist for the Use of Medicinal Herbs*] says: It replenishes the insufficiency of heart qi and treats the irregular menstruation, and supplements the insufficiency of heart.

Ben Cao says: It is mainly used to treat the disorders of the heart and abdomen, the damage caused by the qi stagnation, the exhaustion of the collaterals of the stomach meridian, emaciation and shortness of breath. It is used to treat the heavy sensation in the body and yellow eyes, the fullness of the inferior cardiac branch, the consumptive disease caused by invading fever, the vexation and thirst, stop vomiting, treat crural paralysis, invigorate yin to tonify essence, benefit the rapid digestion of food and the regulation of the middle energizer, nourish the spirit, stabilize the lung qi, comfort the five zang-organs, strengthen the body, benefit complexion, and make women pregnant. In compatibility, Dihuang [地黄, unprocessed rehmannia root, Rehmannia glutinosa Libosch. ex Fisch. et Mey.] and Cheqianzi [车前子, plantain seed, Semen Plantaginis] serve as its assistant herbs. It is averse to Kuandonghua [款冬花, common coltsfoot flower, Flos Farfarae] and Kuhu [苦瓠, leaf of bottle gourd, Folium Lagenariae Sicerariae], restrained by Kushen [苦参, light yellow sophora root, Radix Sophorae Flavescentis] and Qingxiang [青葙, flower of Qingxiang, Flos Qingxiang]. It enters the meridian of hand-taiyin.

Yan Yi [《衍义》, *Extension of the Materia Medica*] says: It treats the lung heat because of its bitter flavor, and it is specially used to purge rather than astringe. Patients with cold physique are forbidden to take it too much. It is used to treat the deficiency-heat of the heart and lung and consumptive diseases. Maimendong [麦门冬, radix ophiopogonis, Ophiopogon japonicus Ker-Gawl], Dihuang [地黄, unprocessed rehmannia root, Rehmannia glutinosa Libosch. ex Fisch. et Mey.], Maren [麻仁, hemp seeds, Cannabis Sativa L.] and Ejiao [阿胶, ass hide glue, Colla Corii Asini] are used together to tonify the meridian and blood, restore the pulse and regulate the heart. Tianmendong [天门冬, asparagus, Radix Asparagi], Maimendong [麦门冬, radix ophiopogonis, Ophiopogon japonicus Ker-Gawl], Wuweizi [五味子, Chinese magnoliavine fruit, Fructus Schisandrae Chinensis] and Gouqizi [枸杞子, barbary wolfberry fruit, Fructus Lycii] are medicinal herbs to activate the pulse.

葳 蕤

气平,味甘。无毒。

《本草》云:主中风暴热,不能动摇,跌筋结肉诸不足,心腹结气,虚热湿毒,腰痛,茎中寒及目痛、眦烂、泪出。久服,去面黑䵟。

《心》云:润肺除热。

Weirui [葳蕤, stem of October clematis, Caulis Clematidis Apiifoliae]

It is mild in property and sweet in flavor. It is nontoxic.

Ben Cao says: It is mainly used to treat the wind attack with sudden high fever, the inability to move, convulsion and the tension of the sinews and muscles, various syndromes of deficiency, the qi stagnation in the heart and abdomen, deficient-heat and damp pathogen, lumbago, cold in penis, eye pain, canthitis and lacrimation. The long-term taking of it can remove blank moles.

Xin [《用药心法》, *Gist for the Use of Medicinal Herbs*] says: It can tonify the lung and eliminate heat.

茵 陈 蒿

气微寒,味苦、平,阴中微阳。无毒。

入足太阳经。

《象》云:除烦热,主风湿热邪结于内。去枝梗,用叶。

《本草》云:主风湿寒热,邪气热结,黄疸,通身发黄,小便不利,除头热,去伏瘕。入足太阳。

仲景茵陈栀子大黄汤,治湿热也。栀子柏皮汤,治燥热也。如苗涝则湿黄,苗旱则燥黄,湿则泻之,燥则润之可也。此二药治阳黄也。韩祗和、李思训治阴黄,茵陈附子汤,大抵以茵陈为君,佐以大黄、附子,各随其寒热也。

《珍》云:治伤寒发黄。

Yinchenhao [茵陈蒿, capillaries, Herba Artemisiae Scopariae]

It is slightly cold, bitter and bland in flavor, pertaining to slight yang within yin. It is nontoxic.

It enters the meridians of foot-taiyang.

Xiang [《药类法象》, *Rules for the Use of Medicinal Herbs*] says: It removes dysphoria and treats wind dampness and heat pathogen in the interior. Get rid of its twig and peduncle, and use its leaves.

Ben Cao says: It is mainly used to treat the diseases caused by the pathogenic wind, dampness, cold, heat, the heat accumulation due to pathogenic qi, yellowish body due to jaundice, and difficult urination. It eliminates fever and mass in the large intestine. It enters the meridian of foot-taiyang.

Zhang Zhongjing used Yinchen Zhizi Dahuan Decoction to treat damp heat and Zhizi Baipi Decoction to treat dryness-heat. If the seedlings are waterlogged, they pertain to damp yellow; if the seedlings are droughty, they pertain to dryness yellow. Purge it if there is dampness and moisten it if there is dryness. The two herbs can be used in the treatment of yang jaundice. Han Zhihe and Li Sixun used Yinchen Fuzi Decoction to treat yin jaundice, in which Yinchen [茵陈, virgate wormwood herb, Herba Artemisiae Scopariae] is used as the sovereign medicinal herb, Dahuang [大黄, rhubarb root and rhizome, Radix et Rhizoma Rhei], and Fuzi [附子, aconite, Radix Aconiti Praeparata] as the assistant herbs according to their cold and heat property.

Zhen [《珍珠囊》, *Pouch of Pearls*] says: It treats cold damage and yellowish syndrome.

艾　叶

气温,味苦,阴中之阳。无毒。

《本草》云:止下痢吐血,下部䘌疮,辟风寒,令人有子。灸百病。重午日,日未出时,不语采。

《心》云:温胃。

Aiye [艾叶, argy wormwood leaf, Folium Artemisiae Argyi]

It is warm in property and bitter in taste, pertaining to yang within yin. It is nontoxic.

Ben Cao says: It can cease dysentery and blood vomiting and the sting sore in the lower part, prevent the pathogenic wind-cold syndrome, and make women conceive. It can be used to treat all kinds of diseases by moxibustion. On May 5th in the lunar calender, it is picked silently before the sun rises.

Xin [《用药心法》, *Gist for the Use of Medicinal Herbs*] says: It can warm the stomach.

白头翁

气寒,味辛、苦,无毒。有毒。

《本草》云:主温疟狂易(音羊)、寒热,症瘕,积聚,瘿气,逐血止痛,疗金疮鼻衄。

《心》云:下焦肾虚,纯苦以坚之。一名野丈人,一名胡王使者。

Baitouweng [白头翁, Chinese pulsatilla root, Radix Pulsatillae]

It is cold in property, and pungent and bitter in taste. It is nontoxic. But it is toxic if not processed properly.

Ben Cao says: It is mainly used to treat warm malaria, mania, cold-heat disease, abdominal conglomeration, accumulation and aggregation and goiter, expel blood stasis, relieve pain, and cure incised wound and nasal hemorrhage.

Xin [《用药心法》, *Gist for the Use of Medicinal Herbs*] says: It can be used to treat the deficiency of the lower energizer and the kidney by its bitterness. It is also called Yezhangren (野丈人) and Huwang Shizhe (胡王使者) in Chinese.

百 合

气平,味甘。无毒。

《本草》云:主邪气腹胀心痛,利大小便,补中益气,除浮肿胪胀,痞满寒热,遍身疼痛,及乳难喉痹,止涕。

仲景治百合病,百合知母汤、百合滑石代赭石汤,有百合鸡子汤、百合地黄汤。或百合病已经汗者,或未经汗下吐者,或病形如初,或病变寒热。并见《活人书》,治伤寒腹中疼,百合一两,炒黄为末。米饮调服。

孙真人云:治百合阴毒,煮百合浓汁,服一升。

Baihe [百合, lily bulb, Lilium Brownii var. Viridulum Baker]

It is mild in property and sweet in flavor. It is nontoxic.

Ben Cao says: It is mainly used to treat the abdominal distension and the heart pain due to evil-qi, promote defecation and urination, tonify the middle internal organs and replenish qi, remove edema and swelling, abdominal distention and fullness, treat cold and heat disease, body pains, difficult lactation and throat impediment, and stop nasal discharge.

Zhang Zhongjing treated lily disease by using Baihe Zhimu Decoction, Baihe Huashi Daizheshi Decoction, Baihe Jizi Decoction and Baihe Dihuang Decoction. They are used to treat lily disease that has been sweated, or not sweated, purged and vomited; or that remains unchanged or transformed into cold-heat disease. These syndromes are recorded in *Huo Ren Shu* [《活人书》, *Book to Safeguard Life*]. The abdominal pain due to cold damage can be cured after taking 1 Liang of Baihe [百合, lily bulb, Lilium brownii var. viridulum Baker], which ought to be fried into powder and mixed with rice porridge.

Sun Zhenren (Sun Simiao) said: The yin toxin of Baihe can be cured after taking 1 Sheng of the Baihe Decoction.

苁 蓉

气温,味甘、咸、酸。无毒。

《本草》云:主五劳七伤,补中,除茎中寒热痛,养五脏,强阴,益精气,多子,妇人症瘕,除膀胱邪气,腰痛,止痢。久服,轻身。

《液》云:命门相火不足,以此补之。

Congrong [苁蓉, desertliving cistanche herb, Herba Cistanches]

It is warm in property, and sweet, salty and sour in taste. It is nontoxic.

Ben Cao says: It is mainly used to treat five kinds of overstrains and seven kinds of damages, tonify the middle energizer, resolve the cold-heat pain in the penis, nourish the five zang-organs, strengthen yin, replenish the essential qi, increase fertility, treat female abdominal mass, remove the pathogenic qi in the bladder, treat lumbago, and stop dysentery. The long-term taking of it will relax the body.

Ye [《汤液本草》, *Materia Medica for Decoctions*] says: It can be used to supplement the insufficiency of ministerial fire in the vital gate.

玄 参

气微寒,味苦、咸。无毒。

《象》云:足少阴肾经之君药也,治本经须用。

《本草》云:主腹中寒热积聚,女子产乳余疾;补肾气,令人目明,主暴中风伤寒身热,肢满、狂邪、忽忽不知人,温疟洒洒,血瘕,下寒血,除胸中气,下水,止烦渴。

易老云:玄参乃枢机之剂,管领诸气,上下肃清而不浊,风药中多用之。故《活人书》治伤寒毒,玄参升麻汤,治汗下吐后毒不散,则知为肃清枢机之剂。以此论之,治空中氤氲之气,无根之火,以玄参为圣药。

Xuanshen [玄参, figwort root, Radix Scrophulariae]

It is slightly cold in property, and bitter and salty in taste. It is nontoxic.

Xiang [《药类法象》, *Rules for the Use of Medicinal Herbs*] says: It is the sovereign medicinal herb for entering the kidney meridian of foot-shaoyin.

Ben Cao says: It is mainly used to treat cold and heat disease, abdominal mass and accumulation and other diseases caused by the lactation of women, replenish the kidney qi, and improve vision. Besides, it is mainly used to treat cold and heat disease due to severe wind strokes, body fever, distension of limbs, manic psychosis, warm malaria and lump due to blood stasis, relieve cold blood, remove the qi stagnation in the chest, promote urination, and cease polydipsia.

Yi Lao (Zhang Yuansu) said: Xuanshen [玄参, figwort root, Radix Scrophulariae] is the chief medicinal herb in charge of all kinds of qi to clear away the turbidity in the upper and lower body and often used in the prescription of treating the wind-syndrome. Therefore, according to *Huo Ren Shu* [《活人书》, *Book to Safeguard Life*], Xuanshen Shengma Decoction is used in the treatment of cold attack to dispel retained cold after sweating and vomiting. So, Xuanshen [玄参, figwort root, Radix Scrophulariae], as a herb to purify and dredge, is regarded as an effective herb to clean up the epidemic pathogen and deficiency fire.

款 冬 花

气温,味甘、辛,纯阳。无毒。

《珍》云:温肺止嗽。

《本草》云:主咳逆上气,善喘,喉痹,诸惊痫寒热邪气,消渴,喘息呼吸。杏仁为之使,得紫菀,良。恶皂荚、硝石、玄参。畏贝母、辛夷、麻黄、黄芪、黄芩、黄连、青葙。

《药性论》云:君。主疗肺气,心促急,热乏,劳咳,连连不绝,涕唾稠粘,肺痿,肺痈吐脓。

《日华子》云:润心肺,益五脏,除烦,补劳劣,消痰止嗽。肺痿吐血,心虚惊悸。

《衍义》云:有人病嗽多日,或教以燃款冬花三两枚,于无风处,以笔管吸其烟,满口则咽之,数日效。

《时习》云:仲景射干汤用之。

Kuandonghua [款冬花, immature flower of common coltsfoot, Flos Farfarae]

It is warm in property, and sweet and pungent in taste, being of pure yang. It is nontoxic.

Zhen [《珍珠囊》, *Pounch of Pearls*] says: It warms the lung and prevents cough.

Ben Cao says: It is mainly used to treat cough due to the counter-flow of qi, frequent panting, throat impediment, various epilepsy, cold-heat disease caused by evil-qi, consumptive-thirst, gasp and respiration. In compatibility, Xingren [杏仁, bitter apricot seed, Semen Armeniacae Amarum] serves as its assistancse, and when used with Ziwan [紫菀, tatariam root, Radix Asteris], it has a better curing effect. It is averse to Zaojia [皂荚, Chinese honey locust, Gleditsia sinensis Lam.], Xiaoshi [硝石, niter, Sal Nitri] and Xuanshen [玄参, figwort root, Radix Scrophulariae] and restrained by Beimu [贝母, fritillaria, Bulbus Fritillariae Thunbergii], Xinyi [辛夷, immature flower of biond magnolia, immature flower of yulan magnolia], Mahuang [麻黄, ephedra, Herba Ephedrae], Huangqi [黄芪, milkvetch root, Radix Astragali seu Hedysari], Huangqin [黄芩, baical skullcap root, Radix Scutellariae], Huanglian [黄连, golden thread, Rhizoma Coptidis] and Qingxiangzi [青葙子, seed of feather cockscomb, Semen Celosiae].

Yao Xing Lun [《药性论》, *Treatise on Medicinal Properties*] says: It is used as the sovereign medicinal herb. It is mainly used to treat lung qi, epigastric stuffiness, fatigue due to heat, cough due to overstrain, thick snot and phlegm, atrophic lung disease, pulmonary abscess and pyemesis.

Ri Hua Zi [《日华子》, *Materia Medica of Ri Hua-Zi*] says: It nourishes the heart and lung, replenishes the five zang-organs, eliminates dysphoria, supplements consumptive diseases, removes phlegm and cough, hematemesis caused by the atrophic lung disease as well as the fright palpitation due to the deficiency of heart.

Yan Yi [《衍义》, *Extension of the Materia Medica*] says: The person who has cough for several days can ignite two or three flowers of Kuandonghua [款冬花, immature flower of common coltsfoot, Flos Farfarae] in the place without wind, and then inhale smog through the pen tube, swallow it when it fills the mouth, and the syndrome will disappear several days later.

According to *Shi Xi* [《时习》, *Constant Practice*], Zhang Zhongjing used it in Shegan Decoction.

紫 参

气微寒,味苦、辛。无毒。

《本草》云:主心腹积聚,寒热邪气,通九窍,利大小便。疗肠胃大热,唾血衄血,肠中聚血,痈肿诸疮,止渴益精。

仲景治痢,紫参汤主之。紫参半斤,甘草二两,水五升,煎紫参取二升。却内甘草,煎取半升,分温三服。

Zishen [紫参, Chinese sage herb, Herba Salviae Chinesnsis]

It is slightly cold in property, bitter and pungent in taste and nontoxic.

Ben Cao says: It is mainly used to treat the disease marked by the accumulation of pathogenic factors as well as cold-heat and evil-qi, free the nine orifices and promote urination and defecation. It is used to treat the severe heat in the intestines and the stomach, blood vomiting, nosebleed, blood stasis in the intestines, carbuncle, ulcer and scabies, and cease thirst and replenish the essence.

Zhang Zhongjing mainly used Zishen Decoction to treat diarrhea. Half Jin of Zishen [紫参, Chinese Sage Herb, Herba Salviae Chinesnsis], two Liang of Gancao [甘草, liquorice root, Glycyrrhiza uralensis Fisch.] and five Sheng of water are decocted together until two Sheng of the decoction are prepared. Then add Gancao [甘草, liquorice root, Glycyrrhiza uralensis Fisch.] to continue decocting until half a Sheng is left. Take it three times each day while it is warm.

苦 参

气寒,味苦,气沉,纯阴。

《心》云:除湿。

《本草》云:主心腹结气,症瘕积聚,黄疸,溺有余沥,逐水,除痈肿,补中,明目止泪。养肝胆气,安五脏,定志益精,利九窍,除伏热肠澼,止渴醒酒,小便黄赤,疗恶疮;下部䘌,平胃气,令人嗜食、轻身。

《衍义》云:有人病遍身风热细疹,痒痛不可任,连胸颈脐腹近阴处皆然,涎痰亦多,夜不得睡。以苦参末一两,皂角二两,水一升,揉滤取汁,银、石器熬成膏,和苦参末为丸,如梧桐子大,食后温水下二十丸至三十丸。次日便愈。

《时习》云:苦参揩齿,久能病腰。

Kushen [苦参, flavescent sophora, Radix Sophorae Flavescentis]

It is cold in property, bitter in taste and heavy in property, pertaining to pure yin.

Xin [《用药心法》, *Gist for the Use of Medicinal Herbs*] says: It is used to remove dampness.

Ben Cao says: It is mainly used to treat the qi stagnation in the heart and abdomen, abdominal mass and the accumulation due to pathogenic factors, jaundice and dribbling after urination. It is also used to expel water, eliminate carbuncle and swelling, tonify the middle internal organs, improve vision and stop tearing. Besides, it is mainly used to nourish the liver and gallbladder qi, comfort the five-zang organs, stabilize the mind and tonify the essence, disinhibit the nine orifices, clear away latent heat and intestinal afflux, stop thirst, and dispel the effects of alcohol and deep-colored urine. It is used to cure the obstinate sore syndrome with dampness-heat in the lower body, calm the stomach qi, make people have a liking for food, and relax the body.

Yan Yi [《衍义》, *Extension of the Materia Medica*] says: It can be used to treat rubella due to wind-heat, with unbearable itching pain and scattered in the chest, neck, umbilicus, abdomen, and the pubes. The patient with such kind of disease suffers from excessive saliva, phlegm and sleeplessness. Prepare 1 Liang of the powder of Kushen [苦参, flavescent sophora, Radix Sophorae Flavescentis], 2 Liang of Zaojiao [皂角, gleditsia, Gleditsiae Fructus], 1 Sheng of water, knead and leach them, stew into paste in the silver or stone utensil, and mix it with powder of Kushen [苦参, flavescent sophora, Radix Sophorae Flavescentis] to make pills as big as Wutongzi [梧桐子, firmiana seed, Firmianae Semen] in size. Take twenty to thirty pills with warm water after dinner, and then the patient will recover the next day.

Shi Xi [《时习》, *Constant Practice*] says: Kushen [苦参, flavescent sophora, Radix Sophorae Flavescentis] can be used to treat dental caries, but the long-term taking of it will cause damage to the waist.

芦　根

气寒，味甘。

《本草》云：主消渴客热，止小便。《金匮玉函》治五噎膈气烦闷，吐逆不下食，芦根五两，锉，水三盏，煮一盏，去渣，服无时。

Lugen [芦根, reed rhizome, Rhizoma Phragmitis]

It is cold in property and sweet in taste.

Ben Cao says: It is mainly used to treat diabetes and acute catarrhal conjunctivitis, and cease urination. According to *Jin Gui Yu Han* [《金匮玉函》, *Annotations on Synopsis of Jade Book of Golden Chamber*], it can be used to treat five kinds of chokes, dysphagia, inability to digest food due to vomiting. Take five Liang of Lugen [芦根, reed rhizome, Rhizoma Phragmitis], file them, decoct them with three cups of water, and concentrate it into one cup, remove the slag, and take it at no definite time.

射 干（又名乌扇）

气平,味苦,微温,有毒。

《本草》云:主咳逆上气,喉闭咽痛,不得消息,散结气,腹中邪逆,食饮大热。疗老血在心脾间,咳唾,言语气臭,散胸中热气。

《衍义》云:治肺气喉痹为佳。

仲景治咽中动气或闭塞,乌扇汤中用。

《时习》云:仲景射干汤用之。

《心》云:去胃痈。

Shegan (also named Wushan) [射干, blackberry lily rhizome, Rhizoma Belamcandae]

It is mild in property and bitter in flavor. It is slightly warm and toxic.

Ben Cao says: It is mainly used to treat cough and dyspnea due to the counter-flow of qi, impediment and the pain of the throat and the inability to breathe, and disperse the qi stagnation, the retention of evil in the abdomen and the severe heat caused by inappropriate diet. It is used to treat the stale blood between the heart and the spleen, cough and phlegm, foul smell while talking and dissipate the heat qi of the chest.

Yan Yi [《衍义》, *Extension of the Materia Medica*] says: It is quite effective to treat the lung qi and pharyngitis.

Zhang Zhongjing used Wushan Decoction to treat the pathogenic qi and the blocking sensation in the throat.

Shi Xi [《时习》, *Constant Practice*] says: Zhang Zhongjing used it in

Shegan Decoction.

Xin [《用药心法》, *Gist for the Use of Medicinal Herbs*] says: It is used to remove stomach carbuncle.

败　酱

气微寒平,味苦、咸。无毒。

入足少阴经,手厥阴经。

《本草》云:主暴热火疮,赤气,疥瘙疽痔,马鞍热气。除痈肿,浮肿结热,风痹不足,产后疾痛。

仲景治肠痈有脓者,薏苡仁附子败酱汤。薏苡仁二十分,附子二分,败酱五分。三物为末。取方寸匕,以水二升,煎取一升,顿服之。小便当下,愈。

Baijiang [败酱, patrinia, Herba Patriniae]

It is slightly cold and mild in property, bitter and salty in flavor, and nontoxic.

It enters the meridians of foot-shaoyin and hand-jueyin.

Ben Cao says: It is mainly used to treat fever blister caused by sudden heat, heat pathogen, scabies, itching, jaundice, hemorrhoids and heat pathogen due to sitting on the saddle. It can remove abscess, dropsy, heat binding, wandering arthritis due to insufficiency, as well as postartum pain.

Zhang Zhongjing used Yiyiren Fuzi Baijiang Decoction to treat the patient suffering from intestinal carbuncle with pus. Grind 20 Fen of Yiyiren [薏苡仁, coix seed, Semen Coicis], 2 Fen of Fuzi [附子, aconite, Radix Aconiti Praeparata] and 5 Fen of Baijiang [败酱, patrinia, Herba Patriniae] into powder, put them in the square-inch-spoon, and add two Sheng of water to decoct them and concentrate it into one Sheng. The patient would recover when urinating after taking it at a draught.

败　蒲

气平。

《本草》云:主筋溢恶疮。

《药性论》云：亦可单用，主破血。取蒲黄、赤芍药、当归、大黄、朴硝同服，治跌扑瘀血。

陈藏器云：《圣惠方》治霍乱。

Baipu [败蒲, cattail, Typha Angustifolia]

It is mild in property.

Ben Cao says: It is mainly used to treat sinew injury and severe sores.

Yao Xing Lun [《药性论》, *Treatise on Medicinal Properties*] says: It is mainly used to treat blood stasis when used alone. When used together with Puhuang [蒲黄, cattail pollen, Pollen Typhae], Chishaoyao [赤芍药, peony root, Radix Paeoniae Rubra], Danggui [当归, Chinese angelica, Radix Angelicae Sinensis], Dahuang [大黄, rhubarb root and rhizome, Radix et Rhizoma Rhei] and Puxiao [朴硝, crystallized sodium sulfate, Natrii Sulfas], it can treat the blood stasis caused by falling down.

Chen Zangqi said: It is recorded to treat cholera in *Sheng Hui Fang* [《太平圣惠方》, *The Great Peace Sagacious Benevolence Formula*].

苇叶

《液》云：同芦，差大耳。

Weiye [苇叶, reed, Phragmites Trins.]

Ye [《汤液本草》, *Materia Medica for Decoctions*] says: It is the same as Luwei [芦苇, reed, Phragmites australs (Cav.) Trin. ex Steud], but without big ear-like blades.

防 己

气寒，味大苦、辛。苦，阴也，平。无毒。

通行十二经。

《象》云：治腰以下至足湿热肿盛，脚气；补膀胱，去留热，通行十二经。去皮用。

《本草》云：主风寒，温疟，热气诸痫。除邪，利大小便，疗水肿、风肿；去膀胱热，伤寒寒热邪气，中风，手脚挛急，止泄；散痈肿恶结，诸蜗疥癣虫疮；通腠理，利九窍。

《药性论》云：汉防己，君。又云：木防己，使。畏女菀、卤咸。去血中湿热。

Fangji［防己, root of fourstamen stephania, Radix Stephaniae Tetrandrae］

It is cold in property, and extremely bitter and pungent in taste. Bitterness pertains to yin, and it is mild in property. It is nontoxic.

It dredges the twelve main meridians.

Xiang［《药类法象》, *Rules for the Use of Medicinal Herbs*］says: It can be used to treat the dampness, the heat and swelling in the part from the waist to the foot, and beriberi, supplement the bladder, clear away heat ratention and dredge the twelve main meridians. It is used after peeling.

Ben Cao says: It is mainly used to treat wind-cold disease, warm malaria and epilepsy caused by heat-qi, eliminate pathogenic qi and promote defecation and urination. Besides, it is mainly used to cure edema and swelling due to wind, clear away the bladder heat, treat cold damage and the cold and heat disease due to pathogenic qi, treat stroke, the spasm of hands and feet, and cease dysentery. In addition, it is used to disperse abscess and severe binding, treat severe sore and scabies caused by worms and bugs, regulate interstices, and remove obstruction from the nine orifices.

Yao Xing Lun［《药性论》, *Treatise on Medicinal Properties*］says: In compatiblity, Hanfangji［汉防己, root of fourstamen stephania, Radix Stephaniae Tetrandrae］serves as the monarch herb. It is also said that Mufangji［木防己, root of fourstamen stephania, Radix Stephaniae Tetrandrae］is used as the assistant herb. It is restrained by Nüwan［女菀, common turczaninowia herb, Turczaninowia fastigiata (Fisch.) DC.］and halogen salt. It removes the dampness and heat in the blood.

牵 牛

气寒,味苦。有小毒。黑白二种。

《本草》云:主下气,疗脚满水肿,除风毒,利小便。

海藏云:以气药引之则入气;以大黄引之则入血。

张文懿云:不可耽嗜,脱人元气。余初亦疑此药不可耽嗜,后见人有酒食病痞,多服食药以导其气,及服藏用神芎丸,及犯牵牛等丸。如初服,即快;药过,再食,其病痞依然。依前又服,其痞随药而效,药过后病复至。以至久服,则脱人元气而犹不知悔,戒之!惟当益脾健胃,使元气生,而自能消腐水谷,其法无以加矣。

《心》云:泻元气,去气中湿热。凡饮食劳倦,皆血受病。若以此药泻之,是血病泻气,使气血俱虚损。所伤虽去,泻元气损人,不知也。经所谓:毋盛盛,毋虚虚,毋绝人长命。此之谓也。用者戒之。白者亦同。

罗谦甫云:牵牛,乃泻气之药,试取尝之,便得辛辣之味;久而嚼之,猛烈雄壮,渐渐不绝,非辛而何!续注:味苦寒,果安在哉。又曰:牵牛感南方热火之化所生者也,血热泻气,差误已甚。若病湿盛,湿气不得施化,致大小便不通,则宜用之耳。湿去,其气周流,所谓五脏有邪,更相平也。经所谓一脏未平,以所胜平之。火能平金,而泻肺气者即此也。然仲景治七种湿证,小便不利,无一药犯牵牛者,仲景岂不知牵牛能泻湿利小便?为湿病之根在下焦,是血分中气病,不可用辛辣气药,泻上焦太阴之气故也。仲景尚不轻用如此,世医一概而用之可乎?又曰:牵牛辛烈,泻人元气,比诸辛药尤甚,以辛之雄烈故也。

Qianniu [牵牛, morning glory, Pharbitis nil (L.) Choisy]

It is cold in property, bitter in taste, and slightly toxic. There are two kinds of Qianniu [牵牛, morning glory, Pharbitis nil (L.) Choisy], namely the black kind and the white kind.

Ben Cao says: It is mainly used to descend qi, treat the edema of feet, remove wind-toxin, and promote urination.

Hai Zang (Wang Haogu) said: It enters qi if guided by the qi-regulating medicinal herb, and enters the blood if guided by Dahuang [大黄, rhubarb root and rhizome, Radix et Rhizoma Rhei].

Zhang Wenyi said: It can not be used addictively, or it may cause damage of the original qi. Initially, I also doubted this point. Later on I saw the patient who suffered from the distention and fullness caused by excessive drinking and eating took medicinal herbs to guide qi, such as Shen Xiong Pills, Qianniu Pills. It took effect quickly for the first time. But distention and fullness still remained when its effect disappeared. If the patient still took it, the syndrome would be cured according to its efficacy, but it would be recurred after its efficacy. Therefore, the long-term taking of it would damage the original qi, which seemed unknown to them. This should be kept on alert. It should be treated by replenishing the spleen and the stomach to generate the original qi so that digestion could be promoted. No method would be better than this one.

Xin [《用药心法》, *Gist for the Use of Medicinal Herbs*] says: It is used to purge the original qi and eliminate the dampness and heat of qi. Improper diet and overstrain can lead to blood diseases. If used as the purgative medicinal herb, it may purge the qi of blood disease and cause the deficiency of qi and blood. Although the disease has been removed, the original qi that is purged can also damage people, which is unknown. *Jing* says: Don't make the excessive syndrome more excessive, or the deficient syndrome more deficient. Don't prevent people from prolonging their life. The patient should keep on the alert when he or she used it. The same is true with the white kind.

Luo Qianfu said: Qianniu [牵牛, Morning glory, Pharbitis nil (L.) Choisy] is the medicinal herb for purging and is pungent in taste at first trial. The long-term chewing of it makes people feel vigorous and mighty incessantly. Is it not because of its pungency? It is also recorded that it is bitter in taste and cold in property, but where do people find the corresponding applicatiom? It is also said that Qianniu [牵牛, Morning glory, Pharbitis nil (L.) Choisy] is grown and transformed from the fire-heat of the southern region, and has the function of purging qi of blood heat, which is absolutely wrong. If the disease pertains to the excessive dampness, which can not be removed and lead to constipation and urinary stoppage, it can be used to treat it. When the dampness is removed, and qi is circulating in the whole body, the so-called removal of the pathogenic factors in the five zang-organs is realized. *Jing* said that the disease can be treated by following the restriction relationship between the organs. The fire can restrict the metal, which is used to clear away the lung qi. However, Zhang Zhongjing treated seven kinds of dampness and dysuria without using Qianniu [牵牛, Morning glory, Pharbitis nil (L.) Choisy]. Did Zhang Zhongjing not know that it can be used to purge dampness and promote urination? The reason is that dampness disease lies in the lower energizer, being a disease related to qi and blood, and the pungent medicinal herb can not be used to purge the taiyin qi in the upper energizer. Even Zhang Zhongjing did not dare to use it like this, how could others do so? It is also said that Qianniu [牵牛, morning glory, Pharbitis nil (L.) Choisy] is pungent and strong, which can purge the primordial qi more effectively than other kinds of pungent medicinal herbs. The reason lies in its extreme pungency.

三　棱

气平，味苦，阴中之阳。无毒。

《象》云：治老癖症瘕结块，妇人血脉不调，心腹刺痛。须炮用。

《珍》云：破积气，损真气，虚者勿用。

《液》云：又治气胀，血脉不调，补五劳，通月经，消瘀血。色白，破血中之气。

Sanleng [三棱, common buried rubber, Rhizoma Sparganii]

It is mild in property and bitter in taste, pertaining to yang within yin. Besides, it is nontoxic.

Xiang [《药类法象》, *Rules for the Use of Medicinal Herbs*] says: It treats chronic ailments, pelvic mass and agglomeration, blood disharmony of women and prickling in the chest and abdomen. It ought to be used after processing.

Zhen [《珍珠囊》, *Pounch of Pearls*] says: It is used to treat pneumatosis and may damage the genuine qi. The patients with asthenia are not allowed to use it.

Ye [《汤液本草》, *Materia Medica for Decoctions*] says: It is also used to treat flatulence and blood disease, supplement the five kinds of consumptive diseases, regulate menstruation, and remove blood stasis. The white kind can be used to break blood stasis.

蓬 莪 术

气温,味苦、辛。无毒。

《象》云:治心膈痛,饮食不消,破痃癖气最良。炮用。

《本草》云:治妇人血气,丈夫贲豚;治心腹痛,中恶疰忤鬼气,霍乱冷气,吐酸水,解毒,饮食不消。酒研服。

《液》云:色黑,破气中之血,入气药发诸香。虽为泄剂,亦能益气,故孙用和治气短不能接续,所以大小七香丸、集香丸散,及汤内多用此也。

Peng'eshu [蓬莪术, zedoary, Curcuma Phaeocaulis Valeton]

It is warm in property, bitter and pungent in taste, and nontoxic.

Xiang [《药类法象》, *Rules for the Use of Medicinal Herbs*] says: It is used to treat the diaphragmatic pain of the heart, the indigestion of food, and it is especially effective to eliminate the abdominal mass. It ought to be used after processing.

Ben Cao says: It is used to treat the blood disease of women and the syndrome of Bentun of men. In addition, it is used to treat the pain in the heart and abdomen, noxious pathogen attack, chronic infectious disease, ghost-like pathogen, cholera, cold qi, stop vomiting sour water, detoxify, and treat the indigestion of food. It can be taken after grinding with liquor.

Ye [《汤液本草》, *Materia Medica for Decoctions*] says: It is black in color, breaking the blood stasis of qi. If used together with the herb to treat qi diseases, it can disperse the fragrance. Although used as the purgative medicinal herb, it can replenish qi. Sun Yonghe used it to treat the panting caused by incontinuons breath. Therefore, it is used to make Large and Small Qixiang Pill, Jixiangwan Powder and it is also used in the decoctions.

草 龙 胆

气寒,味大苦,气味俱厚,阴也。无毒。

《珍》云:纯阴,酒浸上行。

《心》云:除下焦之湿及翳膜之湿。

《象》云：治两目赤肿，睛胀，瘀血高起，疼痛不可忍。以柴胡为主，治眼中疾必用之药也。去芦。

Caolongdan [草龙胆, Chinese gentian, Radix Gentianae]

It is cold in property, and extremely bitter in taste. Both its smell and taste are thick, pertaining to yin. It is nontoxic.

Zhen [《珍珠囊》, *Pouch of Pearls*] says: It is of yang property and can be used to guide the medicinal herb to go upward after its soaking in liquor.

Xin [《用药心法》, *Gist for the Use of Medicinal Herbs*] says: It is used to remove the dampness of the lower energizer as well as that of the lens opacity.

Xiang [《药类法象》, *Rules for the Use of Medicinal Herbs*] says: It is used to treat red and swollen eyes, the acute inflammation of orbit with protrusion of eyeballs, static blood as well as racking pains. Chaihu [柴胡, Chinese thorowax root, Radix Bupleuri] is used as the major herb in the treatment of eye diseases. It is used after removing rhizome.

栝 楼 根

气寒，味苦。味厚，阴也。

《本草》云：主消渴，身热，烦满大热，补虚安中，通月水。消肿毒瘀血，及热狂。

《心》云：止渴，行津液。苦寒，与辛酸同用，导肿气。

《珍》云：苦，纯阴。若心中枯渴者，非此不能除。

Gualougen [栝楼根, root of Mongolian snakegourd, Radix Trichosanthis]

It is cold in property and bitter in taste. Its flavor is thick, pertaining to yin.

Ben Cao says: It is mainly used to treat diabetes, fever, vexation and severe heat, supplement deficiency, harmonize the middle energizer, and regulate the menorrhea. It is used to eliminate pyogenic infections and blood stasis as well as manic psychosis due to heat.

Xin [《用药心法》, *Gist for the Use of Medicinal Herbs*] says: It is used to relieve thirst and regulate the body fluid. The cold and bitter herbs can be used with the herbs with pungency and sourness to remove the qi stagnation due to swelling.

Zhen [《珍珠囊》, *Pouch of Pearls*] says: It is bitter in taste, pertaining to pure yin. The consumptive thirst can not be cured without it.

地　榆

气微寒，味甘、酸。苦而酸，气味俱厚，阴也。

《本草》云：主妇人乳产，七伤，带下，月水不止，血崩之疾。除恶血，止疼痛，肠风泄血。

《象》云：治小儿疳痢。性沉寒，入下焦，治热血痢。去芦。

《心》云：去下焦之血。肠风下血及泻痢下血，须用之。

《珍》云：阳中微阴，治下部血。

Diyu [地榆, root of garden burnet, Radix Sanguisorbae]

It is slightly cold in property, and sweet and sour in taste. It is bitter and sour, and both its flavor and property are thick, pertaining to yin.

Ben Cao says: It is mainly used to treat the convulsion and pain of the breast in women, seven kinds of damage (namely, the damage caused by food, anxiety, drinking, sexual activity, hunger, overstrain and meridians), as well as leucorrhea, menorrhea, and bloody dysentery. It is used to eliminate blood stasis, cease the pain and hemafecia due to the intestinal wind.

Xiang [《药类法象》, *Rules for the Use of Medicinal Herbs*] says: It is used to treat the infantile emaciation. It is cold in nature and enters the lower energizer. It is also used to treat the bloody dysentery due to heat pathogen. It is used after removing rhizome.

Xin [《用药心法》, *Gist for the Use of Medicinal Herbs*] says: It is used to purge the blood stasis of the lower energizer. Besides, it should be used in the treatment of hemafecia due to the intestinal wind and diarrhea.

Zhen [《珍珠囊》, *Pouch of Pearls*] says: It is used to treat the vaginal bleeding, pertaining to mild yin within yang.

紫 草

气寒,味苦。无毒。

《本草》云:主心腹邪气,五疸;补中益气,利九窍,通水道;治腹肿胀满。去土,用茸。

Zicao [紫草, arnebia root, Radix Arnebiae seu Lithospermi]

It is cold in property and bitter in taste. It is nontoxic.

Ben Cao says: It is mainly used to treat the disease of the heart and abdomen and five kinds of jaundice, tonify the middle energizer, replenish qi, disinhibit the nine orifices and unobstruct the waterway in the body, and treat the abdominal flatulence. Its pilose part is used as the medicinal herb while the earth of the root should be removed.

茜 根

气寒,味苦,阴中微阳。

《珍》云:去诸死血。

《药性论》云:主治六极伤心肺,吐血、泻血。

《日华子》云:止鼻洪,月经不止。

Qiangen [茜根, root of Indian madder, Radix Rubiae]

It is cold in property and bitter in taste, pertaining to slight yang within yin.

Zhen [《珍珠囊》, *Pouch of Pearls*] says: It removes the blood stasis.

Yao Xing Lun [《药性论》, *Treatise on Medicinal Properties*] says: It is mainly used to treat the damage of the heart and lung due to six kinds of consumptive and asthenic diseases, hematemesis and blood-draining.

Ri Hua Zi [《日华子》, *Materia Medica of Ri Hua-Zi*] says: It is used to stop serious epistaxis sheding and excessive menorrhea.

菊　花

苦而甘、寒。无毒。

《心》云：去翳膜，明目。

《珍》云：养目血。

《药性论》云：使。治身上诸风。

《日华子》云：治四肢游风，利血脉，心烦，胸膈壅闷。

Juhua [菊花, flower of florists chrysanthemum, Flos Chrysanthemi]

It is bitter and sweet in taste. It is cold in property and nontoxic.

Xin [《用药心法》, *Gist for the Use of Medicinal Herbs*] says：It is used to remove cataract and improve vision.

Zhen [《珍珠囊》, *Pouch of Pearls*] says：It is used to tonify eyes and the blood.

Yao Xing Lun [《药性论》, *Treatise on Medicinal Properties*] says：In compatibility, it can be used as the assistant herb to treat the wind-syndrome in the body.

Ri Hua Zi [《日华子》, *Materia Medica of Ri Hua-Zi*] says：It is used to treat the urticaria of limbs, promote blood circulation, and remove the dysphoria and stuffiness in the chest and diaphragm.

葶　苈

气大寒，味苦、辛。无毒。

《本草》云：主癥瘕积聚结气，饮食寒热，破坚逐邪，通利水道，下膀胱水，伏留热气，及皮间邪水上出，面目浮肿，身暴中风，热痱痒，利小便。久服，令人虚。又云：疗肺壅上气咳嗽，定喘促，除胸中痰饮。

《液》云：苦、甜二味，主治同。仲景用苦，余方或有用甜者，或有不言甜、苦者。大抵苦则下泄，甜则少缓。量病虚实用之，不可不审。《本草》虽云治同，甜、苦之味安得不异？榆白皮为之使。恶僵蚕、石龙芮。仲景葶苈大枣泻肺汤用之。

Tingli [葶苈, Semen Lepidii, Semen Descurainiae]

It is extremely cold in property, bitter and pungent in flavor and nontoxic.

Ben Cao says: It is mainly used to treat the abdominal mass, conglomeration and accumulation with qi stagnation and the disease caused by poor diet and invasion of cold-heat, break hardness, expel pathogenic factors and unobstruct the waterway in the body, promote the water of bladder to flow downwards, clear away latent heat and pathogenic water in skins, treat facial edema, sudden stroke, reddish sudamen, and promote urination. The long-term taking of it will make people feeble. It is also said to be used to treat cough and the reversed flow of qi due to lung obstruction and dyspnea, remove the phlegm and retention of fluid in the chest.

Ye [《汤液本草》, *Materia Medica for Decoctions*] says: The two kinds of taste, bitter and sweet, have similar function in the treatment. Zhang Zhongjing used it by its bitterness, and other prescriptions used it either by its sweetness or without mentioning the two tastes. Generally speaking, bitterness can lead to discharge, and sweetness has the function of relieving. They should be used according to the syndrome differentiation of excess-deficiency of disease. Although it is recorded that they have similar function in *Ben Cao*, how could we not distinguish the difference between bitterness and sweetness? In compatibility, Yupi [榆皮, bark of Chinese elm, Cortex Ulmi Parvifoliae] is used as its assistant herb. It is averse to Jiangcan [僵蚕, stiff silkworm, Bombyx Batryticatus] and Shilongrui [石龙芮, poisonous buttercup herb, Ranunculus sceleratus L.]. Zhang Zhongjing used Tingli [葶苈, Semen Lepidii, Semen Descurainiae] in Tingli Dazao Xiefei Decoction to clear away the lung fire.

王不留行

味苦,阳中之阴。甘平。无毒。

《珍》云:下乳,引导用之。

《药性论》云:治风毒,通血脉。

《日华子》云:治游风风疹,妇人月经不匀。

Wangbuliu Xing [王不留行, cowherb seed, Semen Vaccariae]

It is bitter in taste, pertaining to yin within yang. It is sweet and mild in property. It is nontoxic.

Zhen [《珍珠囊》, *Pouch of Pearls*] says: It is used as the guiding medicinal herb for promoting lactation.

Yao Xing Lun [《药性论》, *Treatise on Medicinal Properties*] says: It is used to treat wind syndrome and disinhibit vessels.

Ri Hua Zi [《日华子》, *Materia Medica of Ri Hua-Zi*] says: It is used to treat urticaria and rubella as well as irregular menstruation.

通 草

气平,味甘、辛,阳也。无毒。灯草同。

《象》云:治阴窍不利,行小水,除水肿闭,治五淋。生用。

《珍》云:泻肺,利小便。甘平,以缓阴血。

《日华子》云:明目退热,催生,下胞,下乳。

Tongcao [通草, ricepaperplant pith, Medulla Tetrapanacis]

It is mild in property, and sweet and pungent in taste, pertaining to yang. It is nontoxic. So is Dengcao [灯草, rush, Juncus effusus L.]

Xiang [《药类法象》, *Rules for the Use of Medicinal Herbs*] says: It is used to treat the disorder of vaginal orifice, activate micturition, remove edema, and treat five types of stranguria. It is used raw.

Zhen [《珍珠囊》, *Pouch of Pearls*] says: It is used to clear away lung heat and promote urination. It is sweet and mild in property, which can relieve the yin blood.

Ri Hua Zi [《日华子》, *Materia Medica of Ri Hua-Zi*] says: It is used to improve vision, bring down fever, hasten parturition, expel afrerbirth, and promote lactation.

木 通

气平,味甘。甘而淡,性平,味薄,阳也。无毒。
《象》云:主小便不利,导小肠热。去皮用。
《心》云:通经利窍。
《本草》云:除脾胃寒热,通利九窍血脉关节,令人不忘;散痈肿诸结不消,堕胎,去虫。

Mutong [木通, akebia stem, Caulis Akebiae]

It is mild in property and sweet in taste. It is mild in nature, with sweet and light flavor, pertaining to yang. It is nontoxic.

Xiang [《药类法象》, *Rules for the Use of Medicinal Herbs*] says: It is mainly used to treat dysuria, and remove the heat of small intestines. It is used after peeling.

Xin [《用药心法》, *Gist for the Use of Medicinal Herbs*] says: It is used to dredge collaterals for promoting aperture.

Ben Cao says: It is used to eliminate the cold-heat in the spleen and stomach, disinhibit the nine orifices, blood vessels and joints, and prevent amnesia. Besides, it is used to remove swollen welling-abscess and nodule, induce abortion, and expel parasite.

瞿 麦

气寒,味苦、辛,阳中微阴也。
《象》云:主关格诸癃结,小便不通;治痈肿,排脓,明目去翳,破胎下闭血,逐膀胱邪热。用穗。
《珍》云:利小便,为君主之用。
《本草》云:出刺,决痈肿,明目去翳;破胎堕子,下闭血;养肾气,逐膀胱邪逆;止霍乱,长毛发。

Qumai [瞿麦, lilac pink herb, Herba Dianthi]

It is cold in property, and bitter and pungent in taste, pertaining to slight yang within yin.

Xiang [《药类法象》, *Rules for the Use of Medicinal Herbs*] says: It is mainly used to treat dysuria and the retention of urine, expel abscess and pus, improve vision, and eliminate nebula. It can also lead to premature rupture of membranes, break blood stasis, remove the heat in the bladder. Its spikes are used as the medicinal herb.

Zhen [《珍珠囊》, *Pouch of Pearls*] says: It is mainly used to promote urination as the monarch herb.

Ben Cao says: It is used to withdraw stab, expel abscess, improve vision, and eliminate nebula. It can also lead to premature rupture of membranes, cause abortion and break blood stasis, replenish the kidney qi, expel the pathogenic factors in the bladder, cease cholera, and promote hair growth.

车前子

气寒,味甘、咸。无毒。

《象》云:主气癃闭。利水道,通小便;除湿痹,肝中风热,冲目赤痛。

《本草》云:主气癃。止痛,利水道,通小便,除湿痹,男子伤中,女子淋沥,不欲食,养肺;强阴益精,令人有子;明目,治目热赤痛;轻身耐老。

东垣云:能利小便而不走气,与茯苓同功。

Cheqianzi [车前子, seed of Asiatic plantain, Semen Plantaginis]

It is cold in property, and sweet and salty in taste. It is nontoxic.

Xiang [《药类法象》, *Rules for the Use of Medicinal Herbs*] says: It is mainly used to treat bronchial septum, disinhibit the waterway in the body, promote urination, eliminate dampness impediment, clear away the wind-heat in the liver, and alleviate epidemic red eyes.

Ben Cao says: It is mainly used to treat bronchial septum, relieve pain, disinhibit the waterway in the body, promote urination, and eliminate dampness impediment. It can be used to treat the male patients who suffer from damage of the middle energizer, the female patients who suffer from dribbling urine. It can improve appetite, and nourish the lung. It is also used to strengthen yin and replenish the essence, make people conceive, improve vision, treat epidemic red eyes, relax the body, and prevent aging.

Li Dongyuan said: It is used to promote urination without losing qi and has the same efficacy as that of Fuling [茯苓, Indian bread, Poria].

石 韦

此一条,与本经无一字同,恐别是一物,有误,姑存之。名远墨子、血见愁、鹿经草也。

《时习》云:今一种作青苔帚,名蚁子槐,作血见愁。又隰州鼓角楼上一种,名血见愁,俱能破瘀血。《时习》补:或人言,紫花如旋风草,但花不白。又有一种,花黄,叶似槐,结角如绿豆,俗呼夹竹梅。

《局方本草》:石韦味苦、甘,平,无毒。主劳热邪气,五癃闭不通;利小便水道,止烦下气,通膀胱满,补五劳,安五脏,去恶风,益精气。

《药性论》云:使。治劳及五淋,胞囊结热不通,膀胱热满。

《日华子》云:治淋遗溺。杏仁为之使,得菖蒲,良。生华阴,又有生古瓦屋上者,名瓦韦,用治淋亦佳。

Shiwei [石韦, shearer's pyrrosia leaf, Folium Pyrrosiae]

There are no same words about this herb recorded in Ben Jing [《本经》, Shennong's Classic of Materia Medica]. It might have been referring to something else, and it is kept tentatively though not correctively. It is also named Yuanmozi, Xuejianchou and Lujingcao.

Shi Xi [《时习》, Constant Practice] says: Presently, there is one kind named Yizihuai, which is used as a broom and considered as Xuejianchou [血见愁, mapleleaf goosefoot herb, Teucrium viscidum Bl.]. Another one is also called mapleleaf goosefoot herb, growing in Gujiao Tower, Xi County, with the function of removing blood stasis. It is supplemented in Shi Xi [《时习》, Constant Practice] that it is said that the purple flower is like Xuanfengcao [旋风草, motherwort herb, Herba Leonuri], but its flowers are not white. Another kind has yellow flowers, with leaves like those of Huai [槐, cladrastis, Cladrastis Radix et Fructus], with fruit like the mung beans and is also named Jiazhumei.

According to *Ju Fang Ben Cao* [《局方本草》, *Materia Medica of Bureau Prescription*], Shiwei [石韦, shearer's pyrrosia leaf, Folium Pyrrosiae] is bitter and sweet in taste, mild in property and nontoxic. It is mainly used to treat heat due to overstrain and pathogenic qi and five kinds of dysuria, promote urination and unobstruct the waterway in the body, cease annoyance and descend qi, dredge the fullness of bladder, tonify five kinds of consumptive diseases, harmonize the five zang-organs, remove the pathogenic factors due to wind, and replenish the essential qi.

Yao Xing Lun [《药性论》, *Treatise on Medicinal Properties*] says: It serves as the assistance in compatibility. It is used to treat overstrain and five types of stranguria, cystic stasis due to heat accumulation as well as the fullness of the bladder due to heat.

Ri Hua Zi [《日华子》, *Materia Medica of Ri Hua-Zi*] says: It is used to treat stranguria and enuresis. Xingren [杏仁, bitter apricot seed, Semen Armeniacae Amarum] serves as its assistant herb. When used with Changpu [菖蒲, bulrush, calamus], it proves to be effective. Another herb, named Wawei [瓦韦, thunberg lepisorus herb, Folium Pyrrosiae], grows in Huayin and on the ancient tile roof, and proves effective in the treatment of gonorrhea.

白附子

阳,微温。

《珍》云:主血痹,行药势。

《本草》云:主心痛血痹,面上百病。行药势。

Baifuzi [白附子, giant typhonium rhizome, Rhizoma Typhonii]

It is of yang property, and slightly warm in property.

Zhen [《珍珠囊》, *Pounch of Pearls*] says: It is mainly used to treat the blood impediment and guide other herbs to the diseased area.

Ben Cao says: It is mainly used to treat heartache and impediment due to the stagnation of blood as well as facial diseases. It is used to guide other herbs to the diseased area.

葫芦巴

苦,纯阴。

《珍》云:治元气虚冷,及肾虚冷。

《本草》云:得槐香子、桃仁,治膀胱气甚效。腹胁胀满,面色青黑,此肾虚证也。

Huluba [葫芦巴, fenugreek seed, Semen Trigonellae]

It is of pure yin in property, and bitter in taste.

Zhen [《珍珠囊》, *Pounch of Pearls*] says: It is used to treat the deficiency cold of the original qi and the kidney.

Ben Cao says: It proves to be effective in the treatment of bladder disease with Taoren [桃仁, peach kernel, Persicae Semen] and Huaixiangzi [槐香子, Huaixiangzi medicinal, materia medica medicinal]. Besides, it is used to treat distension and fullness in the abdomen and hypochondrium, and blue and dark complexion, pertaining to the syndrome of kidney deficiency.

马兜铃

苦,阴中微阳,味苦、寒。无毒。

《珍》云:去肺热,安肺气,补肺。

《本草》云:主咳嗽痰结。

《药性论》云:平。能主肺气上急,坐息不得,主咳逆连连不止。

《日华子》云:治痔瘘疮,以药瓶中,烧,熏病处。入药炙用。是土青木香独行根子也。

《圣惠方》:治五种蛊毒。

《图经》云:亦名土青木香。实,主肺病。根,治气、下膈、止刺痛。

Madouling [马兜铃, root of common aucklandia, Fructus Aristolochiae]

It is bitter in taste, pertaining to mild yang within yin. It is cold in property and nontoxic.

Zhen [《珍珠囊》, *Pouch of Pearls*] says: It is used to clear away the lung heat, comfort the lung qi, and supplement the lung.

Ben Cao says: It is mainly used to treat cough and phlegm binding.

Yao Xing Lun [《药性论》, *Treatise on Medicinal Properties*] says: It is mild in property. It is mainly used to treat the counter-flow of lung qi and frequent cough hindering normal sitting and resting.

Ri Hua Zi [《日华子》, *Materia Medica of Ri Hua-Zi*] says: It is used to treat haemorrhoids. Put it in the cup and ignite it, and then fumigate where haemorrhoids are. It can be used as the medicinal herb for moxibustion. It is the seed of Tuqing Muxiang [土青木香, root of common aucklandia, Radix Aucklandiae] and that of Duxinggen [独行根, root of Lepidium, Lepidium L.].

Sheng Hui Fang [《太平圣惠方》, *The Great Peace Sagacious Benevolence Formulary*] says: It is used to treat five kinds of diseases due to the noxious agents produced by various parasites.

Tu Jing [《图经本草》, *Illustrated Classics of Materia Medica*] says: It is also named Tuqing Muxiang. Its fruit is mainly used to treat lung diseases. Its root can be used to treat qi diseases, remove diaphram stasis, and relieve stabbing pain.

白 及

苦、甘，阳中之阴。味辛、苦，平，微寒。无毒。

《珍》云：止肺涩。白蔹治证同。

《本草》云：主痈肿恶疮、败疽伤阴死肌，胃中邪气，贼风鬼击，痱缓不收，白癣疥虫。

《药性论》云：使。治热结不消，主阴下痿，治面上䵟皰。

Baiji [白及, **Common Bletilla Rubber, Rhizoma Bletillae**]

It is bitter and sweet, pertaining to yin within yang. It is pungent and bitter in taste, mild and slightly cold in property and nontoxic.

Zhen [《珍珠囊》, *Pouch of Pearls*] says: It is a lung astringent medicinal herb and treats the same syndrome as Bailian [白蔹, Japanese ampelopsis root,

Radix Ampelopsis].

Ben Cao says: It is mainly used to treat abscess, severe sore, refractory ulcer, genital injury, necrotic muscles, the pathogenic qi in the stomach, the fulminant disease caused by severe pathogenic factors like ghost attack, and the miliaria difficult to resolve. It is used to eliminate tinea alba and sarcoptic mite.

Yao Xing Lun [《药性论》*Treatise on Medicinal Properties*] says: It is used as a guiding medicinal herb. It is mainly used to treat heat accumulation, impotence, dark complexion and the spots on the face.

天 南 星

味苦、辛。有毒。

《珍》云：治同半夏。

陈藏器云：主金疮伤折淤血。取根，捣傅伤处。

《日华子》云：味辛烈。治扑损淤血，主蛇虫咬，傅疥癣毒疮。

Tiannanxing [天南星, **Jackinthepulpit Tuber, Rhizoma Arisaematis**]

It is bitter and pungent in taste, and toxic.

Zhen [《珍珠囊》, *Pouch of Pearls*] says: It can treat the same diseases as Banxia [半夏, pinellia, Rhizoma Pinelliae].

Chen Cangqi said: It is mainly used to treat the trauma caused by metal, fracture and blood stasis. Collect its root, pound and apply it on the wound.

Ri Hua Zi [《日华子本草》, *Materia Medica of Ri Huazi*] says: It is strongly pungent in taste. It treats the damage due to falling, blood stasis, insect bite, furuncle and carbuncle.

郁 金

味辛、苦，纯阴。

《珍》云：凉心。

《局方本草》云：郁金，味辛、苦，寒，无毒。主血损下气，生肌止血，破恶血，血淋，尿血，金疮。

《药性论》云：单用亦可。治妇人宿血结聚，温醋磨服。

《经验方》云：尿血不定，葱白相合，煎服，效。

《本草》云：生蜀者，佳。胡人谓之马术，亦啖马。药用，治胀痛，破血而补。

Yujin［郁金，Turmeric Root Tuber，Radix Curcumae］

It is pungent and bitter in taste, pertaining to yin.

Zhen［《珍珠囊》，*Pouch of Pearls*］says：It is used to cool the heart.

Ju Fang Ben Cao［《局方本草》，*Materia Medica of Prescriptions of the Bureau of Pharmacy*］says：Yujin［郁金，Turmeric Root Tuber，Radix Curcumae］is pungent and bitter in taste, cold in property, and nontoxic. It is mainly used to treat the loss of blood, descend qi, promote granulation, cease bleeding, eliminate blood stasis, and treat blood stranguria, hematuria and the trauma caused by metal.

Yao Xing Lun［《药性论》，*Treatise on Medicinal Properties*］says：It can be used alone. It treats the blood retention and stasis of women. It should be taken with warm vinegars after grinding.

Jing Yan Fang［《经验方》，*Proved Prescriptions*］says：It is effective to treat the occasional hematuria when decocting with scallion stalk.

Ben Cao says：Those growing in Shu (Sichuan Province) are of good quality. The Northern barbarian tribes call it Mazhu and feed the horses with it. When used as medicine, it treats the distending pain and tonifies through eliminating blood stasis.

佛耳草

气热，味酸。

《象》云：治寒嗽及痰，除肺中寒，大升肺气，少用。款冬花为使。过食损目。

Fo'ercao［佛耳草，Longtube Ground Ivy，Glechoma Longituba (Nakai) Kupr.］

It is heat in property and sour in taste.

Xiang［《药类法象》，*Rules for the Use of Medicinal Herbs*］says：It treats the cough caused by cold and phlegm, eliminates the cold in the lung, and effectively raises the lung qi, which should be used in a small dose. Kuandonghua [款冬花, common coltsfoot flower, Flos Farfarae] serves as the guiding medicinal herb of it. The excessive taking of it damages eyes.

蛇 床

味苦、辛、甘,平。无毒。

《本草》云:主妇人阴中肿痛,男子阴痿湿痒,除痹气,利关节,癫痫恶疮,温中下气,令妇人子脏热,男子阴强。久服轻身。好颜色,令人有子。一名蛇粟、蛇米。五月采,阴干。恶牡丹、巴豆、贝母。

Shechuang [蛇床, Common Cnidium Fruit, Fructus Cnidii]

It is bitter, pungent and sweet in taste, and mild in property. It is nontoxic.

Ben Cao says: It is mainly used to treat uterine swelling and pain, impotence, pruritus due to dampness, impediment, joint disorder, epilepsy and severe sores. It can warm the middle energizer and descend qi, thus keeping the uterus of women warm and the sexual potency of men strong. The long-term taking of it can relax the body, luster the complexion and enable people to conceive. It is also called Shesu and Shemi. It can be collected in May and dried in the shade. It is averse to Mudan [牡丹, Moutan, Cortex Moutan Radicis], Badou [巴豆, Croton Fruit, Fructus Crotonis] and Beimu [贝母, Fritillaria, Bulbus Fritillaria].

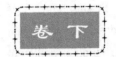

Volume 3

木 部
Tree Herbs

桂（桂心、肉桂、桂枝附）

气热，味甘、苦。有小毒。

入手少阳经。桂枝，入足太阳经。

《本草》云：主温中，利肝肺气，心腹寒热冷疾，霍乱转筋，头痛腰痛，出汗，止烦，止唾，咳嗽鼻齆，能堕胎，坚骨节，通血脉，理疏不足，宣导百药，无所畏。久服，神仙不老。生桂阳，二月、八月、十月采皮，阴干。有菌桂、牡桂、木桂、筒桂、肉桂、板桂、桂心、官桂之类。用者罕有分别。《衍义》所言，不知何缘而得官之名。予考《本草》有出观、宾、宜、韶、钦诸州者，佳。世人以笔画多而懒书之，故只作官也。如写黄檗作黄柏，薑作姜同意。菌桂生交趾山谷，牡桂生南海山谷，木桂生桂阳。从岭至海尽有桂树，惟柳州，象州最多。《本草》所说菌桂、牡桂、板桂，厚薄不同。大抵细薄者为枝、为嫩，厚脂者为肉、为老，处其身者为中也。不必色黄为桂心，但不用皮与里，止用其身中者为桂心。不经水而味薄者，亦名柳桂。易老用此，以治虚人，使不生热也。《衍义》谓桂大热。《素问》谓辛甘发散为阳，故张仲景桂枝汤治伤寒表虚，皆须此药，是专用辛甘之意也。又云：疗寒以热。故知三种之桂，不取菌桂、牡桂者，盖此二种性止温而已，不可以治风寒之病。独有一字桂，《本经》谓辛甘大热，正合《素问》辛甘发散为阳之说，尤知菌桂、牡桂不及也。然《本经》止言桂，而仲景又言桂枝者，盖亦取其枝上皮也，其本身粗厚亦不中用，诸家之说，但各执一己见，终无证据。今又谓之官桂，不知何缘而立名，虑后世以为别物，故于此书之。又有桂心，此则诸桂之心，不若一字桂也。《别说》交广商人所贩者，及医家见用，惟陈藏器之说最是。然菌桂厚实，气味厚重者，宜入治脏及下焦药。轻薄者，宜入治眼目发散药。《本经》

以菌桂养精神，以牡桂利关节。仲景伤寒发汗用桂枝。桂枝者，桂条也，非身干也，取其轻薄而能发散。一种柳桂，乃小嫩枝条也，尤宜入上焦药。仲景汤液用桂枝发表，用肉桂补肾，本乎天者亲上，本乎地者亲下，理之自然，性分之所不可移也。一有差易，为效弥远。岁月既久，习以成弊，宜后世之不及古也。桂心通神，不可言之，至于诸桂数等，皆大小老壮之不同。观，作官也。《本草》所言有小毒，亦从类化。与黄芩、黄连为使，小毒何施；与乌、附为使，止是全得性热；若与有毒者同用，则小毒既去，大毒转甚；与人参、麦门冬、甘草同用，能调中益气，则可久服。可知此药能护荣气而实卫气，则在足太阳经也。桂心，入心，则在手少阴也。若指荣字立说，止是血药，故经言通血脉也。若与巴豆、硇砂、干漆、川山甲、水蛭、虻虫如此有毒之类同用，则小毒化为大毒，其类化可知矣。汤液发汗用桂枝，补肾用肉桂，小柴胡止云加桂何也？《药象》谓肉桂大辛，补下焦热火不足，治沉寒痼冷，及治表虚自汗。春夏二时为禁药。

《珍》云：秋冬治下部腹痛，非桂不能止也。

《心》云：桂枝气味俱轻，故能上行，发散于表；内寒，则肉桂；补阳，则柳桂。桂，辛热散寒经，引导阳气。若正气虚者，以辛润之。散寒邪，治奔豚。

Gui ［桂, Cinnamon bark, Cortex Cinnamomum Cassia］

（also named Guixin, Rougui and Guizhifu）

It is hot in property and sweet and bitter in taste. It is slightly toxic.

It enters the triple energizer meridian of hand-shaoyang. Guizhi ［桂枝, Cinnamon bark, Cortex Cinnamomum Cassia］ enters the bladder meridian of foot-taiyang.

Ben Cao says: It mainly warms the middle, disinhibits liver qi and lung qi, treats the cold-heat disease in the heart and abdomen, cholera cramps, headache and lumbago, promotes sweating, resolves vexation, ceases spittle, stops cough, and frees stuffy nose. It can induce abortion, strengthen the bones and joints, dredge vessels, improve insufficiency, disperse and guide all the medicines without any exception. The long-term taking of it can prolong the lifespan. It grows in Guiyang, and its bark is collected in February, August and October and dried in the shade. There are different kinds such as Jungui, Mugui, Tonggui, Rougui, Bangui, Guixin and Guangui, which are similar in function. *Yan Yi* ［《本草衍义》, *Extension of Materia Medica*］ says that no one knows why it is called

Guangui. The author did the textual research of *Ben Cao* and found that those grow in the states of Guan, Bin, Yi, Shao and Qin are of good quality. People tend to name it as Guangui since it is simple to write. Other examples include 黄檗 [Huangbo, Bark of Amur Corktree, Cortex Phellodendri] written as 黄柏 in Chinese, 薑 [Jiang, Zingiber, Rhizoma Zingiberis] written as 姜 in Chinese. Jungui grows in the valley of Jiaozhi, Mugui in the valley of Nanhai and Mugui in Guiyang. There are many cassia trees distributed from mountains to seasides, most of which are found in the state of Liu and Xiang. Jungui, Mugui and Bangui recorded in *Ben Cao* are different in thickness. Usually the thin ones are from the branches and termed as "tender", while the thick ones are from the barks and termed as "tough". The medium ones are from the trunk. Guixin is one type of Gui with the barks and cores removed and is not necessarily yellow in color. The ones with thin flavor are also called Liugui. Yi Lao (Zhang Yuansu) used it to treat the people with deficiency syndrome without generating heat. *Yan Yi* [《本草衍义》, *Extension of the Materia Medica*] says: Gui is of great heat in nature. *Su Wen* [《素问》, *Plain Conversation*] says: With dispersing function, the pungent and sweet flavor pertains to yang. Thus Zhang Zhongjing's Gui Zhi Decoction treating cold damage and exterior deficiency contains it because of its property of being pungent and sweet. It also says that the cold syndrome can be treated with the medicinal herb of hot nature. Thus it is clear that among the three kinds, Jungui and Mugui with the mild property can not treat wind-cold diseases. Only the Gui, as recorded in *Ben Jing* [《神农本草经》, *Agriculture God's Canon of Materia Medica*], that is pungent, sweet in flavor and extremely hot in hature, corresponds with what is addressed in *Su Wen* [《素问》, *Plain Conversation*] that pungent, sweet flavor and dispersing function pertain to yang, and Jungui or Mugui is inferior to it. *Ben Jing* [《神农本草经》, *Agriculture God's Canon of Materia Medica*] only mentioned Gui, but Zhang Zhongjing mentioned Guizhi, which refers to the bark of the branches instead of the trunk for its being course and tough, and not suitable to use as the medicinal. Different schools hold their own opinions but lack of evidence. Currently it is named as Guangui somehow and I record it here in case the later generations would take it for other things. And there is also Guixin, the core part of Gui, not the same as Gui. *Bie Shuo* [《本草别

说》, Alternative Statements in Materia Medica] says: Among the ones traded by the merchants in the states of Jiao and Guang, and used by the doctors, the statements of Chen Cangqi are the most reasonable ones. As Jungui is thick and strong, with heary and thick property, it is suitable to be used as the medicinal herb for treating zang and lower energizer disorders. The ones that are light and thin are suitable to be used as dispersing medicinal herbs for treating the eye disorders. Ben Jing [《神农本草经》, Agriculture God's Canon of Materia Medica] says: Jungui is used to cultivate spirit and Mugui to disinhibit the joint disorders. Zhang Zhongjing used Guizhi to treat the cold damage by inducing sweating. Guizhi is the branch instead of the trunk, with the light and thin property to disperse. The ones that are called Liugui are twigs, which are especially suitable to treat the disorders of the upper energizer. Zhang Zhongjing often used Guizhi to relieve exterior, and Rougui to tonify the kidney. The property of the two herbs are different according to the rules of the nature, thus their difference can not be ignored in prescription. Otherwise, it may result in wide divergence. As time goes by, people would be accustomed to the improper practice, making the later generations inferior to the ancient people. It is difficult to describe Guixin's function to invigorate the spirit. As to the other kinds of Gui, they all differ in sizes and ages. The Chinese character of 观 (Guan) is used as 官 (Guan). The slight toxicity recorded in Ben Cao is also varied according to different combination. If it is used with Huangqin [黄芩, baical skullcap root, Radix Scutellariae] and Huanglian [黄连, golden thread, Rhizoma Coptidis], it is slightly toxic. If it is combined with Wu [乌, aconite, Aconiti Radix Wutou] and Fu [附, aconite, Aconiti Radix Lateralis Praeparata], it is greatly heat in property. If it is used with toxic ones, the slight toxicity may be counteratal and the heavy toxicity may be increased. If it is used with Renshen [人参, ginseng, Radix Ginseng], Maimendong [麦门冬, radix ophiopogonis, Ophiopogon japonicus Ker-Gawl] and Gancao [甘草, licorice, Radix Glycyrrhea Praeparata], it can regulate the middle and replenish qi, suitable for long-term taking. So the medicinal herb can protect the nutrient qi and consolidate the defense qi, entering the bladder meridian of foot taiyang. Guixin enters the heart and heart meridian of hand shaoyin. It can be regarded as the medicinal herb for promoting blood circulation from the perspective of protecting nutrient qi. Thus *Jing* says it dredges vessels. If it is used with the toxic ones such as Badou [巴豆, Croton Fruit, Fructus Crotonis], Lusha [硇砂, Sal Ammoniac, Sal Ammoniacum], Ganqi [干漆, Dried Lacquer, Resina Toxicodendri], Chuanshanjia [川山甲, Pangolin Scales, Squama Manis], Shuizhi [水蛭, Leech, Hirudo] and Mengchong [虻虫, tabanus, Tabanus], the light toxicity will be transformed into the heavy one. The decoction uses Guizhi to induce sweating and Rougui to tonify the kidney. What is the purpose of adding Gui to Xiaochaihu Decoction? *Yao Xiang* [《药类法象》, *Rules for the Use of Medicinal Herbs*] says: Rougui is strongly pungent, which is used to tonify the insufficiency of heat in the lower energizer, and treat the intractable lingering cold, exterior deficiency and spontaneous sweating. It must be banned to use in spring or summer.

Zhen [《珍珠囊》 *Pouch of Pearls*] says: In autumn and winter, it is only Gui that can stop the pain in the lower abdomen.

Xin [《用药心法》, *Gist for the Use of Medicinal Herbs*] says: Guizhi is light and thin in nature and flavor, thus it can go upward and relieve exterior. Rougui is used to treat the internal cold; Liugui is used to tonify yang. Gui is pungent and hot in nature, dispersing cold and ushering the yang qi. The pungent taste is used to treat the deficiency of healthy qi. It can disperse the pathogenic cold and treat Bentun①.

柏子仁

气平,味甘、辛。无毒。

《本草》云:安主五脏,除风湿痹,益气血。能长生,令人润泽,美颜色,耳目聪明。用之泽润,肾之药也。

《药性论》云:柏子仁,君。恶菊花,畏羊蹄草。能治腰肾中冷,膀胱冷脓宿水;兴阳道,益寿;去头风,治百邪鬼魅,主小儿惊痫。柏子仁,古方十精丸用之。

---

① Ben Tun: name of disease. refering to palpitation underneath the navel similar to a running piglet.

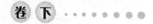

Baiziren［柏子仁, Chinese arborvitae kernel, Semen Platycladi］

It is neutral in property, sweet and pungent in taste, and nontoxic.

Ben Cao says: It is mainly used to treat diseases in the five zang-organs, eliminate the impediment due to wind-dampness, and replenish qi and blood. It can prolong the lifespan, moisten and luster complexion, and improve hearing and eyesight. With the function of moistening, it benefits the kidney.

Yao Xing Lun［《药性论》, *Treatise on Medicinal Properties*］says: Baiziren［柏子仁, Chinese arborvitae kernel, Semen Platycladi］is used as a sovereign medicinal herb. It is averse to Juhua［菊花, chrysanthemums, Dendranthema morifolium Tzvel］and restrained by Yangticao［羊蹄草, emilia, Emiliae Herbacum Radice］. It is used to treat the cold in the waist and the kidney, the pus and fluid retention in the cold bladder, improve the sexual potency, prolong the lifespan, and cure the headache caused by wind pathogen. It mainly treats the pathogenic qi and vicious pathogenic factors like ghost and infantile convulsion. Baiziren［柏子仁, Chinese arborvitae kernel, Semen Platycladi］is used in the ancient prescription called Shijing Pill.

侧 柏 叶

气微温，味苦。无毒。

《本草》云：主吐血、衄血及痢血，崩中赤白。轻身益气，令人耐寒暑。

《药性论》云：侧柏叶苦辛性涩，治冷风历节疼痛，止尿血，与酒相宜。

Cebaiye［侧柏叶, arborvitae leaf, Platycladi Cacumen］

It is slightly warm in property and bitter in taste. It is nontoxic.

Ben Cao says: It mainly treats hematemesis, epistaxis and bloody dysentery, and the metrorrhagia with reddish discharge. It can relax the body, replenish qi and enable people to tolerate cold and summer-heat.

Yao Xing Lun［《药性论》, *Treatise on Medicinal Properties*］says: Cebaiye［侧柏叶, arborvitae leaf, Platycladi Cacumen］is bitter and pungent in taste, and astringent in property. It is used to treat arthralgia due to wind cold and hematuria.

The effectiveness of the medicinal herb can be strengthened when used with liquor.

柏 皮

主火灼烂疮,长毛发。

Baipi［柏皮, arborvitae root bark, Platycladi Radicis Cortex］

It is mainly used to treat the severe sores due to heat, and promote the growth of hair.

槐 实

味苦、酸、咸、寒。无毒。

《珍》云:与桃仁治证同。

《药性论》云:臣。治大热难产。皮煮汁,治淋阴囊坠肿,气瘤。又,槐白皮,治口齿风疳。

《日华子》云:槐子,治丈夫、女人阴疮湿痒;催生,吞七粒。皮,治中风皮肤不仁,喉痹;洗五痔,产门痒痛,及汤火疮。煎膏,止痛,长肉,消痈肿。

Huaishi［槐实, sophora fruit, Sophorae Fructus］

It is bitter, sour and salty in flavor, and cold in nature. It is nontoxic.

Zhen［《珍珠囊》, *Pouch of Pearls*］says: It is used to treat the same syndromes as Taoren［桃仁, peach kernel, Persicae Semen］.

Yao Xing Lun［《药性论》, *Treatise on Medicinal Properties*］says: It is used as a minister medicinal herb. It treats the dystocia due to great heat. The bark is boiled to get liguid which is used to treat stranguria, scrotal swelling and qi tumor. It is also called Huaibaipi［槐白皮, sophora bark Sophorae Cortex（Radicis）］and used to treat the aphtha and ulcerative gingivitis.

Ri Hua Zi［《日华子》, *Materia Medica of Ri Hua-Zi*］says: Huaizi［槐子, sophora fruit, Sophorae Fructus］treats the genital sore and pruritus due to dampness. Taking seven pellets can expedite child delivery. The bark can treat the wind stroke and numbness in the skin, pharyngitis, five kinds of hemorrhoids, itching and pain of the vaginal orifce, and scalds. The soft extract can eliminate pain, promote granulation and dispel abscess.

槐 花

苦,薄阴也。

《珍》云:凉大肠热。

《别录》云:槐花,味苦,无毒。治五痔心痛眼赤,杀腹脏虫及热;治皮肤风,肠风泻血,赤白痢。八月断槐大枝,使生嫩蘖,煮汁酿酒,疗大风痿痹,甚效。槐耳,主五痔心痛,女人阴中疮痛,景天为之使。槐胶,主一切风,化痰。治肝脏风,筋脉抽掣,急风口噤,四肢不收,顽痹或毒风,周身如虫行,或破伤风口眼偏斜,腰膝强硬。槐叶,平,无毒;煎汤,洗小儿惊痫壮热,疥癣丁毒。皮、茎同用,良。

Huaihua [槐花, pagodatree flower, Flos Sophorae]

It is bitter in taste, slight yin in property.

Zhen [《珍珠囊》 *Pouch of Pearls*] says: It can cool the heat in the large intestines.

Bie Lu [《名医别录》, *Miscellaneous Records of Famous Physicians*] says: Huaihua [槐花, pagodatree flower, Flos Sophorae] is bitter in taste and nontoxic. It treats five kinds of hemorrhoids, heart pain and red eye, kills the worms in the abdomen and dispels heat. It treats skin pruritus, bloody stool, and red and white dysentery. Break the thick branches of the tree and let the tender twigs grow in August. Boil it into decoction and make liquor, which can treat wilting and impediment due to the pathogenic wind effectively. Huai'er [槐耳, sophora wood ear, Sophorae Auricularia Auricula] mainly treats five hemorrhoids, the pain in the heart, and the severe sore and pain in the vulva. Jingtian [景天, common stonecrop herb, Herba Hylotelephii Erythrosticti] is used as its guiding medicinal herb. Huaijiao [槐胶, sophora resin, Sophorae Resina] treats all kinds of diseases caused by the pathogenic wind and resolves phlegm. It treats the liver wind, the spasm of sinews, acute wind stroke and lockjaw, flaccidity of the limbs, stubborn impediment and wind toxin sensation of grubs creeping in the skin, or deviated eyes and mouth due to tetanus and the stiffness of the lumbus and knees. Huaiye [槐叶, sophora leaf, Sophorae Folium] is mild in nature and nontoxic. Decocting and bathing in it can treat the infantile malnutrition involving heart, high fever, furuncle scabies and carbuncle. It is effective to use the bark and stalk simultaneously.

蔓荆子

气清,味辛温苦、甘,阳中之阴。太阳经药。

《象》云:治太阳经头痛,头昏闷,除目暗,散风邪药。胃虚人勿服,恐生痰疾。拣净,杵碎用。

《珍》云:凉诸经血,止头痛,主目睛内痛。

《本草》云:恶乌头、石膏。

Manjingzi [蔓荆子, vitex, Viticis Fructus]

It is cold in nature, pungent, bitter and sweet in flavor, pertaining to yin within yang. It enters the taiyang meridian.

Xiang [《药类法象》 *Rules for the Use of Medicinal Herbs*] says: It treats the headache of taiyang meridian, dizziness and heaviness, improves vision and dispels the pathogenic wind. Patients with weak stomach should not take it for it might cause phlegm. Clean it and pound it into pieces befove using.

Zhen [《珍珠囊》 *Pouch of Pearls*] says: It cools the blood in all the channels and stops headache. It mainly treats the pain in eyes.

Ben Cao says: It is averse to Wutou [乌头, aconite, Aconiti Radix Wutou] and Shigao [石膏, gypsum, Gypsum Fibrosum].

大腹子

气微温,味辛。无毒。

《本草》云:主冷热气攻心腹,大肠壅毒,痰膈醋心,并以姜、盐同煎。《时习》谓是气药也。

孙真人云:先酒洗,后大豆汁洗。仲景用。

《日华子》云:下一切气,止霍乱,通大小肠,健脾、开胃、调中。

Dafuzi [大腹子, areca, Arecae Semen]

It is slightly warm in nature and pungent in flavor. It is nontoxic.

Ben Cao says: It mainly treats the disease in the heart and abdomen caused by the cold and heat pathogen, the accumulation of the toxin in the large intestines, the phlegm in the diaphragm and acid regurgitation. It should be decocted with ginger and salt. *Shi Xi* [《时习》, *Constant Practice*] says: It is used as a kind of medicinal treating qi disorders.

Sun Simiao said: Wash it with liquor first and then with the juice of beans. Zhang Zhongjing has used it in his prescription.

Ri Hua Zi [《日华子》, *Materia Medica of Ri Hua-Zi*] says: It descends qi and treats cholera, invigorates the intestines, fortifies the spleen, promotes the appetite and regulates the middle energizer.

酸 枣

气平，味酸。无毒。

《本草》云：主心腹寒热，邪结气聚，四肢酸疼湿痹，烦心不得眠，脐上下痛，血转久泄，虚汗烦渴；补中、益肝气，坚筋骨，助阴气，令人肥健。久服，安五脏、轻身延年。胡洽治振悸不得眠，人参、白术、白茯苓、甘草、生姜、酸枣仁六物煮服。

《圣惠方》：胆虚不眠，寒也。酸枣仁炒香，竹叶汤调服。

《济众方》：胆实多睡，热也。酸枣仁生用，末，茶、姜汁调服。

Suanzao [酸枣, crataegus, Crataegi Fructus]

It is mild in nature and sour in flavor. It is nontoxic.

Ben Cao says: It mainly treats the cold and heat in the heart and abdomen, the accumulation of pathogenic qi, ache limbs and dampness impediment, the insomnia due to heart vexation, the pain around the umbilicus, bloody stools and chronic diarrhea, vacuity sweating, vexation and thirst. It tonifies the middle and boosts the liver qi, strengthens sinews and bones, replenishes yin qi and cultivates health. The long-term taking of it will harmonize the five zang-organs, relax the body and prolong the lifespan. Hu Qia used Renshen [人参, ginseng, Radix Ginseng], Baizhu [白术, largehead atractylodes rhizome, Rhizoma Atractylodis Macrocephalae], Baifuling [白茯苓, white poria, Poria Alba], Gancao [甘草, liquorice root, Glycyrrhiza uralensis Fisch], Shengjiang [生姜, fresh ginger, Rhizoma Zingiberis Recens] and Suanzaoren [酸枣仁, spiny jujube, Ziziphi Spinosi Semen] to treat the insomnia due to fright palpitations.

Shen Hui Fang [《太平圣惠方》, *Taiping Holy Prescriptions for Universal Relief*] says: The insomnia due to gallbladder insufficiency often belongs to cold. It can be treated with stir-frying Suanzaoren and Zhu Ye Decoction.

Ji Zhong Fang [《济众方》, *Prescriptions to Aid the Mass*] says: The somnolence due to gallbladder excess often belongs to heat. Grind Suanzaoren [酸枣仁, spiny jujube, Ziziphi Spinosi Semen] into powder and take it with tea and ginger juice.

胡 椒

气温，味辛。无毒。

《本草》云：主下气、温中、去痰，除脏腑中风冷。向阳者为胡椒，向阴者为荜澄茄。胡椒多服损肺。味辛辣，力大于汉椒。

《衍义》云：去胃中寒痰，吐水，食已即吐，甚验。过剂则走气。大肠寒滑亦用，须各以他药佐之。

Hujiao [胡椒, pepper, Piperis Fructus]

It is warm in nature and pungent in flavor. It is nontoxic.

Ben Cao says: It mainly descends qi, warms the middle, dispels phlegm and eliminates the cold and wind in zang-fu organs. Those growing in the sunshine places are Hujiao [胡椒, pepper, Piperis Fructus] and those growing in the shade are Bichengqie [荜澄茄, cubeb, Litseae Fructus]. The excessive taking of Hujiao [胡椒, pepper, Piperis Fructus] may damage the lung. It is pungent in taste and when used as a medicinal herb, it is more powerful than Hanjiao [汉椒, zanthoxylum, Zanthoxyli Pericarpium].

Yan Yi [《衍义》, *Extension of the Materia Medica*] says: It can eliminate the

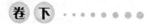

cold phlegm in the stomach, remove water pathogen and promote vomiting right after eating with great effectiveness. The excessive taking of it may dissipate qi. It can also be used to treat the efflux desertion of the large intestines with other medicinal herbs as the assistant.

川　椒

气热温,味大辛。辛温,大热。有毒。

《象》云:主邪气,温中,除寒痹;坚齿发,明目,利五脏。须炒去汗。

《心》云:去汗,辛热,以润心寒。

《本草》云:主邪气逆咳,温中;逐骨节皮肤死肌,寒湿痹痛;下气,除六腑寒冷,伤寒温疟,大风汗不出,心腹留饮,宿食,肠澼下痢,泄精,女子字乳余疾;散风邪瘕结水肿,黄疸,鬼疰蛊毒。耐寒暑,开腠理。闭口者,杀人。恶瓜蒌、防葵。畏雌黄。

Chuanjiao [川椒, zanthoxylum, Zanthoxyli Pericarpium]

It is hot and warm in nature, and strongly pungent in flavor. It is toxic.

Xiang [《药类法象》, *Rules for the Use of Medicinal Herbs*] says: It mainly treats pathogenic qi, warms the middle, and relieves cold impediment, strengthens the teeth and hair, improves eyesight, and harmonizes the five zang-organs. When stir-fried, it can be used to eliminate sweating.

Xin [《用药心法》, *Gist for the Use of Medicinal Herbs*] says: It eliminates sweating. The pungent and hot property can be used to relieve the cold in the heart.

Ben Cao says: It mainly treats the cough with dyspnea due to pathogenic qi, warms the middle, eliminates the necrotic muscles in the bones and skin, the impediment pain due to cold and dampness, lowers qi, eliminates the cold in the six fu-organs, cold damage and warm malaria, absent of sweat due to great wind stroke, water retention in the heart and abdomen, retained food, intestinal afflux and dysentery, prospermia and the diseases caused by breast-feeding, disperses abdominal mass and edema due to wind pathogen, jaundice, disease caused by ghost and monster, parasitic toxin. It enables people to resist cold and summer heat better, and opens striaes and interstices. The ones with no cracks are deadly toxic. It is averse to Gualou [瓜蒌, trichosanthes, Trichosanthis Fructus] and Fangkui [防葵, oreoselinum, Radix Peucedani Praeruptori]. It is restrained by Cihuang [雌黄, orpiment, Auripigmentum].

吴茱萸

气热，味辛、苦，气味俱厚，阳中阴也。辛温大热。有小毒。

入足太阴经、少阴经、厥阴经。

《象》云：食则令人口开目瞪，寒邪所隔，气不得上下。此病不已，令人寒中，腹满膨胀，下利寒气，诸药不可代也。洗去苦味，日干，杵碎用。

《心》云：去胸中逆气。不宜多用，辛热恐损元气。

《珍》云：温中下气，温胃。

《本草》云：主温中下气，止痛，咳逆寒热，除湿血痹，逐风邪，开腠理，去痰冷，腹内绞痛，诸冷实不消，中恶，心腹痛，逆气，利五脏。入足太阴、少阴、厥阴，震坤合见，其色绿。

仲景云：吴茱萸汤、当归四逆汤、大温脾汤及脾胃药，皆用此也。

《衍义》云：此物下气最速，肠虚人服之愈甚。蓼实为之使。恶丹参、硝实、白垩。畏紫石英。

Wuzhuyu [吴茱萸, evodia, Fructus Evodiae]

It is hot in nature, and pungent and bitter in flavor. It is thick in both qi and flavor, pertaining to yin within yang. It is pungent, warm and strongly hot. It is slightly toxic.

It enters the spleen meridian of foot-taiyin, the kidney meridian of foot-shaoyin and the liver meridian of foot-jueyin.

Xiang [《药类法象》, *Rules for the Use of Medicinal Herbs*] says: It can treat the syndrome of food choking with wide-open eyes and the mouth due to qi blockage by cold pathogen. If the disease can not be cured, the patient may suffer from cold stroke, abdominal fullness and distention, diarrhea due to cold. It is of such effectiveness in dispelling the cold qi that no medicinal herbs can replace it. Wash it until it is not bitter anymore, dry it under the sun and pound it for use.

Xin [《用药心法》, *Gist for the Use of Medicinal Herbs*] says: It regulates the counterflow of qi in the chest. The excessive taking of it may damage the original qi due to its pungent and hot property.

Zhen [《珍珠囊》, *Pouch of Pearls*] says: It warms the middle, descends qi and warms the stomach.

Ben Cao says: It is mainly used to warm the middle, descend qi, stop pain, treat cough with dyspnea due to cold and heat, eliminate dampness and blood impediment, expel wind pathogens. It opens striaes and interstices, and disperses cold phlegm. It treats colic in the abdomen, cold excess that is hard to resolve, attack of noxious factor, the pain in the heart and abdomen, the counter-flow of qi, and disinhibits the five zang-organs. It enters the spleen meridian of foot-taiyin, the kidney meridian of foot-shaoyin and the liver meridian of foot-jueyin. It becomes green if the Hexagram Zhen (symbolizing the thunder quake) and the Hexagram Kun (symbolizing the earth) meet with each other.

Zhang Zhongjing said: It is used in Wuzhuyu Decoction, Danggui Sini Decoction, Dawenpi Decoction and other decoctions for the spleen and stomach.

Yan Yi [《衍义》, *Extension of the Materia Medica*] says: It descends qi in short time, especially for the people who are deficient in the intestines. Liaoshi [蓼实, water pepper fruit Polygoni Hydropiperis Fructus] is used as its guiding medicinal herb. It is averse to Danshen [丹参, salvia, Salviae Miltiorrhizae Radix], Xiaoshi [硝石, niter, Nitrum] and Bai'e [白垩, chalk Creta]. It is restrained by Zishiying [紫石英, fluorite, Fluoritum].

山茱萸

气平微温,味酸。无毒。

入足厥阴经、少阴经。

《本草》云:主温中,逐寒湿痹,强阴益精,通九窍,止小便。入足少阴、厥阴。

《圣济经》云:滑则气脱,涩剂所以收之,山茱萸之涩以收其滑。仲景八味丸用为君主,如何涩剂以通九窍。

《雷公》云:用之去核,一斤取肉四两,缓火熬用。能壮元气,秘精。核,能滑精,故去之。

《珍》云：温肝。

《本经》云：止小便利，以其味酸也。观八味丸用为君主，其性味可知矣。

《药性论》亦云：补肾添精。

《日华子》亦云：暖腰膝，助水脏也。

Shanzhuyu [山茱萸, cornus, Fructus Corni]

It is mild and slightly warm in nature and sour in flavor. It is nontoxic.

It enters the liver meridian of foot-jueyin and the kidney meridian of foot-shaoyin.

Ben Cao says: It is mainly used to warm the middle, dispel the impediment due to cold and dampness, improve the sexual potency and replenish essense, free the nine orifices, and stanch urinary incontinence. It enters the kidney meridian of foot-shaoyin and the liver meridian of foot-jueyin.

Sheng Ji Jing [《圣济经》, *Sages' Salvation Classic*] says: The spontaneous seminal emission leads to qi collapse, and the astringent formula is used to astringe it. The astrigency of Shanzhuyu [山茱萸, cornus, Fructus Corni] could astringe the emission. Zhang Zhongjing's Bawei Pill uses it as the sovereign medicinal herb, which is an example of using the astringent formula to free the nine orifices.

Lei Gong [《雷公炮制论》, *Grandfather Lei's Discussion of Herb Preparation*] says: Remove the kernel before using. Take four Liang of the flesh from one Jin, and decoct it with mild fire. It can be used to strengthen the original qi and secure the semen. The kernel should be removed since it can lead to the spontaneous seminal emission.

Zhen [《珍珠囊》, *Pouch of Pearls*] says: It warms the liver.

Ben Jing [《神农本草经》, *Agriculture God's Canon of Materia Medica*] says: It stanches the urinary incontinence for its sour flavor. Since it is used as the sovereign medicinal herb in Bawei Pill, the property could be figured out.

Yao Xing Lun [《药性论》 *Treatise on Medicinal Properties*] also says: It tonifies the kidney and boosts the production of semen.

Ri Hua Zi [《日华子》, *Materia Medica of Ri Hua-Zi*] says: It warms the lumbus and knees, and benefits the water zang-organ.

益 智

气热,味大辛。辛温。无毒。

主君相二火。手足太阴经,足少阴经,本是脾经药。

《象》云:治脾胃中受寒邪,和中益气,治多唾,当于补中药内兼用之,勿多服。去皮用。

《本草》云:主遗精虚漏,小便遗沥,益气安神。补不足,安三焦,调诸气。夜多小便者,取二十四枚。碎之。入盐同煎服,有神效。

《液》云:主君相二火,手、足太阴,足少阴,本是脾药。在集香丸,则入肺;在四君子汤,则入脾;在大凤髓丹,则入肾。脾、肺、肾,互有子母相关。

Yizhi [益智, sharp-leaf glangal fruit, Fructus Alpiniae Oxyphyllae]

It is hot in nature and highly pungent in flavor. It is pungent and warm, and nontoxic.

It governs the sovereign and ministerial fire. It enters the lung meridian of hand-taiyin, the spleen meridian of foot-taiyin and the kidney meridian of foot-shaoyin. It mainly acts on the spleen meridian.

Xiang [《药类法象》, *Rules for the Use of Medicinal Herbs*] says: It treats the coldness in the spleen and stomach, harmonizes the middle and replenishes qi. When treating ptyalism, it should be used together with other medicinal herbs which supplement the middle, and should not be taken excessively. The coat should be removed before using.

Ben Cao says: It mainly treats spontaneous seminal emission and dribbling urination, replenishes qi and tranguilizs the mind. It supplements insufficiency, calms the triple energizer and regulates all kinds of qi. When treating nocturia, pound twenty-four pieces of Yizhi and decoct with salt, it will take magical effect.

Ye [《汤液本草》, *Materia Medica for Decoctions*] says: It governs the sovereign and ministerial fire. It enters the lung meridian of hand-taiyin, the spleen meridian of foot-taiyin and the kidney meridian of foot-shaoyin. It mainly acts on the spleen meridian. It enters the lung channel when used in Jixiang Pill, the spleen channel when used in Sijunzi Decoction, the kidney channel when used in

Dafengsui Pill. The spleen, lung and kidney are in the relationship of child-organ and mother-organ.

厚 朴

气温,味辛,阳中之阴。苦而辛,无毒。

《象》云:能治腹胀,若虚弱,虽腹胀皆斟酌用之。寒胀,是大热药中兼用。结者散之神药。误用脱人元气,切禁之。紫色者,佳。去皮,姜汁制,微炒。

《珍》云:去腹胀,厚肠胃。

《心》云:味厚,阴也。专去腹胀满,去邪气。

《本草》云:主中风,伤寒头痛寒热,惊悸,气血痹,死肌。去三虫,温中益气,消痰下气,疗霍乱及腹痛胀满,胃中冷逆,胸中呕不止,泄痢,淋露;除惊,去留热,心烦满,厚肠胃。

《本经》云:治中风伤寒头痛,温中益气,消痰下气,厚肠胃,去腹胀满。果泄气乎? 果益气乎? 若与枳实、大黄同用则能泄实满,《本经》谓消痰下气者是也;若与橘皮、苍术同用,则能除湿满,《本经》谓温中益气者是也;与解利药同用,则治伤寒头痛;与痢药同用,则厚肠胃。大抵苦温,用苦则泄,用温则补。

《衍义》云:平胃散中之用,最调中,至今盛行。既能温脾胃,又能走冷气。

海藏云:加减随证,如五积散治疗同。

《本草》又云:干姜为使。恶泽泻、寒水石、硝石。

Houpu [厚朴, magnolia bark, Cortex Magnoliae Officinalis]

It is warm in nature and pungent in flavor, pertaining to yin within yang. It is bitter and pungent, and nontoxic.

Xiang [《药类法象》, *Rules for the Use of Medicinal Herbs*] says: It treats the abdominal distention. If the patient is in deficiency, it can also be used with careful consideration. When treating cold distention, it should be used together with the medicinal herb of great heat. It is greatly effective in dissipating accumulations. The wrongly using of it can lead to the collapse of the original qi, which should be prohibited. The purple ones are of good quality. Remove the coat, process it with ginger juice, and then stir-fry it slightly.

Zhen [《珍珠囊》, *Pouch of Pearls*] says: It treats the abdominal distention and strengthens the stomach and intestines.

Xin [《用药心法》, *Gist for the Use of Medicinal Herbs*] says: It is thick in flavor and pertains to yin. It treats the abdominal distention and dispels the pathogenic qi.

Ben Cao says: It mainly treats wind stroke, cold damage and the headache due to cold and heat, fright palpitations, the impediment of qi and blood, and necrotic muscle. It kills three kinds of worms, warms the middle and replenishes qi. It eliminates phlegm and descends qi, treats cholera and pain, the distention and fullness of the abdomen, cold and the counter-flow of qi in the stomach, constant vomiting, diarrhea and strangury. It eliminates fright, lingering heat, relieves vexation and fullness of the heart, and strengthens the stomach and intestines.

Ben Jing [《神农本草经》, *Agriculture God's Canon of Materia Medica*] says: It treats wind stroke, cold damage and headache, warms the middle and replenishes qi, disperses phlegm, descends qi, strengthens the stomach and intestines, and treats distention and fullness of the abdomen. Does it indeed disperse or replenish qi? If it is used together with Zhishi [枳实, immature orange fruit, Fructus Aurantii Immaturus] and Dahuang [大黄, rhubarb root and rhizome, Radix et Rhizoma Rhei], it discharges excess and fullness, which can be used to disperse phlegm and descend qi as recorded in *Ben Jing* [《神农本草经》, *Agriculture God's Canon of Materia Medica*]. If it is used together with Jupi [橘皮, tangerine peel, Citri Reticulatae Pericarpium] and Cangzhu [苍术, atractylodes rhizome, Rhizoma Atractylodis], it eliminates dampness and fullness, which can be used to warm the middle and replenish qi as recorded in *Ben Jing* [《神农本草经》, *Agriculture God's Canon of Materia Medica*]. If it is used together with the medicinal herb with uninhibiting function, it treats cold damage and headache; if it is used with the medicinal herb that treats dysentery, it strengthens the stomach and intestines. It is generally bitter in flavor and warm in nature. The bitter flavor is used to discharge and the warm nature is used to supplement.

Yan Yi [《衍义》, *Extension of the Materia Medica*] says: When used in Pingwei Powder, it is so effective in regulating the middle that it is still very popular today. It not only warms the spleen and stomach but also dissipates the cold qi.

Hai Zang (Wang Haogu) said: It should be tailored according to different syndromes, which is the same as the indications of Wuji Powder.

Ben Cao also says: Ganjiang [干姜, dried ginger, Rhizoma Zingiberis] serves as the guiding medicinal herb of it. It is averse to Zexie [泽泻, oriental waterplantain rhizome, Rhizoma Alismatis], Hanshuishi [寒水石, glauberite, Gypsum seu Calcitum] and Xiaoshi [硝石, niter, Sal Nitri].

丁 香

气温,味辛,纯阳。无毒。

入手太阴经、足阳明经、少阴经。

《象》云:温脾胃,止霍乱,消痃癖,气胀反胃,腹内冷痛,壮阳,暖腰膝,杀酒毒。

《珍》云:去胃中之寒。

《本草》云:主温脾胃,止霍乱,壅胀,风毒诸肿,牙齿疳䘌,能发诸香,能疗反胃,肾气奔豚气,阴痛,壮阳,暖腰膝,消痃癖,除冷劳。

《液》云:与五味子、广术同用,亦治奔豚之气,能泄肺,能补胃,大能疗肾。

Dingxiang [丁香, clove, Flos Caryophylli]

It is warm in nature and pungent in flavor, pertaining to pure yang. It is nontoxic.

It enters the lung meridian of hand-taiyin, the stomach meridian of foot-yangming and the heart meridian of hand-shaoyin.

Xiang [《药类法象》, *Rules for the Use of Medicinal herbs*] says: It warms the spleen and stomach, treats cholera, abdominal mass, distending pain and the regurgitation due to the counter-flow of qi, and the cold and pain in the abdomen. It strengthens yang, warms the lumbus and knees, and removes the liquor toxin.

Zhen [《珍珠囊》 *Pouch of Pearls*] says: It eliminates the cold in the stomach.

Ben Cao says: It mainly warms the spleen and stomach, treats cholera, distention and congestion, the swelling caused by wind toxin and ulcerative gingivitis. It gives off fragrance, treats stomach regurgitation, the kidney qi and Bentun. It can also be used to treat the genital pain and tonify yang. It warms the lumbus and knees, eliminates abdominal mass and treats the consumptive diseases due to cold pathogen.

Ye [《汤液本草》, *Materia Medica for Decoctions*] says: If it is used with Wuweizi [五味子, Chinese magnoliavine fruit, Fructus Schisandrae Chinensis] and Guangshu [广术, Rhioxma Curcumae Aeruginosae, Curcuma Zedoary], it can treat Bentun, purge the lung, tonify the stomach, and it is of great effectiveness in treating the diseases of the kidney.

沉 香

气微温,阳也。

《本草》云:治风水毒肿,去恶气,能调中壮阳,暖腰膝,破症癖冷风麻痹,骨节不任湿风,皮肤痒,心腹痛,气痢,止转筋吐泻。

东垣云:能养诸气,上而至天,下而至泉。用为使,最相宜。

《珍》云:补右命门。

Chenxiang [沉香, aquilaria, Aquilariae Lignum Resinatum]

It is slightly warm in nature, pertaining to yang.

Ben Cao says: It is used to treat the wind edema, dispel the malign qi, regulate the middle and strengthen yang. It warms the lumbus and knees, eliminates abdominal mass and cold wind impediment. It treats the pain of joints due to damp wind, the pruritus of the skin, the pain in the heart and abdomen, and qi dysentery. It can treat cramps, vomiting and diarrhea.

Dong Yuan (Li Gao) said: It cultivates all kinds of qi, from celestial control to terrestrial effect. It is best to be used as a guiding medicinal herb.

Zhen [《珍珠囊》 *Pouch of Pearls*] says: It tonifies the life gate on the right.

乳 香

气味微温,无毒。

《珍》云：定诸经之痛。

Ruxiang [乳香, frankincense, Olibanum]

It is slightly warm in nature and nontoxic.

Zhen [《珍珠囊》, *Pouch of Pearls*] says: It is used to relieve the pain in all the channels.

藿 香

气微温，味甘、辛，阳也。甘苦，纯阳。无毒。

入手足太阴经。

《象》云：治风水，去恶气，治脾胃吐逆，霍乱，心痛。去枝、梗，用叶。

《心》云：芳馨之气，助脾开胃，止呕。

《珍》云：补卫气，益胃进食。

《本草》云：主脾胃呕逆，疗风水毒肿，去恶气，疗霍乱心痛，温中快气；酒口臭，上焦壅，煎汤漱口。入手足太阴。入顺气乌药，则补肺；入黄芪四君子汤，则补脾。

Huoxiang [藿香, Wrinkled Gianthyssop Herb, Agastache Rugosa]

It is slightly warm in nature, sweet and pungent in flavor, pertaining to yang. It is sweet and bitter, pertaining to pure yang. It is nontoxic.

It enters the lung meridian of hand-taiyin and the spleen meridian of foot-taiyin.

Xiang [《药类法象》, *Rules for the Use of Medicinal Herbs*] says: It is used to treat wind edema and dispel malign qi, the vomiting and counter-flow of qi in the spleen and stomach, cholera and the pain in the heart. Remove the branches and sticks, and use the leaves only.

Xin [《用药心法》, *Gist for the Use of Medicinal Herbs*] says: The fragrance is good for the spleen and promotes the appetite. It can stop vomiting.

Zhen [《珍珠囊》, *Pouch of Pearls*] says: It tonifies the defense qi and promotes the appetite.

Ben Cao says: It mainly treats the vomiting and counter-flow of qi in the spleen and stomach. It dispels wind edema and malign qi, and treats cholera and the pain in the heart. It warms the middle and replenishes qi. Rinsing the mouth with its decoction can eliminate the foul smell after drinking due to the congestion in the upper energizer. It enters the lung meridian of hand-taiyin and the spleen meridian of foot-taiyin. It can tonify the lung if used in Shunqiwuyao Decoction and the spleen if used in Huangqisijunzi Decoction.

檀 香

气温,味辛、热。无毒。

入手太阴经,足少阴经,通行阳明经。

《本草》云:主心腹痛,霍乱,中恶鬼气,杀虫。又云:治肾气诸痛,腹痛。消热肿。

东垣云:能调气而清香,引芳香之物,上行至极高之分,最宜橙橘之属,佐以姜、枣,将以葛根、豆蔻、缩砂、益智,通行阳明之经。在胸膈之上,处咽嗌之中,同为理气之药。

《珍》云:主心腹霍乱中恶。引胃气上升,进食。

Tanxiang [檀香, sandalwood, Santali Albi Lignum]

It is warm in nature and pungent in flavor. It is hot and nontoxic.

It enters the lung meridian of hand-taiyin and the kidney meridian of foot-shaoyin, and it dredges yangming meridians.

Ben Cao says: It mainly treats the pain in the heart and abdomen, cholera, the attack of noxious factors and pathogenic factors like ghost. It kills worms. It also says: It treats all the pains due to the kidney qi deficiency and the abdominal pain. It disperses the swelling due to heat.

Dong Yuan (Li Gao) said: It can regulate qi and the fragrance of it can guide other aromatic substances to go upward to their full play. It functions well with the citrus genus. Assisted with ginger and date, Gegen [葛根, kudzuvine root, Radix Puerariae], Doukou [豆蔻, cardamom, Amomi Fructus Rotundus], Suosha [缩砂, Fructus Amomi Xanthioidis, Amomum villosum Lour. Var. xanthioides T. L. Wu et Senjen] and Yizhi [益智, sharp-leaf glangal fruit, Fructus Alpiniae oxyphyllae], it can dredge the yangming meridian. It is a medicinal herb of regulating qi and functions above the chest and diaphragm and up to the throat.

Zhen [《珍珠囊》, *Pouch of Pearls*] says: It is used to treat cholera and the attack of noxious factors in the heart and abdomen. It can guide the stomach qi to ascend and improve the appetite.

苏 合 香

味甘,温。无毒。
《本草》云:主辟恶,杀鬼精物,温疟,蛊毒。痫痓,去三虫,除邪,令人无梦魇。久服,通神明、轻身长年。生中台川谷。
禹锡云:按《梁书》云:中天竺国出苏合香,是诸香汁煎之,非自然一物也。

Suhexiang [苏合香, storax, Styrax]

It is sweet in flavor, warm in nature, and nontoxic.

Ben Cao says: It is used to counteract pathogens, treat diseases caused by pathogenic factors like ghosts, treat warm malaria, the disease caused by worm toxin, convulsion and epilepsy, and kill three kinds of worms. It can eliminate pathogens and avoid being awakened by nightmare. The long-term taking of it will improve the mind, relax the body and prolong the lifespan. It grows in mountains and valleys.

Liu Yuxi said: According to *Liangshu* [《梁书》, *The Historical Events of Liang Dynasty*], the storax produced in the ancient India is generated by mixing all kinds of fragrant juice, and it is not a natural substance.

槟 榔

气温,味辛、苦,味厚气轻,阴中阳也。纯阳,无毒。
《象》云:治后重如神。性如铁石之沉重,能坠诸药至于下极。杵细用。
《心》云:苦以破滞,辛以散邪,专破滞气下行。
《珍》云:破滞气,泄胸中至高之气。
《本草》云:主消谷逐水,除痰癖,下三虫,去伏尸,疗寸白虫。

Binlang [槟榔, areca seed, Semen Arecae]

It is warm in nature, and pungent and bitter in flavor. It is thick in flavor and light in property, pertaining to yang within yin. It pertains to its pungent yang, and it is nontoxic.

Xiang [《药类法象》, *Rules for the Use of Medicinal Herbs*] says: It is of great effectiveness in treating tenesmus. It is heavy in nature like iron, which can guide other medicinal herbs to go downward. Grind it into fine pieces before use.

Xin [《用药心法》, *Gist for the Use of Medicinal Herbs*] says: It can break the stagnation due to its bitter flavor and dissipate pathogen due to its pugent flavor. It is effective to break and descend the stagnant qi.

Zhen [《珍珠囊》, *Pouch of Pearls*] says: It breaks the stagnant qi and discharges the qi in the uppermost part of the chest.

Ben Cao says: It is used to improve digestion and expel water, dispel phlegm aggregation, kill three kinds of worms, treat diseases hidden in the five zang-organs, and kill pinworms.

栀 子

气寒，味微苦。味苦，性大寒，味薄，阴中阳也。无毒。

入手太阴经。

《象》云：治心烦，懊侬而不得眠，心神颠倒欲绝，血滞，小便不利。杵细用。

《心》云：去心中客热，除烦躁，与豉同用。

《珍》云：止渴，去心懊侬烦躁。

《本草》云：主五内邪气，胃中热气，面赤，酒皶皻鼻、白癞、赤癞、疮疡。疗目热赤痛，胸心大小肠大热，心中烦闷，胃中热气。

仲景用栀子治烦，胸为至高之分也。故易老云：轻浮而象肺也，色赤而象火，故能泄肺中之火。《本草》不言吐，仲景用此为吐药。栀子本非吐药，为邪气在上，拒而不下，故令上吐，邪因得以出。经曰：其高者因而越之，此之谓也。或用栀子利小便，实非利小便，清肺也。肺气清而化，膀胱为津液之府，小便得此气化而出也。《本经》谓治大小肠热，辛与庚合，又与丙合，又能泄戊，其先入中州故也。入手太阴。栀子豉汤治烦躁，烦者，气也，躁者，血也。气主肺，血主肾。故用栀子，以治肺烦；用香豉，以治肾躁。躁者，懊恼不得眠也。少气、虚满者，加甘草；若呕哕者，加生姜、橘皮。下后，腹满而烦，栀子厚朴枳实汤；下后，身热微烦，栀子甘草干姜汤。栀子大而长者，染色，不堪入药。皮薄而圆，七棱至九棱者，名山栀子，所谓越桃者是也。

《衍义》云：仲景治伤寒，发汗下吐后，虚烦不得眠。若剧者，必反复颠倒，心中懊恼，以栀子豉汤治虚烦。故不用大黄，以有寒毒故也。栀子虽寒无毒，治胃中热气。既亡血，亡津液，脏腑无润养，内生虚热，非此不可降。又，治心经留热，小便赤涩，去皮山栀子（火煨），大黄、连翘、甘草（炙）等分，末之。水煎三钱匕，服之无不效。

仲景《伤寒论》及古今诸名医，治发黄皆用栀子、茵陈、香豉、甘草四物，等分，作汤饮之。又治大病起，劳复，皆用栀子、鼠矢等汤，并利小便而愈。其方极多，不可悉载。用仁，去心胸中热，用皮，去肌表热。

Zhizi［栀子, gardenia, Gardeniae Fructus］

It is cold in nature and slightly bitter in flavor. It is thin in flavor, pertaining to yang within yin. It is nontoxic.

It enters the lung meridian of hand-taiyin.

Xiang［《药类法象》, *Rules for the Use of Medicinal Herbs*］says： It is used to treat vexation, the insomnia due to anguish, confused mind, blood stasis and inhibited urination. Pound it into powder before use.

Xin［《用药心法》, *Gist for the Use of Medicinal Herbs*］says： It eliminates invading fever in the heart, vexation and agitation. It is used together with fermented soybean.

Zhen［《珍珠囊》, *Pouch of Pearls*］says： It quenches thirst and relieves vexation and the agitation in the heart.

Ben Cao says： It mainly treats the pathogenic qi in the five zang-organs, the heat in the stomach, red face, rosacea, white and red leprosy and sores. It treats the redness and the pain of eyes due to heat, the sever heat in the chest, heart, large intestines and small intestines, the vexation and oppression in the heart, and the heat in the stomach.

Zhang Zhongjing treated the vexation in the chest with Zhizi［栀子, gardenia, Gardeniae Fructus］, which is of great effectiveness. The chest is the uppermost part of the body. Thus Yi Lao (Zhang Yuansu) said: The light and floating nature resembles the dispersing function of the lung, and the red color resembles fire, thus it can discharge the lung heat. The function of emetic is not recorded in *Ben Cao*, while Zhang Zhongjing used it as the emetic medicinal. Zhizi [栀子, gardenia, Gardeniae Fructus] generally did not serve as the emetic medicinal, for the pathogenic qi lying in the upper part and not going downward, thus to induce vomit from the upper part can dispel the pathogenic qi. *Jing* says: If the pathogenic factors have accumulatal in the upper part, it can be treated with the method of vomiting. Zhizi [栀子, gardenia, Gardeniae Fructus] is used to promote urination, but actually it is the function of clearing the lung that works. The lung qi is clear and can be transformed, and the bladder is the house of fluids, from which the urine is transformed and discharged. *Ben Jing* says: It treats the heat in the large intestines and small intestines. Xin[①] corresponds well with Geng and Bing, and discharges Wu, because it enters the central part of the body firstly. It enters the lung meridian of hand-taiyin. Zhizichi Decoction is used to treat the vexation due to qi disorder and the agitation due to blood disorder. Qi governs the lung and blood governs the kidney. Thus Zhizi [栀子, gardenia, Gardeniae Fructus] is used to treat the vexation of the lung and Xiangchi [香豉, fermented soybean, Semen Sojae Preparatum] is used to treat the agitation of the kidney. Agitation is due to anguish, which further leads to insomnia. If the patient feels short of breath and fullenss in the chest, Gancao [甘草, liquorice root, Glycyrrhiza uralensis Fisch] can be added. If there is vomiting, Shengjiang [生姜, fresh ginger, Rhizoma Zingiberis Recens] and tangerine peel can be added. If the patient suffers from fullness and rexation after giving purgation, Zhizi Houpu Zhishi Decoction can be used. If the patient suffers from fever and slight rexation, Zhizi Gancao Ganjiang Decocfian can be used. Zhizi [栀子, gardenia, Gardeniae Fructus], which is large and long and dyed, can not be used as medicinal herbs. The one with thin skin, round shape and seven or nine ribs is called Shanzhizi [山

---

① Xin (辛) is one of the ten heavenly stems in traditional Chinese lunar calendar, which is of yin property and also connects with the lung correspondingly. The following three stems of Geng (庚), Bing (丙) and Wu (戊) are of yang property and connect with large intestines, small intestines and the stomach correspondingly.

栀子, cape jasmine fruit, Fructus Gardeniae] or Yuetao [越桃, gardenia, Gardeniae Fructus].

Yan Yi [《衍义》, *Extension*, *of the Materia Medica*] says: Zhang Zhongjing often used perspiration, emesis and purgation to treat cold damage which may lead to dysphoria due to deficienay and insomnia. If severe, the pattient will tumble on bed, feeling anguished, which can be terated by Zhizichi Decoction. Dahuang [大黄, rhubarb root and rhizome, Radix et Rhizoma Rhei] can not be used since it has cold toxin. Zhizi [栀子, gardenia, Gardeniae Fructus] is cold but with no toxin, which can be used to treat the heat in the stomach. For the syndromes as blood exhaustion, fluid exhaustion, failure of nourishment in zang-fu organs, deficiency heat arising internally, this medicinal herb is necessary to be used in the treatment. Moreover, it can treat the lingering heat in the heart channel and inhibited reddish urine. Put together the same does of Shanzhizi [山栀子, cape jasmine fruit, Fructus Gardeniae] without skin, (remove the bark roasted), Dahuang [大黄, rhubarb root and rhizome, Radix et Rhizoma Rhei], Lianqiao [连翘, weeping forsythia, Forsythia suspensa Vahl] and Gancao [甘草, liquorice root, Glycyrrhiza uralensis Fisch] (burnt), and then pound them into powder. Decoct and take three Qian Bi of the mixture. It is always effective.

Zhongjing's *Shang Han Lun* [《伤寒论》, *On Cold Damage*] and other famous doctors from the ancient times to present all treated jaundice with the decoction composed of Zhizi [栀子, gardenia, Gardeniae Fructus], Yinchen [茵陈, virgate wormwood herb, Herba Artemisiae Scopariae], Xiangchi [香豉, fermented soybean, Semen Sojae the Preparatum] and Gancao [甘草, liquorice root, Glycyrrhiza uralensis Fisch], which are of the same dose. The decoction consisting Zhizi [栀子, gardenia, Gardeniae Fructus] and Shushi [鼠矢, cornus, Corni Fructus] are used to treat severe diseases and overfatigue relapse, which could promote urination and cure the diseases. The prescriptions are in such a large number that we can not record all of them. The kernel is used to relieve the heat in the heart and chest, and the peel to relieve the heat of muscles and the skin.

黄 柏

气寒,味苦。苦厚微辛,阴中之阳,降也。无毒。

足太阳经引经药,足少阴经之剂。

《象》云:治肾水膀胱不足,诸痿厥,脚膝无力,于黄芪汤中少加用之,使两膝中气力涌出,痿即去矣。蜜炒此一味,为细末,治口疮如神。瘫痪必用之药。

《珍》云:泻膀胱之热,利下窍。

《心》云:太阳经引经药,泻膀胱经火,补本经及肾不足。苦寒安蛔,疗下虚焦,坚肾。经曰:苦以坚之。

《本草》云:主五脏,肠胃中结热,黄疸,肠痔,止泄痢,女子漏下赤白,阴伤蚀疮,疗惊气,在皮间肌肤热赤起,目热赤痛,口疮。久服,通神。

《液》云:足少阴剂,肾苦燥,故肾停湿也,栀子、黄芩入肺,黄连入心,黄柏入肾,燥湿所归,各从其类也。《活人书》解毒汤,上下内外通治之。恶干漆。

Huangbo [黄柏, bark of amur corktree, Cortex Phellodendri]

It is cold in nature and bitter in flavor. It is strongly bitter and slightly pungent, pertaining to yang within yin. It has descending functional tendency and it is nontoxic.

It is the channel ushering the drug of the bladder meridian of foot-taiyang, and it enters the kidney meridian of foot-shaoyin.

Xiang [《药类法象》 *Rules for the Use of Medicinal Herbs*] says: It is used to treat the edema due to the dysfunction of the kidney and the insufficiency of the bladder, the flaccidity and fatigue in the knees and feet. If used together with Huangqi Decoction, it can induce the gush of strength of the knees and cure flaccidity. Stir-fry it with honey and grind it into powder, which is of great effectiveness in treating the aphtha. It is an essential medicinal herb for treating paralysis.

Zhen [《珍珠囊》 *Pouch of Pearls*] says: It drains the heat of the bladder and frees lower orifices.

Xin [《用药心法》, *Gist for the Use of Medicinal Herbs*] says: It is the channel ushering the herb of the taiyang channel. It can reduce the heat in the bladder channel and supplement the insufficiency of the bladder and kidney channel. It is cold and bitter, expels the intestinal ascarid, treats the deficiency of the lower energizer and strengthens the kidney. *Jing* says: The bitterness is suitable to strengthen the kidney.

Ben Cao says: It is used to eliminate the heat accumulation in the five zang-organs and the stomach and intestines, jaundice, intestine hemorrhoids, stop diarrhea and dysentery, metrostaxis with reddish discharge, genital ulceration and sore, relieve fright, eliminate the heat in the skin and relieve red and painful eyes and aphtha. The long-term taking of it may improve the spirit.

Ye[《汤液本草》, *Materia Medica for Decoctions*] says: It enters the kidney meridian of foot-shaoyin. The kidney tends to suffer from dryness and retain dampness. Zhizi[栀子, gardenia, Gardeniae Fructus] and Huangqin[黄芩, baical skullcap root, Radix Scutellariae] enter the lung, Huanglian[黄连, golden thread, Rhizoma Coptidis] enters the heart, and Huangbo[黄柏, bark of amur corktree, Cortex Phellodendri] enters the kidney. They can treat dryness or dampness according to their properties. *Huo Ren Shu*[《活人书》, *Book to Safeguard Life*] says: It is used in the decoction for detoxication, and treats all kinds of diseases. It is averse to Ganqi[干漆, Dried Lacquer, Resina Toxicodendri].

枳 实

气寒，味苦、酸、咸，纯阴。无毒。

《象》云：除寒热，破结实，消痰癖，治心下痞，逆气胁痛。麸炒用。

《心》云：洁古用去脾经积血。故能去心下痞，脾无积血，则心下不痞。治心下痞，散气消宿食。苦寒，炙用，破水积，以泄里除风。

《珍》云：去胃中湿。

《本草》云：主大风在皮肤中，如麻豆苦痒。除寒热结，止痢，长肌肉利五脏，益气轻身。除胸胁痰癖，逐停水，破结实，消胀满，心下急，痞痛，逆气，胁风痛。安胃气，止溏泄，明目。生河内川泽，商州者，佳。益气，则佐之以人参、干姜、白术。破气，则佐之以大黄、牵牛、芒硝。此《本经》所以言益气，而复言消痞也。非白术，不能去湿；非枳实，不能除痞。壳主高而实主下。高者主气；下者主血。主气者，在胸膈；主血者，在心腹。仲景治心下坚大如盘，水饮所作，枳实白术汤主之。枳实七枚，术三两，水一斗，煎取三升，分三服。腹中软即消。

《衍义》云：枳实、枳壳，一物也。小则性酷而速，大则性祥而缓，故仲景治伤寒仓卒之病，承气汤中用枳实，此其意也。皆取其疏通决泄，破结实之意。他方但导败风壅之气，可常服者，故用枳壳。故胸中痞，有桔梗枳壳汤；心下痞，有枳实白术汤。高低之分，易老详定为的也。

Zhishi [枳实, immature orange fruit, Fructus Aurantii Immaturus]

It is cold in nature, bitter, sour and salty in flavor. It pertains to pure yin. It is nontoxic.

Xiang [《药类法象》, *Rules for the Use of Medicinal Herbs*] says: It is used to eliminate cold-heat, resolve mass and disperse phlegm aggregation. It treats the epigastric stuffiness and the pain of hypochondrium due to the counter-flow of qi. It can be used by stir-frying with bran.

Xin [《用药心法》, *Gist for the Use of Medicinal Herbs*] says: Jiegu (Zhang Yuansu) used it to eliminate the blood accumulation in the spleen channel. When the blood accumulation in the spleen is eliminated, the epigastric stuffiness disappears. It is used to treat epigastric stuffiness, disperse qi and promote the digestion of retained food. It is bitter in flavor and cold in nature. Processed by stir-frying with liquid adjuvant, it can break water accumulation, discharge the interior and dispel wind.

Zhen [《珍珠囊》, *Pouch of Pearls*] says: It eliminates the dampness in the stomach.

Ben Cao says: It is mainly used to treat the disease marked by pain and the pruritus caused by the invasion of severe wind into the skin like sesames and soybeans in the skin. It eliminates heat-cold retention, stanches dysentery, promotes granulation, harmonize the five zang-organs, replenishes qi and relaxes the body. It dispels the phlegm aggregation in the chest and rib-side, expels water retention, resolves mass and disperses distention and fullness. It treats the epigastric distress and stuffiness, the counter-flow of qi and the pain caused by wind invasion into the rib-side. It regulates the qi in the stomach, stanches the sloppy diarrhea, and improves eyesight. It grows in Henei, mountains and pools, and those produced in Shang State are of good quality. If it is used for replenishing qi, it should be assisted with Renshen [人参, ginseng, Radix Ginseng], Ganjiang [干姜, dried ginger, Rhizoma Zingiberis] and Baizhu [白术, argehead atractylodes rhizome, Rhizoma Atractylodis Macrocephalae]. If it is used to break qi, it should be combined with Dahuang [大黄, rhubarb root and rhizome, Radix et Rhizoma

Rhei], Qianniu [牵牛, morning glory, Pharbitidis Semen] and Mangxiao [芒硝, crystallized sodium sulfate, Natrii Sulfas]. This is what is recorded in *Ben Jing* [《神农本草经》, *Agriculture God's Canon of Materia Medica*] that it replenishes qi and disperses stuffiness. Baizhu [白术, argehead atractylodes rhizome, Rhizoma Atractylodis Macrocephalae] is essential in eliminating dampness; Zhishi [枳实, immature orange fruit, Fructus Aurantii Immaturus] is essential in removing mass. Zhiqiao [枳壳, bitter orange, Fructus Aurantii] mainly functions in the upper part and Zhishi [枳实, immature orange fruit, Fructus Aurantii Immaturus] excels in the lower part, with the former governing qi and the latter governing blood. The ones governing qi act on the chest and diaphragm; the ones governing blood act on the heart and abdomen. Zhang Zhongjing treated hardness below the heart which is caused by fluid retention with Zhishi Baizhu Decoction. Take seven pieces of Zhishi and three Liang of Baizhu, decoct them with one Dou of water, and get three Sheng of the decoction, take one Sheng each time and three times a day. This can resolve the abdominal mass effectively.

Yan Yi [《衍义》 *Extension of the Materia Medica*] says: Zhishi [枳实, immature orange fruit, Fructus Aurantii Immaturus] and Zhiqiao [枳壳, orange fruit, Fructus Aurantii] are the same herbs. The small ones are of drastic effects while the big ones are of mild effects. Thus Zhang Zhongjing treated the urgent diseases like the cold damage with Chengqi Decoction which contains Zhishi [枳实, immature orange fruit, Fructus Aurantii Immaturus], in which the functions of freeing, dredging, discharging and breaking mass are used. The prescription with Zhiqiao [枳壳, orange fruit, Fructus Aurantii] can disperse qi congestion, and it is suitable for long-term taking. Jiegeng Zhiqiao Decoction is used to treat the stuffiness in the chest, and Zhishi Baizhu Decoction is used to treat the epigastric stuffiness. Yi Lao (Zhang Yuansu) has presented the specific statements of the different applications.

枳 壳

气寒，味苦。苦而酸，微寒，味薄气厚，阳也。阴中微阳。无毒。

《象》云：治脾胃痞塞，泄肺气。麸炒用。

《心》云：利胸中气，胜湿化痰。勿多用，损胸中至高之气。

《珍》云：破气。

《本草》云：主风痒麻痹，通利关节，劳气咳嗽，背膊闷倦，散留结，胸膈痰滞，逐水，消胀满，大肠风，安胃，止风痛。

《药性论》云：枳壳，使。味苦、辛。治遍身风疹，肌中如麻豆恶痒。壳，高，主皮毛、胸膈之病；实，低，主心胃之病。其主治大同小异。

Zhiqiao［枳壳, orange fruit, Fructus Aurantii］

It is cold in nature, and bitter and sour in flavor. It is thin in flavor and thick in property, pertaining to yang. It pertains to yang within yin, and it is nontoxic.

Xiang［《药类法象》, *Rules for the Use of Medicinal Herbs*］says：It treats the stuffiness in the spleen and stomach and discharges the lung qi. It can be used by stir-frying with bran.

Xin［《用药心法》, *Gist for the Use of Medicinal Herbs*］says：It disinhibits the qi in the chest, eliminates dampness and resolves phlegm. The excessive taking is not recommended for it can damage the qi in the high position of the chest.

Zhen［《珍珠囊》, *Pouch of Pearls*］says：It breaks the stagnant qi.

Ben Cao says：It is used to treat the pruritus and numbness due to pathogenic wind, free the joint, and it can also deal with the cough caused by the consumption of qi, and the oppression and fatigue in the back and arms. It dissipates qi accumulation, the phlegm stagnation in the chest and diaphragm, expels water, disperses distention and fullness, removes wind in the large intestine, harmonizes the stomach, and stanches the pain due to the invasion of wind.

Yao Xing Lun［《药性论》*Treatise on Medicinal Properties*］says：Zhiqiao［枳壳, orange fruit, Fructus Aurantii］is often used as a guiding medicinal herb. It is bitter and pungent in flavor. It is used to treat the wind papules around the body and the disease marked by pain and the pruritus like sesames and soybeans in the skin. Zhiqiao［枳壳, orange fruit, Fructus Aurantii］, with the higher functional tendency, is used to treat the diseases in the skin, hair, the chest and diaphragm；Zhishi［枳实, immature orange fruit, Fructus Aurantii Immaturus］, with the lower functional tendency, is used to treat the diseases of the heart and stomach. Their main indications are similar.

牡 丹 皮

气寒,味苦、辛。阴中微阳。辛苦微寒。无毒。

手厥阴经,足少阴经。

《象》云:治肠胃积血,及衄血、吐血必用之药。

《珍》云:凉骨蒸。

《本草》云:主寒热中风,瘛疭,痉,惊痫邪气。除症坚、淤血留舍肠胃。安五脏,疗痈疮,除时气头痛,客热,五劳之气,腰痛,风噤,癫疾。

易老云:治神志不足。神不足者,手少阴;志不足者,足少阴。故仲景八味丸用之。牡丹乃天地之精,群花之首。叶为阳,发生;花为阴,成实;丹为赤,即火。故能泄阴中之火。牡丹皮,手厥阴,足少阴,治无汗骨蒸;地骨皮,足少阴,手少阳,治有汗骨蒸也。

Mudanpi［牡丹皮, tree peony root bark, Cortex Moutan Radicis］

It is cold in nature, and bitter and pungent in flavor, pertaining to yang within yin. It is pungent and bitter in flavor, slightly cold in nature, and nontoxic.

It enters the pericardium meridian of hand-jueyin and the kidney meridian of foot-shaoyin.

Xiang［《药类法象》, *Rules for the Use of Medicinal Herbs*］says: It treats the blood accumulation in intestines and the stomach, and it is the essential medicinal for epistaxis and hematemesis.

Zhen［《珍珠囊》, *Pouch of Pearls*］says: It treats the hectic fever due to yin deficiency.

Ben Cao says: It mainly treats cold-heat stroke, convulsion, spasm and the epilepsy due to the pathogenic qi. It eliminates the fixed mass and the blood stasis in intestines and the stomach. It harmonizes the five zang-organs and cures abscess. It can be used to treat the headache caused by the seasonal qi, invading fever, five kinds of strain, the pain in the waist, the clenched jaw due to wind and epilepsy.

Yi Lao (Zhang Yuansu) said: It treats the insufficiency of spirit. For the patients who are insufficient in spirit, the disease lies in the heart meridian of hand-shaoyin; for those who are insufficient in mind, the disease lies in the kidney meridian of foot-shaoyin. It is used in Zhang Zhongjing's Bawei Pill. Mudan [牡丹, moutan, Cortex Moutan Radicis] is the essence of the heaven and the king, and the head of all the flowers. The leaves pertain to yang, sprouting; the flowers pertain to yin, yielding fruits; 丹 (dan) in Chinese means red, representing fire. Thus it is used to discharge the heat of the yin syndrome. Mudanpi [牡丹皮, tree peony root bark, Cortex Moutan Radicis] enters the pericardium meridian of hand-jueyin and the kidney meridian of foot-shaoyin, and treats the hectic fever without sweat; Digupi [地骨皮, Chinese wolfberry root-bark, Cortex Lycii] enters the kidney meridian of foot-shaoyin and the triple energizer meridian of hand-shaoyang, and treats the hectic fever with sweat.

地 骨 皮

气寒,味苦,阴也。大寒,无毒。

足少阴经,手少阳经。

《象》云:解骨蒸肌热,主风痹湿,消渴,坚筋骨。去骨,用根皮。

《心》云:去肌热及骨中之热。

《珍》云:凉血、凉骨。

《本草》云:主五内邪气,热中消渴,周痹风湿,下胸胁气,客热头痛。补内伤大劳嘘吸,坚筋骨,强阴,利大小肠。

《药性论》云:根皮细锉,面拌,熟煮吞之。主肾家风,益精气。

《衍义》云:枸杞当用梗皮,地骨当用根皮,枸杞子当用其红实。实,微寒;皮,寒;根,大寒。

Digupi [地骨皮, Chinese wolfberry root-bark, Cortex Lycii]

It is cold in nature and bitter in flavor, pertaining to yin. It is extremely cold in property and nontoxic.

It enters the kidney meridian of foot-shaoyin and the triple energizer meridian of hand-shaoyang.

Xiang [《药类法象》, *Rules for the Use of Medicinal Herbs*] says: It treats the hectic fever and the heat in the flesh. It treats the impediment due to wind dampness, consumptive thirst. It strengthens sinews and bones. Only the root and bark can be used.

Xin [《用药心法》, *Gist for the Use of Medicinal Herbs*] says: It eliminates the heat in the flesh and bones.

Zhen [《珍珠囊》, *Pouch of Pearls*] says: It cools the blood and bones.

Ben Cao says: It is mainly used to expel the pathogenic qi in the five zang-organs, treat heat stroke, consumptive thirst, and the impediment due to wind-dampness. It regulates the counter-flow of qi below the chest and rid-side. It is used to treat the headache due to invading heat. It supplements internal damage, exhaustion and qi consumption. It strengthens sinews and bones, improves the potency of men, and disinhibits the large intestines and small intestines.

Yao Xing Lun [《药性论》, *Treatise on Medicinal Properties*] says: Pound the root and bark into fine powder, mix it with flour, then boil and take it. It can treat the pathogenic wind in the kidney and boost essence and qi.

Yan Yi [《衍义》, *Extension of the Materia Medica*] says: The stalk bark of Gouqi [枸杞, fruit of barbary wolfberry, Fructus Lycii] is used, so is the root bark of Digu [地骨, lycium bark, Lycii Cortex] and the red fruit of Gouqizi [枸杞子, lycium, Lycii Fructus]. The fruit is slightly cold, the bark is cold, and the root is strongly cold in property.

猪 苓

气平,味甘、苦,甘寒。甘苦而淡,甘重于苦,阳也。无毒。

入足太阳经、少阴经。

《象》云:除湿。此诸淡渗药大燥,亡津液,无湿证勿服。去皮用。

《心》云:苦以泄滞,甘以助阳,淡以利窍。故能除湿,利小便。

《珍》云:利小便。

《本草》云:主痎疟,解毒蛊疰不详。利水道,能疗妊娠淋。又治从脚上至腹肿,小便不利。仲景,少阴渴者猪苓汤。入足太阳、少阴。

《衍义》云:行水之功多,久服必损肾气,昏人目。果欲久服者,更宜详审。

Zhuling [猪苓, zhuling, Polyporus Umbellatus]

It is mild in nature, and sweet and bitter in flavor. It is cold in property. It is sweet, bitter and bland, and its sweetness is greater than its bitterness. It pertains to yang, and it is nontoxic.

It enters the bladder meridian of foot-taiyang and the heart meridian of hand-shaoyin.

Xiang [《药类法象》, *Rules for the Use of Medicinal Herbs*] says: It can eliminate dampness. The bland medicinal herbs are strongly dry, which may damage fluid. Thus it should not be taken without the syndromes of dampness. Use it after removing the skin.

Xin [《用药心法》, *Gist for the Use of Medicinal Herbs*] says: The bitterness can discharge stagnation, the sweetness can reinforce yang and the blandness can disinhibit the orifices. Thus it can dispel dampness and promote urination.

Zhen [《珍珠囊》, *Pouch of Pearls*] says: It is used to promote urination.

Ben Cao says: It is used to treat malaria, resolve toxin and treat the severe syndrome caused by worm toxin. It frees the waterways and treats the strangury in pregnancy. It also treats the swelling from the abdomen to feet, and the inhibited urination. Zhang zhongjing used Zhuling Decoction to treat the thirst caused by the pathogenic heat invading the meridian-shaoyin. It enters the bladder meridian of foot-taiyang and the heart meridian of hand-shaoyin.

Yan Yi [《衍义》, *Extension of the Materia Medica*] says: It functions well in moving water, thus the long-term taking of it can damage the kidney qi and damage the eyesight. Be cautious if one needs long-term taking of it.

茯苓

气平，味淡。味甘而淡，阳也。无毒。

白者，入手太阴经、足太阳经、少阳经；赤者，入足太阴经、手太阳经、少阴经。

《象》云：止渴，利小便，除湿益燥，和中益气，利腰脐间血为主。治小便不通，溺黄或赤而不利。如小便利或数服之，则大损人目。如汗多人服之，损真气，夭人寿。医云赤泻白补，上古无此说。去皮用。

《心》云：淡能利窍，甘以助阳，除湿之圣药也。味甘平，补阳，益脾逐水。湿淫所胜，小便不利。淡味渗，泄阳也。治水缓脾，生精导气。

《珍》云：甘，纯阳。渗泄止渴。

《本草》云：主胸胁逆气，忧恚惊邪恐悸，心下结痛，寒热烦满，咳逆，口焦舌干。利小便，止消渴，好唾，大腹淋沥，消膈中痰水，水肿，淋结。开胸腑，调脏气，伐肾邪，长阴，益气力，保神守中。

《液》云：入足少阴，手足太阳。色白者，入辛壬癸；赤者，入丙丁。伐肾邪，小便多，能止之；小便涩，能利之。与车前子相似，虽利小便而不走气。酒浸，与光明朱砂同用，能秘真。味甘、平，如何是利小便。

Fuling [茯苓, Indian bread, Poria]

It is mild in property, and sweet and bland in taste. It pertains to yang, and it is nontoxic.

The white one enters the lung meridian of hand-taiyin, the bladder meridian of foot-taiyang and the gallbladder meridian of foot-shaoyang; the red one enters the spleen meridian of foot-taiyin, the small intestine meridian of hand-taiyang and the heart meridian of hand-shaoyin.

Xiang [《药类法象》, *Rules for the Use of Medicinal Herbs*] says: It ceases thirst and promotes urination. It eliminates dampness, moistens dryness, harmonizes the middle energizer, replenishes qi and disinhibits the blood circulation between the waist and the umbilicus. It treats the yellowish or red urination and the inhibited urination. If people without the inhibited urination syndrome take it, it can damage the eyesight. If the people who sweat a lot take it, it can damage the genuine qi and shorten the lifespan. Some doctors say that the red ones drain and the white ones supplement, while there was no such statement in the ancient times. Use it after removing the skin.

Xin [《用药心法》, *Gist for the Use of Medicinal Herbs*] says: The blandness disinhibits orifices and the sweetness reinforces yang, thus it is an effective medicinal herb for dispelling dampness. Being sweet in taste and mild in property, it can be used to supplement yang, tonify the spleen and expel water. It can treat the syndrome of excessive dampness and inhibited urination. The bland medicinal eliminating dampness pertains to yang. It is used to treat severe edema, tonify the spleen, generate the essence and guide qi.

Zhen [《珍珠囊》, *Pouch of Pearls*] says: It is sweet, and it pertains to yang. It promotes urination, drains dampness and ceases thirst.

Ben Cao says: It is used to treat the counter-flow of qi from the chest and ribside, relieve anxiety, fright and palpitation, remove the epigastric accumulation and pain, eliminate vexation and the fullness due to cold-heat, cease the cough with dyspnea, and dispel the parchment of the mouth and the dryness of the tongue. It is used to promote urination, eliminate dispersion-thirst and copious spittle. It treats the swollen abdomen and dribbling urine, and disperses the phlegm in the diaphragm, edema and strangury accumulation. It opens the chest, regulates the visceral qi, dispels the pathogens in the kidney, replenishes yin, increases energy, preserves spirit and guards the middle energizer.

Ye [《汤液本草》, *Materia Medica for Decoctions*] says: It enters the kidney meridian of foot-shaoyin, the small intestine meridian of hand-taiyang and the bladder meridian of foot-taiyang. The white ones enter Xin, Ren and Gui; the red ones enter Bing and Ding①. It dispels the pathogens in the kidney. It stanches the dribbling urination and promotes the inhibited urination. It has the similar function as Cheqianzi [车前子, plantain seed, Semen Plantaginis], which promotes urination but will not discharge qi. Immersing it in liquor and using it together with Cinnabar can secure the original qi. It is sweet in taste and mild in property, thus it can promote urination.

茯 神

阳也，味甘。无毒。

《珍》云：治风眩心虚，非此不能安。

《药性论》云：君，主惊痫，安神定志，补虚乏。主心下急痛坚满，人虚而小便不利者。

Fushen [茯神, root poria, Poria cum Pini Radice]

It pertains to yang, and it is sweet in taste and nontoxic.

Zhen [《珍珠囊》, *Pouch of Pearls*] says: It is essential in treating the

---

① Xin (辛), Ren (壬), Gui (癸), Bing (丙), Ding (丁): These five are from the ten heavenly stems in the traditional Chinese lunar calendar, which also connects with the lung, the urinary bladder, the kidney, the small intestines and the heart respectively.

dizziness due to the pathogenic wind and the heart deficiency.

Yao Xing Lun [《药性论》, *Treatise on Medicinal Properties*] says: It is used as a sovereign medicinal herb which treats fright epilepsy, calms spirit and mind, and supplements the deficiency and weakness of the body. It is used to treat epigastric distress, pain and fullness, and inhibit the urination due to deficiency.

乌 药

气温,味辛。无毒。

入足阳明经、少阴经。

《本草》云:主中恶心腹痛,蛊毒,疰忤鬼气,宿食不消,天行疫瘴,膀胱、肾间冷气,攻冲背膂。妇人血气,小儿腹中诸虫。又云:去猫涎,极妙。乌药叶及根,嫩时采,作茶片炙碾煎服,能补中益气,偏止小便滑数。

Wuyao [乌药, lindera, Linderae Radix]

It is warm in property, pungent in taste, and nontoxic.

It enters the stomach meridian of foot-yangming and the heart meridian of hand-shaoyin.

Ben Cao says: It mainly treats the pain in the heart and abdomen due to the attack of noxious factors, the disease due to noxious agents produced by various parasites, the noxious pathogen attack, spectral pathogenic factors, and the indigestion of retained food. It eliminates the warm disease and stagnation, and the cold qi in the bladder and kidney which can strike the back. It treats the blood diseases of women and eliminates the parasite from children's abdomen. It is also said that it functions well in eliminating the salivation of cat. The leaf and root of Wuyao [乌药, lindera, Linderae Radix] should be collected when they are tender. Fry and grind it into pieces like tea and boil it, which can supplement the middle energizer, replenish qi, and stanch slippery and frequent urination.

干 漆

气温、平,味辛。有毒。

《本草》云：主绝伤，补中，续筋骨，填髓脑，安五脏。治五缓六急，风寒湿痹。疗咳嗽，消淤血痞结腰痛，女子疝瘕，利小肠，去蛔虫。生漆，去长虫，半夏为之使。畏鸡子。忌油脂。

Ganqi［干漆，Dried Lacquer，Resina Toxicodendri］

It is warm and mild in property, and pungent in taste. It is toxic.

Ben Cao says：It is mainly used to treat severe damages, supplement the middle energizer, remedy the severe injury of sinews and bones, enrich the brains, and harmonize the five zang-organs. It is used to treat five kinds of retardations, six kinds of extreme syndromes and the wind-cold dampness impediment. It treats cough, disperses blood stasis, conglomeration and accumulation and the pain in the waist, the mounting-conglomeration of women, disinhibits the small intestines, and kills ascarid. Raw lacquer can kill roundworms, with Banxia［半夏, pinellia tuber, Rhizoma Pinelliae］served as its guiding medicinal herb. It is restrained by eggs and incompatible with lard.

皂 荚

气温，味辛、咸。有小毒。

引入厥阴经药。

《本草》云：主风痹死肌邪气，风头泪出，利九窍，疗腹胀满，消谷，除咳嗽。治囊缩，妇人胞不落，明目，益精，可为沐药，不入汤。

《日华子》云：通关节，除湿风，消痰，杀劳虫，治骨蒸，开胃，破坚癥，腹中痛，能堕胎。柏实为之使。恶麦门冬。畏空青、人参、苦参。

仲景治咳逆上气，唾浊，但坐不得卧，皂荚丸主之。杵末，一物蜜丸桐子大，用枣汤服一丸，日三夜一。

《活人书》：治阴毒，正阳散内用皂荚，引入厥阴也。用之有蜜炙、酥炙、烧灰之异，等分依方。

Zaojia［皂荚，gymnocladus fruit, Gymnocladi Fructus］

It is warm in property, and pungent and salty in taste. It is slightly toxic.

It enters the liver meridian of foot-jueyin.

Ben Cao says: It is mainly used to treat wind impediment, muscle necrosis and pathogenic qi, the headache with tearing due to the invasion of pathogenic wind, disinhibit the nine orifices, eliminate distention and the fullness of the abdomen, improve digestion, and eliminate cough. It treats the retracted scrotum and the retention of the placenta of women, improves vision, and boosts the essence. It can be used in bathing, but not in decoction.

Ri Hua Zi [《日华子》, *Materia Medica of Ri Hua-Zi*] says: It disinhibits the joints, eliminates dampness and wind, disperses phlegm, kills worms, treats the hectic fever due to yin deficiency, increases the appetite, breaks the abdominal mass and conglomeration, relieves the pain in the abdomen, and induces abortion. Baishi, [柏实, arborvitae seed, Platycladi Semen] is used as its guiding medicinal herb. It is averse to Maimendong [麦门冬, radix ophiopogonis, Ophiopogon japonicus Ker-Gawl]. It is restrained by Kongqing [空青, hollow azurite, Azuritum Vacuum], Renshen [人参, ginseng, Radix Ginseng] and Kushen [苦参, flavescent sophora, Sophorae Flavescentis Radix].

The syndrome of cough with dyspnea, the counter-flow of qi and the turbid spittle making peeple unable to lie down to sleep, was treated with Zaojia Pill by Zhang Zhongjing. Pestle it to powder and make it honeyed pills as big as phoenix tree seeds, and take it with Jujube soup three times a day and one time a night.

Huo Ren Shu [《活人书》, *Book to Safeguard Life*] says: It can be used to eliminate the turbid yin pathogen. Zaojia [皂荚, gymnocladus fruit, Gymnocladi Fructus] is used in Zhengyang Powder, and it enters the liver meridian of foot-jueyin. It could be used after being stir-fried with honey or butter, or burned to ash in accordance with the prescriptions.

竹 叶

气平,味辛。又苦大寒,辛平。无毒。

《本草》云:主咳逆上气,溢筋急,恶疡,杀小虫。除烦热,风痉,喉痹,呕吐。仲景竹叶汤用淡竹叶。

《心》云:除烦热,缓皮而益气。

《珍》云:阴中微阳,凉心经。

Zhuye [竹叶, bamboo leaf, Lophatheri Folium]

It is mild in property, and pungent and bitter in taste. It is strongly cold in property and nontoxic.

Ben Cao says: It is mainly used to treat the cough with dyspnea and the counter-flow of qi, the spasm of sinews and severe sores, and kill small worms. It dispels vexing fever, tetanus, throat impediment and vomiting. Danzhuye [淡竹叶, lophatherum, Lophatheri Herba] is used in Zhang Zhongjing's Zhuye Decoction.

Xin [《用药心法》, *Gist for the Use of Medicinal Herbs*] says: It eliminates vexing fever, relieves fatigue and replenishes qi.

Zhen [《珍珠囊》, *Pouch of Pearls*] says: It pertains to yang within yin, and it cools the heart channel.

竹 茹

气微寒,味苦。

《本草》云:主呕哕,温气寒热,吐血,崩中。溢筋。

Zhuru [竹茹, bamboo shavings, Bumbusae Caulis in Taenia]

It is slightly cold in property and bitter in taste.

Ben Cao says: It is mainly used to treat retching, the cold-heat syndrome due to the pathogenic qi, blood ejection, and vaginal bleeding and the spasm of sinews.

淡 竹 叶

气寒,味辛、平。

《本草》云:主胸中痰热,咳逆上气。

《药性论》云:淡竹叶主吐血,热毒风,压丹石药毒,止渴。

《日华子》云:淡竹及根,消痰,治热狂烦闷,中风失音不语,壮热头痛,头风,并怀孕妇人头旋倒地,止惊悸,温疫迷闷,小儿惊痫天吊。茎叶同用(见《局方本草》,今录附于此)。

Danzhuye [淡竹叶, lophatherum, Lophatheri Herba]

It is cold in property, pungent in taste and mild in nature.

Ben Cao says: It is mainly used to treat the phlegm-heat in the chest, the cough with dyspnea and the counter-flow of qi.

Yao Xing Lun [《药性论》, *Treatise on Medicinal Properties*] says: Danzhuye [淡竹叶, lophatherum, Lophatheri Herba] is mainly used to treat blood ejection, eliminate heat toxin, suppress the toxicity of elixir and relieve thirst.

Ri Hua Zi [《日华子》, *Materia Medica of Ri Hua-Zi*] says: Danzhuye [淡竹叶, lophatherum, Lophatheri Herba] and its root could be used to disperse phlegm, treat heat mania, vexation and oppression, loss of voice due to wind stroke, high fever, headache, the head disorder due to the invasion of wind and the dizziness of pregnant women leading to falling, eliminate fright palpitation, epidemic disease, infantile convulsion, epilepsy and convulsion. The stalks and leaves have the similar functions. (From *Ju Fang Ben Cao* [《局方本草》, *Materia Medica of Prescriptions of the Bureau of Pharmacy*], and it is recorded here today.)

茗苦荼

气微寒,味苦、甘。无毒。

入手足厥阴经。

《液》云:腊茶是也。清头目,利小便,消热渴,下气消食,令人少睡。中风昏愦,多睡不醒,宜用此。入手足厥阴。茗苦荼,苦、甘微寒。无毒。主瘘疮,利小便,去痰热渴,治阴证汤药内,用此,去格拒之寒。及治伏阳,大意相似。茶苦,《经》云:苦以泄之,其体下行,如何是清头目。

Mingkucha [茗苦荼, bitter tea, Camellia assamica (Mast.) Chang var. kucha Chang et Wang]

It is slightly cold in property, and bitter and sweet in taste. It is nontoxic.

It enters the pericardium meridian of hand-jueyin and the liver meridian of foot-jueyin.

Ye [《汤液本草》, *Materia Medica for Decoctions*] says: It is also called Lacha [腊茶, tea, Theae Folium]. It is used to clear the heat in the head and eyes, promote urination, disperse the thirst due to heat, descend qi, digest food, and reduce somnolence. It could be used to treat wind stroke, confusion of the mind, and somnolence. It enters the pericardium meridian of hand-jueyin and the liver meridian of foot-jueyin. It is bitter and sweet in taste and slightly cold in property. It is nontoxic. It is mainly used to treat fistula, promote urination, disperse phlegm and the thirst due to heat. It could be used in decoction for the yin syndrome to dispel the repulsion cold. It is similar in treating the pathogenic heat in the body. The tea is bitter. *Jing* says: The bitterness has the function of discharging and conducting downward, thus it could clear the heat in the head and eyes.

秦 皮

气寒，味苦。无毒。

《液》云：主热利下重，下焦虚。《经》云：以苦坚之。故用白头翁、黄柏、秦皮，苦之剂也。治风寒湿痹，目中青翳白膜，男子少精，妇人带下，小儿惊痫，宜作汤洗目，俗呼为白梣木。取皮渍水，浸出青蓝色，与紫草同用，以增光晕尤佳。大戟为之使。恶吴茱萸。

Qinpi [秦皮, ash, Fraxini Cortex]

It is cold in property, bitter in taste, and nontoxic.

Ye [《汤液本草》, *Materia Medica for Decoctions*] says: It is mainly used to treat the dysentery with rectal heaviness and deficiency in the lower energizer. *Jing* says: Bitterness is used to consolidate. Thus Baitouweng [白头翁, pulsatilla Pulsatillae Radix], Huangbo [黄柏, bark of amur corktree, Cortex Phellodendri] and Qinpi [秦皮, ash, Fraxini Cortex] are the medicinal herbs to fortify with bitterness. It is used to treat the damp impediment due to wind-cold, the green-blue screen and white membrane in eyes, the scant semen of men, the vaginal discharge of women, and the infantile convulsion and epilepsy. It is suitable to be made into decoction to wash eyes. It is usually called Baixunmu. Take the bark and immerse it in water till it becomes green-blue. Using it together with Zicao [紫草, arnebia root, Radix Lithospermi] can make it more bright and effective. Daji [大戟, euphorbia, Euphorbiae seu Knoxiae Radix] serves as its guiding medicinal herb, and it is averse to Wuzhuyu [吴茱萸, evodia, Fructus Evodiae].

桑白皮

气寒,味苦。酸,甘而辛,甘厚辛薄。无毒。

入手太阴经。

《象》云:主伤中五劳羸瘦,补虚益气,除肺气,止唾血、热渴,消水肿,利水道。

《心》云:甘以固元气,辛以泄肺气之有余。

《本草》云:治伤中五劳六极羸瘦,崩中脉绝,补虚益气。去肺中水气,唾血热渴,水肿,腹满胪胀,利水道,去寸白,可缝金疮。出土者,杀人。续断、麻子、桂心为之使。忌铁铅。

Sangbaipi [桑白皮, white mulberry root-bark, Cortex Mori]

It is cold in property and bitter in taste. It is sour, sweet and pungent. Its sweetness is greater than its pungency. It is nontoxic.

It enters the lung meridian of hand-taiyin.

Xiang [《药类法象》, *Rules for the Use of Medicinal Herbs*] says: It is mainly used to treat the five taxations with emaciation, supplement vacuity, replenish qi, remove the excessive lung qi, stanch the spitting of blood, remove the thirst due to heat, disperse edema, and free the waterways.

Xin [《用药心法》, *Gist for the Use of Medicinal Herbs*] says: The sweetness can consolidate the original qi, and the pungency can discharge the excessive lung qi.

Ben Cao says: It is used to treat middle damage, five overstrains, six extremes, emaciation, profuse vaginal bleeding, weak pulse, supplement deficiency and replenish qi. It is used to eliminate the fluid retention in the lung, blood spitting, the thirst due to heat, edema, abdominal fullness, free the waterways, eliminate the pinworm and sew trauma caused by metal. It may be harmful to people if growing out of the earth. Xuduan [续断, dipsacus, Dipsaci Radix], Mazi [麻子, cannabis fruit, Cannabis Fructus] and Guixin [桂心, shaved cinnamon bark, Cinnamomi Cortex Rasus] are used as its guiding medicinal herbs. It contraindicates the iron and the lead.

梓 白 皮

气寒,味苦。无毒。

《本草》云:主热,去三虫,治目中疾。生河内山谷,今近道皆有之。木似梧桐。

Zibaipi [梓白皮, root-bark of ovate catalpa, Cortex Catalpae Ovatae Radicis]

It is cold in property, bitter in taste, and nontoxic.

Ben Cao says: It is mainly used to treat fever and eliminate three kinds of worms. It treats the illness in eyes. It grows in mountains and valleys, and today it can be found in places nearby. The plant resembles firmiana.

紫 葳（即凌霄花）

气微寒,味酸。无毒。

《本草》云:主妇人产乳余疾,崩中,症瘕血闭,寒热羸瘦,养胎。茎、叶味苦,无毒。主痿蹶,益气。

《日华子》云:根,治热身风痒,游风风疹。治淤血带下,花、叶功用同。又云:凌霄花,治酒齄,热毒风刺,妇人血膈游风,崩中带下。

《衍义》云:木也,紫葳花是也。畏卤咸。

Ziwei [紫葳, campsis flower, Campsis Flos] (also called Lingxiaohua)

It is slightly cold in property and sour in taste. It is nontoxic.

Ben Cao says: It is mainly used to treat the remnant disease after the delivery of babies, profuse vaginal bleeding, abdominal mass, blood block, cold-heat disease and emaciation, and nourish the fetus. The stalks and leaves are bitter in taste and nontoxic. It is mainly used to treat the flaccidity of legs and replenish qi.

Ri Hua Zi [《日华子》, *Materia Medica of Ri Hua-Zi*] says: The root is used to treat the pruritus due to severe heat, and the urticaria. It is used to treat blood stasis and vaginal discharge. The function of its flowers and leaves is the same. It is also said that Lingxiaohua is used to treat rosacea, heat toxin, the pruritus due to wind, the blood occlusion due to urticaria, metrostaxis and leukorrhea.

Yan Yi [《衍义》, *Extension of the Materia Medica*] says: Ziwei [紫葳, campsis flower, Campsis Flos] belongs to the tree category. It is restrained by salt.

诃 黎 勒

气温,味苦。苦而酸,性平,味厚,阴也,降也。苦重酸轻。无毒。

《象》云:主腹胀满,不下饮食;消痰下气,通利津液,破胸膈结气;治久痢赤白,肠风。去核,捣细用。

《心》云:经曰肺苦气上逆,急食苦以泄之,以酸补之。苦重泻气,酸轻不能补肺,故嗽药中不用。俗名诃子、随风子。

《本草》云:主冷气,心腹满,下食。仲景治气痢,以诃黎勒十枚,面裹,煻灰火中煨之。令面黄熟,去核,细研为末,和粥饮顿服。

《衍义》云:气虚人亦宜缓缓煨熟,少服。此物能涩肠而又泄气,盖其味苦涩故尔。其子未熟时,风飘堕者,谓之随风子。

Helile [诃黎勒, chebule, Terminalia Chebula Retz.]

It is warm in property and bitter in taste. It is bitter and sour, mild in property and thick in flavor. It pertains to yin and descends. It is heavy in bitterness, light in sourness, and nontoxic.

Xiang [《药类法象》, *Rules for the Use of Medicinal Herbs*] says: It is mainly used to treat distention and the fullness of the abdomen, indigestion, disperse phlegm, descend qi, disinhibit fluid, break the qi accumulation in the chest and diaphragm, and treat the chronic dysentery with bloody leucorrhea and the intestinal wind. Remove the kernel and pound it into powder before usage.

Xin [《用药心法》, *Gist for the Use of Medicinal Herbs*] says: According to *Jing*, the counter-flow of the bitter qi in the lung can be discharged with bitter medicinal herbs, and supplemented with sour medicinal herbs. Being heavy in bitterness, it can drain qi, while being light in sourness, it can not supplement the lung, thus it can not be used in the medicinal herb for cough. It is commonly referred to as Kezi [诃子, medicine terminalia fruit, Fructus Chebulae] or Suifengzi [随风子, chebule, Chebulae Fructus].

Ben Cao says: It is mainly used to treat the cold qi, the fullness of the heart and abdomen, and digest food. Zhang Zhongjing used ten pieces of it to treat the qi dysentery. Wrap it with flour and bake it in the hot ash. When the flour is yellowish and done, remove the kernel and grind it into powder, and take it with porridge during the meal time.

Yan Yi [《衍义》, *Extension of the Materia Medica*] says: Bake it slowly till it is done, take a small amount each time to treat qi deficiency. It can astringe the intestines and discharge qi for its bitter and astringent taste. The fruits that are not ripe and flow down with wind are called Suifengzi [随风子, chebule, Chebulae Fructus].

杜 仲

味辛、甘、平、温，无毒。阳也，降也。

《本草》云：主腰脊痛，补中益精气，坚筋骨，强志；除阴下湿痒，小便余沥，脚中酸疼，不欲践地。久服，轻身、耐老。恶蛇脱皮、玄参。

《日华子》云：暖，治肾劳，腰脊挛，入药炙用。

Duzhong [杜仲, eucommia, Eucommiae Cortex]

It is pungent and sweet in taste, mild and warm in property, and nontoxic. It pertains to yang and descends.

Ben Cao says: It is mainly used to treat the pain in the lumbar spine, supplement the middle energizer, boost the essence, consolidate sinews and bones, and strengthen the mind; it eliminates the genital pruritus due to dampness, the dribbling urination, the aching pain in the feet causing people unable to step on the ground. The long-term taking of it can relax the body and prevent aging. It is averse to Shetui [蛇蜕, snake slough, Periostracum Serpentis] and Xuanshen [玄

参, figwort root, Radix Scrophulariae].

Ri Hua Zi [《日华子》, *Materia Medica of Ri Hua-Zi*] says: Since it has the function of warming, it is used to treat the taxation of the kidney and the hypertonicity of the lumbar spine. It can be used in moxibustion.

琥 珀

气平,味甘,阳也。
《珍》云:利小便,清肺。
《本草》云:安五脏,定魂魄,消淤血,通五淋。杵细用。
《药性论》云:君。治产后血疹痛。
《日华子》云:疗蛊毒,壮心,明目磨翳。止心痛、癫邪,破症结。

Hupo [琥珀, Amber, Ambrum]

It is mild in property and sweet in taste, pertaining to yang.

Zhen [《珍珠囊》, *Pouch of Pearls*] says: It promotes urination and clears the lung.

Ben Cao says: It is used to harmonize the five zang-organs, pacify the ethereal soul and the corporeal soul, disperse blood stasis and free five stranguries. Pound it into powder before use.

Yao Xing Lun [《药性论》, *Treatise on Medicinal Properties*] says: It is used as a sovereign medicinal herb. It is used to treat the pain caused by blood papules after delivery.

Ri Hua Zi [《日华子》, *Materia Medica of Ri Hua-Zi*] says: It is used to treat the parasitic toxin, strengthen the heart, brighten the eyes and remove the eye screens. It is used to remove the pain in the heart, epilepsy and break concretions and accumulations.

郁 李 仁

味苦、辛,阴中之阳。辛、苦,阴也。
《珍》云:破血润燥。

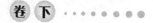

《本草》云：郁李根主齿龈肿，龋齿坚齿，去百虫。

《药性论》云：根，治齿痛，宣结气，破积聚。

《日华子》云：根凉，无毒，治小儿发热，作汤浴。风蚛牙，浓煎含之。

Yuliren [郁李仁, bush cherry kernel, Pruni Semen]

It is bitter and pungent in taste, pertaining to yang within yin.

Zhen [《珍珠囊》, *Pouch of Pearls*] says: It is used to break blood stasis and moisten dryness.

Ben Cao says: The root is mainly used to treat the swollen gum and caries, strengthen the teeth and kill all kinds of worms.

Yao Xing Lun [《药性论》, *Treatise on Medicinal Properties*] says: The root can be used to treat toothache, remove qi stagnation and break accumulations and gatherings.

Ri Hua Zi [《日华子》, *Materia Medica of Ri Hua-Zi*] says: The root is cold in property and nontoxic. It is used to treat the infantile fever in the form of medicated bath. Keeping the dense decoction in the mouth can treat the decay of teeth.

巴 豆

气温，味辛，生温，熟寒。有大毒。

《本草》云：主伤寒温疟寒热，破症瘕结聚，坚积留饮，痰癖，大腹水胀。荡涤五脏六腑，开通闭塞。利水谷道，去恶肉，除鬼毒蛊疰邪物，杀虫鱼。疗女子月闭，烂胎，金疮脓血不利，丈夫阴癞。杀斑猫毒，健脾开胃。

易老云：斩关夺门之将，大宜详悉，不可轻用。

《雷公》云：得火则良，若急治，为水谷道路之剂，去皮心膜油，生用。若缓治，为消坚磨积之剂，炒烟去，令紫黑，研用。可以通肠，可以止泄，世所不知也。仲景治百病客忤，备急丸主之。巴豆、杏仁例，及加减寒热佐使，五色并余例，并见《元戎》。

《珍》云：去胃中寒湿。

Badou [巴豆, croton, Crotonis Fructus]

It is mild in property and pungent in taste. The raw ones are warm and the ripe ones are cold in property. It is greatly toxic.

Ben Cao says: It is mainly used to treat cold damage, warm malaria and cold-heat disease, break abdominal mass, remove hard accumulation and persistent fluid retention, phlegm aggregation, and the water distention in the abdomen. It clears the five zang-organs and frees the six fu-organs, and opens the blocking, promotes the digestion of food, dispels the severely damaged muscles, expels the pathogenic factors like ghost, parasitic toxin and pathogens, and kills worms and fish. It is used to treat the menstrual block of women, abort the dead fetus, treat the trauma caused by metal, pus and blood, and the impotence of men. It dispels the toxin of Banmao [斑猫, mylabris, Mylabris], invigorates the spleen and promotes the appetite.

Yi Lao (Zhang Yuansu) said: The medicinal herb plays the leading role in treating diseases, which should be known clearly before use.

Lei Gong [《雷公炮制论》, *Grandfather Lei's Discussion of Herb Preparation*] says: The processed ones are of good quality. If it is used to treat emergent diseases, it functions to clear the route of digestion. Remove the skin and kernel before using it. If it is used to treat chronic diseases, it functions to disperse the hard accumulations. Bake it till the color is dark purple and grind it. It can be used to free the intestine and stanch diarrhea, which is unknown by people. Zhang Zhongjing used Beiji Pill to treat various diseases including the infantile fright. The formula includes Badou [巴豆, croton, Crotonis Fructus] and Xingren [杏仁, bitter apricot seed, Semen Armeniacae Amarum], and other cold-heat assistant and guiding medicinal herbs, which is also recorded in *Yuan Rong* [《医垒元戎》, *Medicinal Administration as Military Commander*].

Zhen [《珍珠囊》, *Pouch of Pearls*] says: It eliminates the dampness and cold in the stomach.

芫 花

气温,味辛、苦。有小毒。

《本草》云:主咳逆上气,喉鸣喘急,咽肿短气,蛊毒鬼疟,痈肿疝瘕。杀虫鱼。消胸中痰水,喜(音去)唾,水肿,五水在五脏、皮肤及腰痛。下寒毒、肉毒。

久服令人虚。仲景治太阳中风,胁下痛,呕逆者,可攻,十枣汤主之。

《液》云:胡洽治痰癖饮,加以大黄、甘草,五物同煎。以相反主之,欲其大吐也。治之大略,水者,肺、肾、胃三经所主,有五脏、六腑、十二经之部分,上而头,中而四肢,下而腰脐,外而皮毛,中而肌肉,内而筋骨。脉有尺寸之殊,浮沉之异,不可轻泻,当知病在何经何脏,误用则害深。然大意泄湿,内云五物者,即甘遂、大戟、芫花、大黄、甘草也。

Yanhua [芫花, genkwa, Genkwa Flos]

It is warm in property, and pungent and bitter in taste. It is slightly toxic.

Ben Cao says: It is mainly used to treat the cough with dyspnea and the counter-flow of qi, the laryngeal stridor, the swelling of the throat, shortness of breath, the parasitic toxin, the severe malaria, the abscess and hernia with conglomeration. It kills worms and fish. It disperses the phlegm in the chest, removes saliva, edema, five kinds of fluid in the five zang-organs and skin, and the pain in the waist. It dispels cold toxin and flesh toxin. The long-term taking of it will make people weak. Zhang Zhongjing mainly used Shizao Decoction to treat the taiyang wind-invasion syndrome, the pain in the rib-side and vomiting.

Ye [《汤液本草》, *Materia Medica for Decoctions*] says: Hu Qia used five kinds of medicinal herbs including Dahuang [大黄, rhubarb root and rhizome, Radix et Rhizoma Rhei] and Gancao [甘草, liquorice root, Glycyrrhiza uralensis Fisch.] to treat the phlegm aggregation. The purpose of using the medicinal in antagonism is to cause the severe vomiting of the patient. The general strategy of treating diseases is to know that the channels of the lung, kidney and stomach govern water, which is distributed in the five zang-organs, six fu-organs and twelve channels. The head is in the upper part; limbs, the middle; waist and umbilicus, the lower; hair and skin, the exterior; muscle, the middle, and sinews and bones, the interior of the body. Since the pulse manifestations are completely different in Chi and Cun pulse, floating and deep pulse, thus purging method should be cautiously considered before its being taken. The location of the diseases should be made clear and the misuse of treatment method can lead to serious damage. To discharge dampness, Gansui [甘遂, kansui, Kansui Radix], Daji [大戟, euphorbia, Euphorbiae seu Knoxiae Radix], Yanhua [芫花, genkwa,

Genkwa Flos], Dahuang [大黄, rhubarb root and rhizome, Radix et Rhizoma Rhei] and Gancao [甘草, liquorice root, Glycyrrhiza uralensis Fisch] are generally used.

苏 木

气平，味甘、咸。甘而酸、辛，性平。甘胜于酸辛，阳中之阴也。无毒。
《本草》云：主破血，产后血胀闷欲死者。排脓止痛，消痈肿瘀血，妇人月水不调及血晕口噤。
《心》云：性平，甘胜于酸辛。去风，与防风同用。
《珍》云：破死血。

Sumu [苏木, sappan wood, Lignum Sappan]

It is mild in property, and sweet and salty in taste. It is sweet, sour and pungent. Its sweetness is greater than sourness and pungency. It pertains to yin within yang, and it is nontoxic.

Ben Cao says: It is mainly used to break blood stasis, postpartum distention and the oppression of blood. It is used to expel pus and relieve pain, dispel abscess and static blood, and regulate menstruation, treat anemic fainting and clenched jaw.

Xin [《用药心法》, *Gist for the Use of Medicinal Herbs*] says: It is mild in property, and its sweetness is greater than sourness and pungency. It can be used together with Fangfeng [防风, divaricate saposhnikovia root, Radix Saposhnikoviae] to disperse wind.

Zhen [《珍珠囊》, *Pouch of Pearls*] says: It is used to break blood stasis.

川楝子

气寒，味苦、平。有小毒。
《本草》云：治伤寒大热烦躁，杀三虫疥疡，利小便。杵细用。
《珍》云：入心，主上下部腹痛。

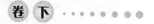

Chuanlianzi [川楝子, szechwan chinaberry fruit, Fructus Meliae Toosendan]

It is cold and mild in property, and bitter in taste. It is slightly toxic.

Ben Cao says: It is used to treat the cold damage, and the vexation and agitation due to great heat, eliminate three kinds of parasitic worms, scabies and ulcer, and promote urination. Pound it into powder before use.

Zhen [《珍珠囊》, *Pouch of Pearls*] says: It enters the heart and is mainly used to treat the abdominal pain in the upper and lower part.

金 铃 子

酸苦,阴中之阳。

《珍》云:心暴痛,非此不能除,即川楝子也。

Jinlingzi [金铃子, toosendan, Toosendan Fructus]

It is sour and bitter, pertaining to yang within yin.

Zhen [《珍珠囊》, *Pouch of Pearls*] says: It is essential in treating the great pain in the heart. It is also called Chuanlianzi [川楝子, szechwan chinaberry fruit, Fructus Meliae Toosendan].

没 药

味苦、平。无毒。

《本草》云:主破血止痛,疗金疮杖疮,诸恶疮,痔漏卒下血,目中翳,晕痛,肤赤。生波斯国,似安息香,其块大小不定,黑色。

Moyao [没药, myrrh, Myrrha]

It is bitter in taste and mild in property. It is nontoxic.

Ben Cao says: It is mainly used to break blood stasis, relieve pain, treat the trauma caused by metal or beat, all kinds of malign sores, the bleeding due to hemorrhoids, and eliminate the screens in eyes, dizziness, pain and the red skin.

It grows in Persia, and it is similar to Anxixiang [安息香, benzoin, Benzoinum]. It is of various sizes and is black.

梧 桐 泪

味咸。
《珍》云：瘰疬，非此不能除。
《本草》云：味咸、苦，大寒，无毒。主大毒热，心腹烦满，水和服之取吐。又主牛马急黄，黑汗，水研三二两，灌之，立瘥。
《日华子》云：治风虫牙齿痛，杀火毒并面毒。
《海药》云：主风疳䘌，齿牙疼痛，骨槽风劳。能软一切物。多服，令人吐也。又为金银焊药。

Wutonglei [梧桐泪, tear of fermiana platanifolia, Firmiana Platanifolia (L. f.) Marsili]

It is salty in taste.

Zhen [《珍珠囊》, *Pouch of Pearls*] says: It is essential to treat scrofula.

Ben Cao says: It is salty and bitter in taste, strongly cold and nontoxic. It is mainly used to treat the strong toxic heat, and the vexation and fullness in the heart and abdomen. Its mixture with water will make people vomit. It is also used to treat the acute jaundice and the dark sweat of cattle and horses. Grind two or three Liang, mix it with water, and feed the cattle and horses with it, which can ease the syndromes instantly.

Ri Hua Zi [《日华子》, *Materia Medica of Ri Hua-Zi*] says: It is used to treat the tooth decay and toothache, and eliminate the fire toxin and the facial toxin.

Hai Yao [《海药本草》, *Herbal Foundation of Overseas*] says: It is mainly used to treat ulcerative gingivitis, toothache and maxillary osteomyelitis. It has the function of softening. The excessive taking of it can make people vomit. It can also be used to weld gold and silver.

桑东南根

《时习》云：根暖，无毒。研汁，治小儿天吊，惊痫客忤，及傅鹅口疮，大效。

Sangdongnan Gen [桑东南根, root of white mulberry, Cortex Mori]

Shi Xi [《时习》, *Constant Practice*] says: The root is warm in property and nontoxic. Grind it into juice and it can be used to treat the rolled-up eyes of infants, the fright epilepsy and the infantile fright. It is very effective in treating thrush.

果 部
Fruit Herbs

大 枣

气温,味甘,气厚,阳也。无毒。

《珍》云:味甘,补经不足,以缓阴血。

《液》云:主养脾气,补津液,强志。三年陈者,核中仁,主腹痛,恶气卒疰忤,治心悬。《经》云:助十二经脉,治心腹邪气,和百药,通九窍,补不足气。生者多食,令人腹胀注泄。蒸熟食,补肠胃,肥中益气。中满者勿食甘,甘者令人中满,故大建中汤,心下痞者,减饴、枣,与甘草同例。

Dazao [大枣, Chinese date, Fructus Jujubae]

It is warm in property, sweet in taste and thick in nature. It pertains to yang, and it is nontoxic.

Zhen [《珍珠囊》, *Pouch of Pearls*] says: It is sweet in taste. It can be used to supplement the insufficiency of channels and the yin blood.

Ye [《汤液本草》, *Materia Medica for Decoctions*] says: It is mainly used to nourish the spleen qi, supplement the fluids and strengthen the mind. The seeds in the kernel which have been kept for three years are mainly used to treat the abdominal pain, the malign qi and the chronic infectious disease, and relieve the suspension of the stomach. *Jing* says: Harmonizing varieties of medicinal herbs, it is used to assist twelve channels, eliminate the pathogenic qi in the heart and abdomen, free the nine orifices, and supplement the insufficiency of qi. The excessive taking of the raw ones can cause abdominal distention and diarrhea. The steamed ones can supplement the stomach and intestines, tonify the middle energizer and replenish qi. Patients with abdominal fullness must not take sweet herbs because it can make the situation worse. Thus when Dajianzhong Decoction is used to treat the epigastric stuffiness, the amount of malt sugar and jujube should be reduced, so is Gancao [甘草, liquorice root, Glycyrrhiza Uralensis Fisch].

生 枣

味甘、辛。

多食，令人多寒热，羸瘦者不可食。叶，覆麻黄能令出汗。生河东平泽，杀乌头毒。

Shengzao [生枣, fresh jujube, Fructus Ziziphi Jujubae]

It is sweet and pungent in taste.

The excessive taking of it can cause the cold-heat syndrome, and it should not be taken by people with emaciation syndrome. The leaves, used together with Mahuang [麻黄, ephedra, Herba Ephedrae], can promote sweat. It grows along the river in He Dong. It eliminates the toxin of Wutou [乌头, common monkshood, Aconitum carmichaeli Debx].

陈 皮

气温，味微苦。辛而苦，味厚，阴也。无毒。

《象》云：能益气。加青皮，减半，去滞气，推陈致新。若补脾胃，不去白；若理胸中肺气，须去白。

《心》云：导胸中滞气，除客气。有白术，则补脾胃；无白术，则泻脾胃。然勿多用也。

《珍》云：益气利肺。有甘草，则补肺；无甘草，则泻肺。

《本草》云：主胸中痰热逆气，利水谷，下气，止呕咳。除膀胱留热停水，五淋，利小便。主脾不能消谷，气冲胸中，吐逆霍乱，止泻，去寸白虫。能除痰，解酒毒。海藏治酒毒，葛根陈皮茯苓甘草生姜汤。手太阴气逆，上而不下，宜以此

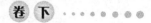

顺之。陈皮、白檀为之使。其芳香之气,清奇之味,可以夺橙也。

Chenpi [陈皮, dried tangerine peel, Pericarpium Citri Reticulatae]

It is warm in property and slightly bitter in taste. It is pungent, bitter and thick in flavor. It pertains to yin, and it is nontoxic.

Xiang [《药类法象》, *Rules for the Use of Medicinal Herbs*] says: It is used to replenish qi. Add Qingpi [青皮, immature tangerine peel, Pericarpium Citri Reticulatae Viride] into it and reduce its amount by half, which can eliminate the qi stagnation and promote the discharge of waste. For supplementing the spleen and stomach, keep the tangerine pith; for rectifying the lung qi, remove the tangerine pith.

Xin [《用药心法》, *Gist for the Use of Medicinal Herbs*] says: It could free the stagnant qi in the chest and eliminate the exogenous pathogenic qi. With Baizhu [白术, argehead atractylodes rhizome, Rhizoma Atractylodis Macrocephalae], it can supplement the spleen and stomach; without it, it can drain them. However, do not use it excessively.

Zhen [《珍珠囊》, *Pouch of Pearls*] says: It is used to replenish qi and disinhibit the lung. With Gancao [甘草, liquorice root, Glycyrrhiza uralensis Fisch], it can supplement the lung; without it, it can drain the lung.

Ben Cao says: It is mainly used to treat the phlegm-heat and the counter-flow of qi in the chest, promote the digestion of food, descend qi and stanch vomiting and cough. It removes the stagnant heat and water in the bladder and five stranguries. It promotes urination. It is mainly used to treat the spleen that does not digest, the qi surging into the chest, vomiting and cholera. It stanches diarrhea and kills pinworms. It dispels phlegm and resolves the liquor toxin. Hai Zang (Wang Haogu) used the decoction of Gegen [葛根, kudzuvine root, Radix Puerariae], Chenpi [陈皮, dried tangerine peel, Pericarpium Citri Reticulatae], Fuling [茯苓, Indian bread, Poria], Gancao [甘草, liquorice root, Glycyrrhiza uralensis Fisch] and Shengjiang [生姜, fresh ginger, Rhizoma Zingiberis Recens] to resolve the liquor toxin. It can also be used to smooth the qi counter-flow in the lung meridian of hand-taiyin. Chenpi [陈皮, dried tangerine peel, Pericarpium Citri Reticulatae] and Baitan [白檀, sapphire-berry sweetleaf, Symplocoris

Paniculatae Radix] are used as its guiding medicinal herbs. Its fragrant aroma and the fresh taste excel oranges.

青 皮

气温，味辛。苦而辛，性寒，气厚，阴也。

足厥阴经引经药，又入手少阳经。

《象》云：主气滞，消食，破积结膈气。去穰。

《心》云：厥阴经引经药也。有滞气则破滞气，无滞气则损真气。

《液》云：主气滞，下食，破积结及膈气。或云与陈皮一种。青皮小而未成熟，成熟而大者橘也，色红故名红皮。日久者佳，故名陈皮。如枳实、枳壳一种，实小而青，未穰；壳大而黄紫色，已穰。故壳高而治胸膈；实低而治心下。与陈皮治高，青皮治低同义。又云：陈皮、青皮二种，枳实、枳壳亦有二种。

Qingpi [青皮, immature tangerine peel, Pericarpium Citri Reticulatae Viride]

It is warm in property and pungent in taste. It is bitter and pungent in taste, cold in property and thick in nature. It pertains to yin.

It is a channel ushering drug which functions in the liver meridian of foot-jueyin, and it enters the triple energizer meridian of hand-shaoyang.

Xiang [《药类法象》, *Rules for the Use of Medicinal Herbs*] says: It is mainly used to treat qi stagnation, digest food, and break the accumulation and diaphragm qi. Remove the pulp before use.

Xin [《用药心法》, *Gist for the Use of Medicinal Herbs*] says: It is a channel ushering drug which functions in the liver meridian of foot-jueyin. If there is the stagnant qi in the patient, it can break it; but if not, it can damage the genuine qi.

Ye [《汤液本草》, *Materia Medica for Decoctions*] say: It is mainly used to treat qi stagnation, digest food, and break accumulation and diaphragm qi. It is also said that it is the same as Chenpi [陈皮, dried tangerine peel, Pericarpium Citri Reticulatae]. Qingpi [青皮, immature tangerine peel, Pericarpium Citri Reticulatae Viride] is the small and unripe kind, while the ripe and big kind is orange, and due to the reddish color, it is called Hongpi [红皮, cork-leaved snowbell, Styracis Suberifoliae Folium seu Radix]. The aged ones are of good quality, thus they are called Chenpi [陈皮, dried tangerine peel, Pericarpium Citri Reticulatae]. Zhishi [枳实, immature orange fruit, Fructus Aurantii Immaturus] and Zhiqiao [枳壳, orange fruit, Fructus Aurantii] are actually the same fruits in different stages. Zhishi is small and green, with no pulp yet; Zhiqiao is big and yellowish purple, with pulp already. Thus Zhiqiao, with the floating nature, is used to treat the diseases in the upper part, such as the chest and diaphragm; while Zhishi, with the sinking nature, is used to treat the diseases in the lower part, such as epigastrium. In this aspect, it is similar to Chenpi [陈皮, dried tangerine peel, Pericarpium Citri Reticulatae] and Qingpi [青皮, immature tangerine peel, Pericarpium Citri Reticulatae Viride]. It is also said that Chenpi [陈皮, dried tangerine peel, Pericarpium Citri Reticulatae] and Qingpi [青皮, immature tangerine peel, Pericarpium Citri Reticulatae Viride] are two different kinds of medicinal herbs, so are Zhishi [枳实, immature orange fruit, Fructus Aurantii Immaturus] and Zhiqiao [枳壳, orange fruit, Fructus Aurantii].

桃 仁

气温，味苦、甘，性平，苦重于甘，阴中阳也。无毒。

入手、足厥阴经。

《象》云：治大便血结、血秘、血燥，通润大便。七宣丸中，专治血结破血。以汤浸，去皮尖，研如泥用。

《心》云：苦以泄滞血，甘以生新血，故凝血须用。又去血中之热。

《本草》云：主瘀血血闭，症瘕邪气，杀小虫，止咳逆上气，消心下坚，除卒暴击血，通月水，止痛破血。入手足厥阴。

《衍义》云：老人虚秘，与柏子仁、大麻仁、松子仁等分。同研，溶白蜡和丸如桐子大。以少黄丹汤下，仲景治中焦畜血用之。

Taoren [桃仁, peach seed, Semen Persicae]

It is warm and mild in property, and bitter and sweet in taste. Its bitterness is greater than sweetness, pertaining to yang within yin. It is nontoxic.

It enters the meridian of the hand and foot-jueyin.

Xiang [《药类法象》, *Rules for the Use of Medicinal Herbs*] says: It is commonly used in treating hematochezia, constipation and blood dryness, and purging the stool. If made into Qixuan Pill, it is effective in treating hematochezia. It is usually immersed in decoction or ground into powder with skin and tip removed.

Xin [《用药心法》, *Gist for the Use of Medicinal Herbs*] says: Bitterness is used to relieve the blood stagnation while sweetness is good for generating the new blood. Therefore, Taoren [桃仁, peach seed, Semen Persicae] can be used to coagulate blood, which is also beneficial to remove the heat in blood.

Ben Cao says: It is mainly used to treat the blood stasis, the blockage of blood and the abdominal conglomeration caused by evil-qi, kill insects, stop the cough with dyspnea and the counter-flow of qi, break the lumps below the heart, eliminate the sudden and violent bleeding, promote menstruation, cease pain and promote the blood circulation. It enters the meridian of the hand and foot jueyin.

Yan Yi [《本草衍义》, *Extension of the Materia Medica*] says: If the old people have constipation due to deficiency, they can prepare the same amount of Taoren [桃仁, peach seed, Semen Persicae], Chinese arborvitae kernels, cannabis seeds and pine nut seeds respectively. After being ground, they can be dissolved in bleached beeswax and made into pills as big as the jatropha, which needs to be taken with Huangdan Decoction. It was used by Zhang Zhongjing to treat the blood stasis in the middle energizer.

杏 仁

气温,味甘、苦,冷利。有小毒。

入手太阴经。

《象》云:除肺燥,治风燥在胸膈间。麸炒,去皮尖用。

《心》云:散结润燥,散肺之风及热,是以风热嗽者用之。

《本草》云:主咳逆上气雷鸣,喉痹,下气,产乳金疮,寒心豚,惊痛,心下烦热,风气往来,时行头痛,解肌,消心下急,杀狗毒,破气,入手太阴。王朝奉治伤寒气上喘冲逆者,麻黄汤内加杏仁、陈皮;若气不喘冲逆者,减杏仁、陈皮。知其能泻肺也。

东垣云:杏仁下喘,用治气也。桃仁疗狂,用治血也。桃、杏仁俱治大便秘,当以气血分之。昼则难便,行阳气也;夜则难便,行阴血也。大肠虽属庚,为白肠,以昼夜言之,气血不可不分也。年虚人大便燥秘、不可过泄者,脉浮在气,杏仁、陈皮;脉沉在血,桃仁、陈皮。所以俱用陈皮者,以其手阳明病,与手太阴俱为表里也。贲门上主往来,魄门下主收闭,故王氏言肺与大肠为通道也。

Xingren [杏仁, bitter apricot seed, Semen Armeniacae Amarum]

It is warm in property, sweet and bitter in taste, cold in nature, and slightly toxic.

It enters the meridian of the hand-taiyin.

Xiang [《药类法象》, *Rules for the Use of Medicinal Herbs*] says: It can remove the lung dryness and the wind dryness in the chest and diaphragm. It is usually stir-fried with bran, skin and tip removed.

Xin [《用药心法》, *Gist for the Use of Medicinal Herbs*] says: It is used to resolve nodule, moisten dryness, and disperse the wind and heat in the lung. It is suitable to be taken by the patients who suffer from the cough caused by wind and heat.

Ben Cao says: It is mainly used to treat the cough with dyspnea and the counter-flow of qi, the thunderous sound in the throat and the throat impediment. It is also helpful to descend qi, cure the disease after the delivery of babies, treat the injuries caused by metal and the pathogenic cold that damages the heart, alleviate the pain caused by shock, eliminate the vexing fever below the heart, stop the alternate attacks of wind and qi, alleviate the epidemic exogenous headache, expel the pathogenic factors from muscles, and resolve the fullness and dull pain in the upper abdomen. It is in mutual suppression with Goudu [狗毒, Willowleaf Rhizome, Rhizoma Cynanchi Stauntonii], and breaks qi. It enters the meridian of the hand-taiyin. Wang Chaofeng treated patients with dyspnea and the qi counter-flow caused by the cold damage through putting Xingren [杏仁, bitter apricot seed, Semen Armeniacae Amarum] and Chenpi [陈皮, Tangerine Peel, Pericarpium Citri Reticulatae] into Mahuang Decoction. If the patient has the syndrome of the adverse flow of qi without dyspnea, the amount of Xingren [杏仁, bitter apricot seed, Semen Armeniacae Amarum] and Chenpi [陈皮, Tangerine Peel, Pericarpium Citri Reticulatae] should be reduced. The function is known to clear away the lung heat.

Li Dongyuan said: Xingren [杏仁, bitter apricot seed, Semen Armeniacae Amarum] is effective to alleviate dyspnea and treat the diseases related with qi. As Taoren [桃仁, peach seed, Semen Persicae] is useful in treating mania, it can be used to cure the diseases related with blood. Although both Taoren [桃仁, peach seed, Semen Persicae] and Xingren [杏仁, bitter apricot seed, Semen Armeniacae Amarum] can treat constipation, syndromes should be distinguished clearly whether it is the disorder of qi or blood. If patients have constipation in the daytime, the yang qi should be conducted. If patients have constipation at night, the yin blood should be conducted. Large intestines rank the seventh in heavenly stems and earthly branches, being white intestines. Therefore, taking day and night into consideration, it is necessary to distinguish between qi and blood syndromes. For the weak people who have constipation but can not endure the excessive defecation and the floating pulse due to the qi deficiency, Xingren [杏仁, bitter apricot seed, Semen Armeniacae Amarum] and Chenpi [陈皮, Tangerine Peel, Pericarpium Citri Reticulatae] are recommended. While for those who have deep pulse due to the blood deficiency, Taoren [桃仁, peach seed, Semen Persicae] and Chenpi [陈皮, Tangerine Peel, Pericarpium Citri Reticulatae] are advised. The reason why Chenpi [陈皮, Tangerine Peel, Pericarpium Citri Reticulatae] is adopted in both cases is that the large intestines meridian of hand-yangming pertains to the large intestines and linked with the lung; the lung meridian of hand-taiyin pertains to the lung and linked with the large intestines. Cardia, located at the upper part of gastric cavity, is mainly responsible for transporting food from the mouth through the esophagus into the stomach while anus, located at the lower part to the pylorus, and claims the ending of food digestion. Therefore, Wang Haogu says the lung and large intestines serve as passages connected with each other.

乌 梅

气平，味酸。酸温，阳也。无毒。

《象》云：主下气，除热烦满，安心调中，治痢止渴。以盐为白梅，亦入除痰药。去核用。

《心》云：收肺气。

《本草》云：主肢体痛，偏枯不仁，死肌。去青黑痣恶疾，止下痢，好唾口干，去骨间热。又方，治一切恶疮肉出，以乌梅烧为灰，杵末，敷上，恶肉立尽。仲景治吐蛔下利，乌梅丸。

Wumei［乌梅, smoked plum, Fructus Mume］

It is mild in property and sour in taste. Being of sour in nature and warm in property, it pertains to yang. It is nontoxic.

Xiang［《药类法象》, *Rules for the Use of Medicinal Herbs*］says：It is mainly used to descend qi, and eliminate heat, vexation and fullness. It is also effective to tranquilize patients, coordinate the cold-heat in their spleens and stomachs, relieve diarrhea and thirst. The salted and dried one is called white plum, which is also included in drugs to remove sputum. It should be used after removing the seed.

Xin［《用药心法》, *Gist for the Use of Medicinal Herbs*］says：It is effective to restore the lung qi.

Ben Cao says：It can be used to treat the pain in limbs, hemiplegia, the numbness of limbs and the muscle necrosis. It also treats the melanotic nevus, diarrhea, the excessive spittle, the dryness in mouth, and the heat of bones. Another prescription shows that it can erode all kinds of vicious muscles if burned into ash, pestled into powder and compressed on the sore. Wumei Pill was adopted by Zhang Zhongjing to cure the vomiting of roundworms and diarrhea.

木　瓜

气温，味酸。

入手足太阴经。

《本草》云：治脚气湿痹，邪气霍乱，大吐下，转筋不止。益肺而去湿，和胃而滋脾。

《衍义》云：木瓜得木之正，故入筋。以铅白霜涂之，则失酸味，受金制也。此物入肝，故益筋与血。病腰肾脚膝无力，此物不可缺也。

东垣云：气脱则能收，气滞则能和。

雷公云：调荣卫，助谷气是也。

Mugua［木瓜，common floweringqince fruit, Fructus Chaenomelis］

It is warm in property and sour in taste.

It enters the meridian of the hand and foot taiyin.

Ben Cao says: It is used to treat beriberi, the impediment due to dampness, the pathogenic qi, cholera, severe vomiting and diarrhea, and persistent spasm. It is used to replenish the lung, expel dampness, harmonize the stomach and nourish the spleen.

Yan Yi ［《本草衍义》, *Extension of the Materia Medica*］ says: Mugua ［木瓜, chaenomeles, Chaenomelis Fructus］ pertains to the wood among the five elements to which the liver belongs, so it enters the sinews. If coated with lead frost, Mugua ［木瓜, chaenomeles, Chaenomelis Fructus］ will lose the sour taste since the wood is inhibited by metal. As it enters the liver, it benefits sinews and blood. It is indispensable for treating the diseases of the waist and kidney, and the lassitude in feet and knees.

Li Dongyuan said: For the patients who have the exhaustion of qi, it can help restore qi; while for those who have qi stagnation, it can harmonize qi.

Lei Gong (Lei Xiao) said: Mugua ［木瓜, chaenomeles, Chaenomelis Fructus］ is useful to regulate the nutrient qi and the defensive qi, which is good for the stomach qi.

甘李根白皮

《时习》云：根皮大寒，主消渴，止心烦，气逆奔豚。仲景奔豚汤中用之。

Ganligen Baipi ［甘李根白皮, root-bark of Japanese plum, Prunus Salicina Lindl］

Shi Xi ［《时习》, *Constant Practice*］ says: It is great cold in property, mainly used to treat diabetes, dysphoria, qi counter-flow and Bentun. Zhang Zhongjing included it into his Bentun Decoction.

菜　部
Vegetable Herbs

荆 芥 穗

气温，味辛、苦。

《本草》云：辟邪毒，利血脉，通宣五脏不足气，能发汗，除劳渴。杵，和醋封毒肿。去枝梗，手搓碎用，治产后血晕如神。动渴疾，多食，熏五脏神，破结气。

Jingjiesui [荆芥穗, schizonepetae spica, Herba Schizonepetae]

It is warm in property, and pungent and bitter in taste.

Ben Cao says: It can be used to remove the evil toxin, unblock the blood and vessels, regulate and disperse the deficient qi in the five zang-organs, induce diaphoresis, and remove thirst. After being pestled, it can be used to treat the toxic swelling together with vinegar. Remove the peduncles and rub into pieces, Jingjiesui [荆芥穗, schizonepetae spica, Herba Schizonepetae] is very effective to treat the postpartum hemorrhagic syncope. It also treats thirst and polyphagia. It can fumigate the spirit of the five zang-organs and break the qi stagnation.

生 姜

气温，味辛。辛而甘，微温，气味俱轻，阳也。无毒。

《象》云：主伤寒头痛鼻塞，咳逆上气，止呕吐，治痰嗽。生与干同治。与半夏等分，治心下急痛，剪细用。

《心》云：能制半夏、厚朴之毒。发散风寒，益元气，大枣同用。辛温，与芍药同用，温经散寒，呕家之圣药也。辛以散之，呕为气不散也。此药能行阳而散气。

《珍》云：益脾胃、散风寒。久服，去臭气、通神明。

孙真人云：为呕家之圣药。

或问东垣曰：生姜辛温入肺，如何是入胃口？曰：俗皆以心下为胃口者，非也。咽门之下，受有形之物，系胃之系，便为胃口。与肺同处，故入肺而开胃口也。又问曰：人云夜间勿食生姜，食则令人闭气，何也？曰：生姜辛温，主开发，夜则气本收敛，反食之，开发其气，则违天道，是以不宜食。此以平人论之可也，若有病则不然。姜屑比之干姜，不热；比之生姜，不润。以干生姜代干姜者，以其不僭故也。

《本草》云：秦椒为之使。杀半夏、莨菪毒。恶黄芩、黄连、天鼠粪。

Shengjiang [生姜, fresh ginger, Rhizoma Zingiberis Recens]

It is warm in property and pungent in taste. Being pungent and sweet, slightly warm in nature with mild odor, it pertains to yang. It is nontoxic.

Xiang [《药类法象》, *Rules for the Use of Medicinal Herbs*] says: It is mainly used to treat headache and the nasal congestion due to the cold damage, the cough with dyspnea and the counter-flow of qi, vomitings, and the cough with phlegm. Both fresh gingers and dried gingers are effective in the treatment. If used in equal amount with Banxia [半夏, pinellia, Rhizoma Pinelliae], Shengjiang [生姜, fresh ginger, Rhizoma Zingiberis Recens] can treat the sharp pain below the heart after being sliced into strips.

Xin [《用药心法》, *Gist for the Use of Medicinal Herbs*] says: It is often added in the processing of Banxia [半夏, pinellia, Rhizoma Pinelliae] and Houpu [厚朴, magnolia bark, Cortex Magnoliae Officinalis] in order to remove their toxin. It is good for dispersing the wind-cold, and activating the primordial qi if taken together with Dazao [大枣, Chinese date, Fructus Jujubae]. As it is pungent in taste and warm in nature, Shengjiang [生姜, fresh ginger, Rhizoma Zingiberis Recens] is used to warm meridians and disperse cold if taken together with Shaoyao [芍药, Chinese herbaceous peony, Paeonia lactiflora Pall]. It is also one of the most effective medicinal herbs to cure vomiting because it is pungent in taste, and effective to disperse as the cause for vomiting is ascribed to the detention of qi. Shengjiang [生姜, fresh ginger, Rhizoma Zingiberis Recens] is used to activate yang and disperse qi.

Zhen [《珍珠囊》, *Pounch of Pearls*] says: It benefits the spleen and the stomach, and dissipates the wind-cold syndrome. The Long-term taking of it can expel the fetid odor, and cultivate spirit and mentality.

Sun Zhenren (Sun Simiao) said: It is one of the most effective medicinal herbs to cure vomiting.

Someone asked Li Dongyuan: Shengjiang [生姜, fresh ginger, Rhizoma Zingiberis Recens] is pungent in taste and warm in nature, entering the lung. Why do you say it enters the stomach? He answered: It is generally known that the stomach is located below the heart, but that is not true. The part that is below fauces and receives visible things, belonging to the stomach, is called cardia. The stomach connects with the lung; therefore, if Shengjiang [生姜, fresh ginger, Rhizoma Zingiberis Recens] enters the lung, it will stimulate the appetite. Someone asked again: As the old saying goes, Shengjiang [生姜, fresh ginger, Rhizoma Zingiberis Recens] is forbidden to eat at night. If eaten at night, the qi blocking may occur. Can you explain it? He answered: Shengjiang [生姜, fresh ginger, Rhizoma Zingiberis Recens] is pungent and warm with the function of dispersing qi. However, qi astringes at night. If people take Shengjiang [生姜, fresh ginger, Rhizoma Zingiberis Recens] at night, their qi will disperse, which violates the law of nature. As a result, it is not suitable to eat at night. Nevertheless, the above saying is applied to the healthy people rather than patients. Compared with Ganjiang [干姜, dry ginger, Rhizoma Zingiberis], ginger crumbs are not so hot; compared with Shengjiang [生姜, fresh ginger, Rhizoma Zingiberis Recens], they are not so moist. Ganjiang [干姜, dry ginger, Rhizoma Zingiberis] can be replaced by dried fresh gingers, because they are moderate in nature.

Ben Cao says: Qinjiao [秦椒, hot pepper, Capsici Fructus] is its assistance. It counteracts the toxin in Banxia [半夏, pinellia, Rhizoma Pinelliae] and Langdang [莨菪, henbane seed, Semen Hyoscyami]. It is averse to Huangling [黄芩, baical skullcap root, Radix Scutellariae], Huanglian [黄连, golden thread, Rhizoma Coptidis] and Tianshufen [天鼠粪, bat faeces, Feaces Vespertilio].

干 姜

气热,味大辛。辛,大热,味薄气厚,阳中之阴也。辛、温。无毒。

《象》云:治沉寒痼冷,肾中无阳,脉气欲绝,黑附子为引,用水煎二物,名姜附汤。亦治中焦有寒。水洗,慢火炮。

《心》云:发散寒邪,如多用则耗散元气,辛以散之,是壮火食气故也,须以生甘草缓之。辛热,散里寒,散阴寒。肺寒,与五味同用,治嗽,以胜寒蛔。此正气虚者,散寒,与人参同补药,温胃腹中寒,其平以辛热。

《珍》云:寒淫所胜,以辛散之。经炮则味苦。

《本草》云:主胸满,咳逆上气,温中止血,出汗。逐风湿痹,肠澼下利,寒冷腹痛,中恶霍乱,胀满,风邪诸毒,皮肤间结气,止唾血。生者尤良。主胸满,温脾燥胃,所以理中,其实主气而泄脾。

易老云:干姜能补下焦,去寒,故四逆汤用之。干姜本味辛,及见火候,稍苦,故止而不移,所以能治里寒。非若附子行而不止也。理中汤用此者,以其四顺也。

或云:干姜味辛热,人言补脾,今言泄而不言补者,何也?东垣谓:泄之一字,非泄脾之正气也,是泄脾中寒湿之邪,故以姜辛热之剂燥之,故曰泄脾也。

Ganjiang [干姜, dry ginger, Rhizoma Zingiberis]

It is hot in property and pungent in taste. It is pungent, greatly hot with light taste and strong smell, pertaining to yin within yang. It is pungent and warm, and nontoxic.

Xiang [《药类法象》, *Rules for the Use of Medicinal Herbs*] says: It is used to treat the lingering cold, the loss of yang in the kidney, and the exhaustion of the meridian qi. Heifuzi [黑附子, aconite, Radix Aconiti Praeparata] is its assistance. Decoct them together, and one can get Jiangfu Decoction. It is also used to treat the cold in the middle energizer. Clean it and then process it with mild fire.

Xin [《用药心法》, *Gist for the Use of Medicinal Herbs*] says: It can be used to disperse cold. However, if overtaken, it can consume and dissipate the primordial qi. Pungency is mainly for dispersing because the sthenic fire leads to the consumption of yin qi. Therefore, raw Gancao [甘草, liquorice root, Glycyrrhiza uralensis Fisch] can be used to relieve the symptom. Being pungent in taste and warm in nature, Ganjiang [干姜, dry ginger, Rhizoma Zingiberis] is effective to treat both the interior cold and the yin cold. If the lung is attacked by cold, Ganjiang [干姜, dry ginger, Rhizoma Zingiberis] should be taken together with herbs with five tastes in order to cure cough and beat the ascaris caused by cold. For the people who suffer qi deficiency, it can be used to disperse cold if taken with Renshen [人参, ginseng, Radix Ginseng] as a tonic. It is also effective to warm the stomach with its pungency and heat.

Zhen [《珍珠囊》, *Pounch of Pearls*] says: Excessive cold should be dispersed by pungency. After being processed, Ganjiang [干姜, dry ginger, Rhizoma Zingiberis] becomes bitter.

Ben Cao says: It is mainly used to treat the chest fullness, stop the cough with dyspnea and the counter-flow of qi, warm the middle internal organs, cease bleeding, and promote sweating. It is used to eliminate the wind impediment due to dampness, the intestinal afflux and dysentery, the abdominal pain caused by cold, the cholera affected by the pathogenic qi, the abdominal distension, the various toxins due to the wind pathogen, the qi stagnation in skin, and the spitting of blood. The fresh ginger functions better. Ganjiang [干姜, dry ginger, Rhizoma Zingiberis] is mainly used to treat the fullness of the chest, warm the spleen and dry the stomach. Therefore, it regulates the middle energizer by dominating qi and relieving the spleen.

Yi Lao (Zhang Yuansu) said: Ganjiang [干姜, dry ginger, Rhizoma Zingiberis] can nourish the lower energizer, and remove cold, thereby it is included in Sini Decoction. Ganjiang [干姜, dry ginger, Rhizoma Zingiberis] is pungent in flavor. If it is heated by fire, it becomes slightly bitter. Therefore, it is effective to treat the interior cold and prevent its transformation. Only Fuzi [附子, aconite, Radix Aconiti Praeparata] can achieve the similar effect. The reason why it is put into Lizhong Decoction relies on its four functions of regulation.

Someone asked: Ganjiang [干姜, dry ginger, Rhizoma Zingiberis] is pungent in taste and hot in nature. It was said that it could invigorate the spleen while nowadays people stress the function of discharging without mentioning the function of invigoration. Why is that? Li Dongyuan said: The word "discharging" here does not mean the discharging of the healthy qi in the spleen but the discharging of cold and dampness in it. Therefore, the spleen discharging actually refers to drying the dampness with its pungency and heat.

薄 荷

气温,味辛、苦,辛、凉。无毒。

手太阴经、厥阴经药。

《象》云:能发汗,通骨节,解劳乏。与薤相宜。新病瘥人,勿多食,令虚汗出不止。去枝梗,搓碎用。

《心》云:上行之药。

陈士良云:能引诸药入荣卫,又主风气壅并。

Bohe [薄荷, peppermint, Herba Menthae]

It is warm in property, pungent and bitter in flavor, and pungent and cold in nature. It is nontoxic.

It is the medicinal herb for the meridian of the hand-taiyin and the meridian of the hand-jueyin.

Xiang [《药类法象》, *Rules for the Use of Medicinal Herbs*] says: It is effective to induce sweating, regulate joints and relieve vexation. It can be taken with Xie [薤, bulb of longstamen onion, Bulbus Allii Macrostemi]. For the patients who have just recovered from diseases, it should not be overtaken because it may cause the persistent sweating due to debility. It should be smashed for use with twigs and peduncles removed.

Xin [《用药心法》, *Gist for the Use of Medicinal Herbs*] says: It is an ascending medicinal herb.

Chen Shiliang said: It can lead medicinal herbs to enter the nutrient qi and the defense qi, and treat the stagnation due to wind pathogen.

葱 白

气温,味辛。无毒。

入手太阴经、足阳明经。

《液》云:以通上下之阳也。《活人书》:伤寒头痛如破,连须葱白汤主之。

《心》云:通阳气,辛而甘,气厚味薄,阳也。发散风邪。

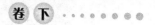

《本草》云：葱实，主明目，补中不足。其茎白，平。可作汤，主伤寒寒热出汗，中风面目肿，伤寒骨肉痛，喉痹不通，安胎，归目，除肝邪气，安中，利五脏，益目精，杀百药毒。葱根，主伤寒头痛。葱汁，平温，主溺血，解黎芦毒。

Congbai [葱白, scallion white, Allii Fistulosi Bulbus Recens]

It is warm in property and pungent in taste. It is nontoxic.

It enters the meridian of the hand-taiyin and the meridian of the foot-yangming.

Ye [《汤液本草》, *Materia Medica for Decoctions*] says：It is used to regulate the passageway between the upper and the lower of yang. *Huo Ren Shu* [《活人书》, *Book to Safeguard Life*] says：For the patients who suffer from the severe headache due to cold damage, Lianxu Congbai Decoction is effective.

Xin [《用药心法》, *Gist for the Use of Medicinal Herbs*] says：It regulates the yang qi, and it is pungent and sweet in taste with strong smell and light taste. It pertains to yang. It can be used to disperse the wind pathogen.

Ben Cao says：Congshi [葱实, fistular onion seed, Semen Allil Fistulosi] is mainly used to brighten eyes and supplement the middle energizer. The stalk of it is white and smooth. The stalk can be used to make soup, mainly for treating the sweating caused by cold damage, the facial swelling due to stroke, the pain in bones and flesh due to cold, and the throat impediment. It is also effective to prevent miscarriage. As it pertains to eyes, it can remove the pathogenic qi in the liver, calm the middle energizer, benefit the five zang-organs, supplement eyes, and remove the toxin of various herbs. The root of scallion is mainly used to treat the headache caused by cold damage. Being mild and warm, the succus of scallion is mainly used to treat the hematuria and toxin in Lilu [黎芦, falsehellebore root and rhizome, Veratrum Nigrum].

韭 白

气温，味辛，微酸。无毒。

《本草》云：归心，安五脏，除胃中热，利病人，可久食。子，主梦泄精，溺白。根，养发。阴中变为阳。

Jiubai [韭白, Chinese chive stalk, Allium tuberosum Rottb. ex Spreng]

It is warm in property, pungent and sour in taste. It is nontoxic.

Ben Cao says: It enters the heart meridian, tranquilizes the five zang-organs, removes heat in the stomach, and benefits patients; therefore, it can be taken for a long term. The seed of Jiubai [韭白, Chinese chive stalk, Allium tuberosum Rottb. ex Spreng] is mainly used to treat the seminal emission at night and turbid urine. The root of it is effective to nourish hair. It invigorates yang by nourishing yin.

薤 白

气温,味苦、辛。无毒。

入手阳明经。

《本草》云:主金疮疮败。轻身不饥,耐老。除寒热,去水气,温中散结,利病人。诸疮中风寒水肿,以此涂之。下重者,气滞也。四逆散加此,以泄气滞。

《心》云:治泄痢下重,下焦气滞,泄滞气。

Xiebai [薤白, longstamen onion bulb, Bulbus Allii Macrostemonis]

It is warm in property, and bitter and pungent in taste. It is nontoxic.

It enters the meridian of the hand-yangming.

Ben Cao says: It is mainly used to cure incised wounds and festered sores. It can relax the body and make patients rarely feel hungry, and it is anti-aging. It is effective to remove cold and heat, treat edema, resolve nodule, warm the middle internal organs, and benefit patients. Those sores and edema caused by wind and cold may be treated by applying Xiebai [薤白, longstamen onion bulb, Bulbus Allii Macrostemonis] on the wound. Rectal tenesmus is usually caused by the qi stagnation. Therefore, Xiebai [薤白, longstamen onion bulb, Bulbus Allii Macrostemonis] can be added in Sini Powder to treat qi stagnation.

Xin [《用药心法》, *Gist for the Use of Medicinal Herbs*] says: It is effective to treat the dysentery and rectal tenesmus, the qi stagnation in the lower energizer and purge qi stagnation.

瓜 蒂

气寒,味苦。有毒。

《本草》云:治大水,身面四肢浮肿,下水,杀蛊毒。咳逆上气,及食诸果,病在胸腹中者,皆吐下之。去鼻中息肉,疗黄疸,鼻中出黄水。除偏头疼,有神,头目有湿,宜此。瓜蒂苦,以治胸中寒,与白虎同例,俱见知母条下。与麝香、细辛同为使。治久不闻香臭。仲景钤方:瓜蒂一十四个,丁香一个,黍米四十九粒,为末,含水搐一字,取下。

Guadi [瓜蒂, muskmelon fruit pedicel, Pediculus Melo]

It is cold in property and bitter in taste. It is toxic.

Ben Cao says: It is used to treat serious fluid retention, edema of the body, face and limbs. It is also used to discharge water and treat the disease due to the noxious agents produced by various parasites. For the patients who suffer from cough, the counter-flow of qi and the disorder in the chest and abdomen due to improper eating of fruits, Guadi [瓜蒂, muskmelon fruit pedicel, Pediculus Melo] can be used to induce vomiting so as to remove its toxin. It is also used to treat nasal polyp, jaundice, and the yellow liquid in the nose. It is suitable to remove migraine, benefit spirit, treat the dampness in the head and eyes. Guadi [瓜蒂, muskmelon fruit pedicel, Pediculus Melo], bitter in taste, is used to treat the cold in the chest with the same function as Baihu [白虎, gypsum, Gypsum Fibrosum], and more detailed information can be found under the entry of Zhimu [知母, common anemarrhena rhizome, Rhizoma Anemarrhenae]. Guadi [瓜蒂, muskmelon fruit pedicel, Pediculus Melo] serves as the assistance together with Shexiang [麝香, musk, Moschus] and Xixin [细辛, asarum, Asarum Sieboldii Miq]. It is often used to treat the loss of olfactory sense. Zhang Zhongjing prescribed a formula: Put 14 Guadi [瓜蒂, muskmelon fruit pedicel, Pediculus Melo], 1 Dingxiang [丁香, clove, Flos Caryophylli] and 49 grains of Shusi [黍米, broomcorn millet fruit, Semen Panici Miliacei] together, and then smash them into power. Mix a very small amount of it into water and have a gargle with that.

冬葵子

气寒,味甘。无毒。

《本草》云:主五脏六腑寒热羸瘦,五癃,利小便。疗妇人乳难内闭。久服,坚筋骨,长肌肉,轻身。

《衍义》云:性滑利,不益人。患痈疖,毒热内攻,未出脓者,水吞三五粒,遂作窍,脓出。

Dong Kuizi [冬葵子, cluster mallow fruit, Fructus Malvae]

It is cold in property and sweet in taste. It is nontoxic.

Ben Cao says: It is mainly used to treat the emaciation due to the cold and heat in the five zang-organs and six fu-organs, treat urinary diseases and promote urination. It is effective to treat the difficult lactation and the internal blockade of women. The long-term taking of it may strengthen the tendons and bones, the muscles, and relax the body.

Yan Yi [《本草衍义》, *Extension of the Materia Medica*] says: It is slippery in nature, and not helpful to human health. The carbuncle furuncle due to the heat in the body and to be headed can be treated by swallowing three to five Dong Kuizi [冬葵子, cluster mallow fruit, Fructus Malvae] to dredge orifices and expel pus.

蜀葵花

冷,阴中之阳。

《珍》云:赤者,治赤带;白者,治白带;赤治血燥,白治气燥。

Shukuihua [蜀葵花, Flower of Hollyhock, Althaea Rosea]

It is cold in property, pertaining to yang within yin.

Zhen [《珍珠囊》, *Pounch of Pearls*] says: The red Shukuihua [蜀葵花, Flower of Hollyhock, Althaea Rosea] is used to treat the leukorrhea with bloody discharge while the white one is for leucorrhea. The red one is used to treat the blood dryness and the white one to treat qi dryness respectively.

香 薷

味辛,微温。

《本草》云:主霍乱腹痛吐下,散水肿。

Xiangru [香薷, Chinese mosla, Herba Moslae]

It is pungent in taste and slightly mild in nature.

Ben Cao says: It is mainly used to treat the abdominal pain, vomiting and the diarrhea caused by cholera, and it is also effective to disperse edema.

炊单布

《液》云:仲景治坠马,及一切筋骨损方中用。《时习》补入。

Chuidanbu [炊单布, gauze, Gaze]

Ye [《汤液本草》, *Materia Medica for Decoctions*] says: Zhang Zhongjing used it to treat the injuries caused by falling off the horse, and in formulas to treat all kinds of damages of tendons and bones. *Shi Xi* [《时习》, *Constant Practice*] added an entry for it.

米谷部
Rice and Grain Herbs

粳 米

气微寒,味甘、苦。甘平。无毒。

入手太阴经、少阴经。

《液》云:主益气,止烦、止渴、止泄。与熟鸡头相合,作粥食之,可以益精强志,耳目聪明。本草诸家共言益脾胃,如何白虎汤用之入肺?以其阳明为胃之经,色为西方之白,故入肺也。然治阳明之经,即在胃也。色白,味甘寒,入手太阴。又少阴证桃花汤用此，甘以补正气；竹叶石膏汤用此，甘以益不足。

《衍义》云：平和五脏，补益胃气，其功莫逮。然稍生，则复不益脾；过熟，则佳。

Jingmi［粳米，rice，Oryza Sativa L.］

It is slightly cold in property, sweet and bitter in flavor, and sweet and mild in nature. It is nontoxic.

It enters the meridian of the hand-taiyin and the meridian of the foot-shaoyin.

Ye［《汤液本草》, *Materia Medica for Decoctions*］says: It is mainly used to replenish qi, resolve vexation, relieve thirst, and stop diarrhea. When made into porridge combined with the cooked chicken head, Jingmi［粳米，rice，Oryza Sativa L.］is good to strengthen the essence and mind, and improve hearing and eyesight. As almost all schools of medicinal herbs hold that it benefits the spleen and the stomach, how does it enter the lung when it is used in Baihu Decoction? The reason is that the meridian of the hand yangming pertains to the stomach channel. Meanwhile, the color of Jingmi［粳米，rice，Oryza Sativa L.］is white, so it corresponds to west and metal in the five elements, thereby it enters the lung. Therefore, the key to treat the disease in the meridian of yangming lies in the stomach. As it is white in color, sweet in taste and cold in nature, it enters the meridian of the hand-taiyin. Put into Taohua Decoction, Jingmi［粳米，rice，Oryza Sativa L.］is used to treat the meridian of the foot-shaoyin, with its sweetness to replenish the healthy qi; put into Zhuye Shigao Decoction, it is used to benefit the qi deficiency with its sweetness.

Yan Yi［《本草衍义》, *Extension of the Materia Medica*］says: It is very effective to moderate the five zang-organs and benefit the stomach qi. However, if it is not fully cooked, it can not invigorate the spleen. So it should be fully cooked to function well.

赤小豆

气温，味辛、甘、酸，阴中之阳。无毒。

《本草》云：主下水，排脓，寒热热中消渴。止泄，利小便，吐逆卒澼下胀满。

又治水肿,通健脾胃。赤小豆,食之行小便,久食则虚人,令人黑瘦枯燥。赤小豆花,治宿酒渴病,即腐婢也。花有腐气,故以名之。与葛花末,服方寸匕,饮酒不知醉。气味平辛。大豆黄卷,是以生豆为蘖,待其芽出,便曝干用。方书名黄卷皮,产妇药中用之,性平。

Chixiaodou [赤小豆, red phaseolus bean, Semen Phaseoli]

It is warm in property, pungent in flavor, and sweet and sour in taste, pertaining to yang within yin. It is nontoxic.

Ben Cao says: It is mainly used to discharge water, expel pus, treat the consumptive thirst with the typical syndrome of polyphagia, polydispia, polyuria, weariness, emaciation and heat. It is used to stop diarrhea, promote urination, help vomiting and discharging so as to relieve the abdominal distension.

It is also effective to treat edema, invigorate the spleen and the stomach. If taken occasionally, Chixiaodou [赤小豆, red phaseolus bean, Semen Phaseoli] is helpful to promote urination. However, the long-term of taking it may weaken people and bring about black complexion, emaciation and dryness. The flowers of Chixiaodou [赤小豆, red phaseolus bean, Semen Phaseoli] are used to treat the thirst due to katzenjammer. It is called Fubi [腐婢, Stem or leaf of Japanese Premna, Premna microphylla Turcz]. The naming is ascribed to the putrid smell of that flower. If taken with powder of Gehua [葛花, flower of lobed kudzuvine, Flos Puerariae] by about one spoon, you will not feel drunk any more. It is mild in property and pungent in flavor. Dadouhuang Juan [大豆黄卷, soybean sprout, Semen GlycinesSiccus] takes raw beans as ferment. After sprouting, its buds are exposed to sunlight, dried and reserved. It is named Huangjuanpi in medical formulary. It can be used in medicines taken by maternal patient, as it is mild in property.

黑 大 豆

气平,味甘。

《本草》云:涂痈疖。煮汁饮,杀鬼毒,止痛,解乌头毒,除胃中热痹,伤中淋露,逐水胀,下瘀血。久服,令人身重。炒令黑,烟未断,热投酒中,治风痹瘫痪,口噤,产后诸风。食罢,生服半掬,去心胸烦热,明目镇心,不忘。恶五参、龙胆。得前胡、乌喙、杏仁、牡蛎良。

Heidadou [黑大豆, black soybean, Glycine Max (L.) Merr.]

It is mild in property and sweet in taste.

Ben Cao says: It can be applied to the carbuncle furuncle. When it is boiled in decoction, it is effective to expel the pathogenic factors like ghosts, relieve pain, treat the toxin of Wutou [乌头, common monkshood, Aconitum carmichaeli Debx.], remove the heat impediment in the stomach, treat gonorrhoea and water distention, and remove the static blood. The long-term taking of it may cause the heaviness of the body. Frying till its color becomes brown, and putting it into alcoholic drinks while it still smokes can treat the paralysis due to wind impediment, clenched jaw, and various wind diseases after delivery. After dinner, patients are recommended to take a half handful of raw Heidadou [黑大豆, black soybean, Glycine max (L.) Merr.], as it is effective to remove the vexing fever in the chest, brighten eyes, calm the mind, and prevent amnesia. It is averse to five types of ginsengs and Longdan [龙胆, root of rough gentian, Radix Gentianae]. It functions better with Qianhu [前胡, radix peucedani, Peucedanum praeruptorum Dunn], Wuhui [乌喙, prepared common monkshood daughter root, radix aconiti lateralis preparata], Xingren [杏仁, bitter apricot seed, Semen Armeniacae Amarum], and Muli [牡蛎, oyster shell, Concha Ostreae].

大麦蘖

气温,味甘、咸。无毒。

《象》云:补脾胃虚,宽肠胃。先杵细,炒黄,取面用。

《本草》云:能消化宿食,破症结冷气,去心腹胀满,开胃,止霍乱,除烦去痰,治产后秘结,鼓胀不通。大麦蘖并神曲二药,气虚人宜服,以代戊己,腐熟水谷。与豆蔻、缩砂、木瓜、芍药、五味子、乌梅为之使。

Damainie [大麦蘖, barley sprout, Hordei Fructus Germinatus]

It is warm in property, and sweet and salty in flavor. It is nontoxic.

Xiang [《药类法象》, *Rules for the Use of Medicinal Herbs*] says: It is effective to replenish the deficiency of the spleen and stomach, and invigorate the stomach and intestine. Pestle it first, then fry it till yellow, and keep the powder for usage.

Ben Cao says: It can be used to remove the retention of food in the gastrointestinal tract, break concretions and binds due to the cold qi, remove the abdominal distension in the heart and abdomen, promote the appetite, stop cholera, eliminate dysphoria and disperse phlegm, treat the constipation after delivery, and cure the blockage caused by tympanites. Damainie [大麦蘖, barley sprout, Hordei Fructus Germinatus] and Shenqu [神曲, medicated leaven, Massa Medicata Fermentata] are good to treat qi deficiency, as they can decompose foodstuff in replace of Wuji Wan (Fifth and Sixth Heavenly Stem Pill). Doukou [豆蔻, Katsumada's galangal seed, Alpiniae Katsumadai Semen], Suosha [缩砂, fructus amomi xanthioidis, Amomum Villosum Lour. Var. Xanthioides T. L. Wu et Senjen], Mugua [木瓜, common floweringqince fruit, Fructus Chaenomelis], Shaoyao [芍药, Chinese herbaceous peony, Paeonia lactiflora Pall.], Wuweizi [五味子, Chinese magnoliavine fruit, Fructus Schisandrae Chinensis] and Wumei [乌梅, smoked plum, Fructus Mume] can serve as its assistance.

小 麦

气微寒，味甘。无毒。

《本草》云：除热，止燥渴咽干，利小便，养肝气，止漏血、唾血。青蒿散有小麦百粒，治大人、小儿骨蒸肌热，妇人劳热。

Xiaomai [小麦, wheat, Triticum Aestivum]

It is slightly cold in property and sweet in taste. It is nontoxic.

Ben Cao says: It eliminates heat, relieves thirst and the dryness of the throat, promotes urination, and nourishes the liver qi, stops the metrostaxis and spitting of blood. Qinghao Powder, containing one hundred grains of Xiaomai [小麦, wheat, Triticum aestivum], is used to treat the hectic fever and heat in the muscles of adults and infants, and the consumptive fever in women.

神 曲

气暖,味甘。

入足阳明经。

《象》云:消食,治脾胃食不化,须于脾胃药中少加之。微炒黄用。

《珍》云:益胃气。

《本草》云:疗脏腑中风气,调中下气,开胃消宿食,主霍乱,心膈气痰逆,除烦,破症结及补虚,去冷气,除肠胃中塞,不下食。令人好颜色。落胎,下鬼胎。又能治小儿腹坚大如盘,胸中满,胎动不安,或腰痛抢心,下血不止。火炒以助天五之气,入足阳明。

Shenqu [神曲, medicated leaven, Massa Medicata Fermentata]

It is warm in property and sweet in flavor.

It enters the meridian of the foot-yangming.

Xiang [《药类法象》, *Rules for the Use of Medicinal Herbs*] says: It is good for digestion. Add a small amount of it in the medicine when it is used to treat the indigestion in the spleen and stomach. Fry it mildly till it becomes brown and keep it for later use.

Zhen [《珍珠囊》, *Pounch of Pearls*] says: It is beneficial for the stomach qi.

Ben Cao says: Shenqu [神曲, medicated leaven, Massa Medicata Fermentata] is used to treat the wind pathogen in the viscera, regulate the spleen and stomach and descend qi, promote the appetite and eliminate the abiding food, cure cholera, treat the counter-flow of qi and phlegm between the heart and the diaphragm, eliminate vexation, break binding and nodules and replenish deficiency, remove the cold qi and blockage in the stomach and intestines, and relieve the retention of food. It may benefit the complexion. It can cause abortion especially the deformed one. It is also used to treat the infant's abdominal hardness resulting in plate-sized abdomin, the fullness in the chest, the fetal irritability, the pain in the loins prodding the heart, and metrorrhagia. It can be fried with fire to assist the five kinds of smell. It enters the meridian of the foot-yangming.

酒

气大热,味苦、甘、辛。有毒。

《本草》云:主行药势,杀百邪恶毒气。能行诸经不止,与附子相同。味辛者能散,味苦者能下,味甘者居中而缓也。为导引,可以通行一身之表,至极高之分。若味淡者,则利小便而速下。大海或凝,惟酒不冰。三人晨行,遇大寒,一人食粥者,病;一人腹空者,死;一人饮酒者,安。则知其大热也。

Jiu [酒, liquor, Vinum]

It is greatly hot in property, and bitter, sweet and pungent in flavor. It is toxic.

Ben Cao says: It is mainly used to promote the effect of medicine, treat various evil and toxic pathogens. It is effective to activate all meridians with the same effect as Fuzi [附子, aconite, Radix Aconiti Praeparata]. It is used to disperse if pungent in flavor, descend if bitter in flavor, and moderate if sweet in flavor. As a kind of guiding medicinal, it can circulate through the exterior of the human body to an extreme extent. For the kind with bland flavor, it is used to promote urination. The ocean may coagulate while Jiu [酒, liquor, Vinum] would never freeze. It is said there were three people walking in the frigid morning, and the one who ate porridge sickened, the one with an empty stomach died, but the one who drank some liquor survived. Therefore, Jiu [酒, liquor, Vinum] is greatly hot in property.

苦 酒 (一名醋,一名醯)

气温,味酸。无毒。

《液》云:敛咽疮,主消痈肿,散水气,杀邪毒。余初录《本草》苦酒条。《本经》一名醯,又一名苦酒,如为一物也。及读《金匮》治黄疸,有麻黄醇酒汤:上以美清酒五升,煮二升,苦酒也。前治黄汗,有黄芪芍药桂枝苦酒汤。

Kujiu [苦酒, vinegar, Acetum] (also named Cu or Xi)

It is warm in property and sour in taste. It is nontoxic.

Ye [《汤液本草》, *Materia Medica for Decoctions*] says: It is used to restrain pharyngeal ulcer, dispel abscess and retained fluid, and kill evil-toxin. It is the first time to record the entry of Kujiu [苦酒, vinegar, acetum] from *Ben Cao* in this book. There were Xi [醯, vinegar, Acetum]) and Kujiu [苦酒, vinegar, Acetum] mentioned in *Ben Jing* [《神农本草经》, *Agriculture God's Canon of Materia Medica*), and they looked like the same thing. After reading *Jin Kui* [《金匮要略》, *Synopsis of Golden Chamber*], I found that Mahuang Chunjiu Decoction is effective to cure jaundice. The decoction is boiled together with 5 Sheng of Qingjiu [清酒, clear wine, Vinum Clarum], with 2 Sheng of it left, and then it became Kujiu [苦酒, vinegar, Acetum]. The yellow sweat that has been mentioned previously is treated by Huangqi Shaoyao Guizhi Kujiu Decoction made up by Huangqi [黄芪, milkvetch root, Radix Astragali seu Hedysari], Shaoyao [芍药, Chinese herbaceous peony, Paeonia Lactiflora Pall.], Guizhi [桂枝, Cinnamon bark, Cortex Cinnamomum Cassia] and Kujiu [苦酒, vinegar, Acetum].

饴（即胶饴）

气温，味甘。无毒。

入足太阴经药。

《液》云：补虚乏，止渴，去血。以其色紫凝如深琥珀色，谓之胶饴。色白而枯者，非胶饴，即饧糖也，不入药用。中满不宜用，呕家切忌。为足太阴经药。仲景谓，呕家不可用建中汤，以甘故也。

Yi [饴, malt sugar, Maltosum] (also named Jiaoyi)

It is warm in property and sweet in flavor. It is nontoxic.

It enters the meridian of the foot taiyin.

Ye [《汤液本草》, *Materia Medica for Decoctions*] says: It is used to replenish deficiency and lassitude, relieve thirst, and remove blood stasis. Jiaoyi [胶饴, malt sugar, Maltosum] is named after its purple color and deep amber color when it is coagulated. If it is white and dry, it is not Jiaoyi [胶饴, malt sugar, Maltosum] but malt sugar, which is not used as a medicinal herb. It is neither appropriate for the patients who suffer from fullness in the chest, nor for those who vomit. It belongs to the medicinal herb that enters the meridian of the foot taiyin. Zhang Zhongjing once said, those who vomited could not take Jianzhong Decoction due to its sweet taste.

香 豉

气寒,味苦,阴也。无毒。

《象》云:治伤寒头痛,烦躁满闷。生用。

《珍》云:去心中懊侬。

《本草》云:主伤寒头痛,寒热。伤寒初觉头痛,内热脉洪,起一二日,便作此加减葱豉汤:葱白一虎口,豉一升,绵裹。以水三升,煎取一升,顿服取汗。若不汗,加葛根三两,水五升,煮二升,分二服。又不汗,加麻黄三两,去节。

Xiangchi [香豉, fermented soybean, Semen Sojae Preparatum]

It is cold in property and bitter in taste, pertaining to yin. It is nontoxic.

Xiang [《药类法象》, *Rules for the Use of Medicinal Herbs*] says: It is used to treat the headache due to the cold damage, and the dysphoria and fullness in the chest. Take it directly without any processing.

Zhen [《珍珠囊》, *Pouch of Pearls*] says: It is used to expel vexation.

Ben Cao says: It is mainly used to treat the headache due to the cold damage, alternate cold and heat. If the patients who are attacked by the cold damage begin to have headache, internal heat and surging pulse, Cong Chi Decoction is recommended one or two days later, which includes a handful of Congbai [葱白, scallion white, Allii Fistulosi Bulbus Recens] and 1 Sheng of Xiangchi [香豉, fermented soybean, Semen Sojae Preparatum] wrapped in cotton. Put them in 3 Sheng of water, and then decoct them till 1 Sheng is left. Take it at a draught to promote sweat. If there is no sweat, 3 Liang of Gegen [葛根, kudzuvine root, Radix Puerariae] should be added. Then boil them in 5 Sheng of water until 2 Sheng is left, and then take 1 Sheng at a time, twice a day. If there is still no sweat, 3 Liang of Mahuang [麻黄, ephedra, Herba Ephedrae] can be added with its nodes removed.

玉石部
Jade Herbs

石 膏

气寒,味甘、辛,微寒。大寒,无毒。

入手太阴经、少阳经,足阳明经。

《象》云:治足阳明经中热,发热,恶热,燥热,日晡潮热,自汗,小便滑赤,大渴引饮,肌肉壮热,苦头痛之药,白虎汤是也。善治本经头痛,若无余证,勿用。

《心》云:细理白泽者良,甘寒。胃经大寒药,润肺除热,发散阴邪,缓脾益气。

《珍》云:辛甘,阴中之阳。止阳明经头痛。胃弱不可服。下牙痛,须用香白芷。

《本草》云:主中风寒热,心下逆气,惊喘,口干舌焦,不能息,腹中坚痛,除邪鬼,产乳金疮。除时气头痛,身热,三焦大热,皮肤热,肠胃中膈气。解肌发汗,止消渴烦逆,腹胀,暴气喘息,咽热。亦可作浴汤。

太上云:石膏发汗。辛寒,入手太阴也。

东垣云:微寒,足阳明也。又治三焦皮肤大热,手少阳也。仲景治伤寒阳明证,身热,目痛鼻干,不得卧。身已前,胃之经也;胸,胃肺之室。邪在阳明,肺受火制,故用辛寒以清肺,所以号为白虎汤也。鸡子为之使。恶莽草、马目毒公。

《药性论》云:石膏,使。恶巴豆。《唐本》注:疗风去热,解肌。

Shigao [石膏, gypsum, Gypsum Fibrosum]

It is cold in property, sweet and pungent in taste, and slightly cold in nature. It is greatly cold in property and nontoxic.

It enters the meridians of the hand-taiyin, hand-shaoyang, and foot-yangming.

Xiang [《药类法象》, *Rules for the Use of Medicinal Herbs*] says: Baihu Decoction is effective to treat the heat in the chest and abdomen that pertains to the meridian of foot-yangming, fever, aversion to heat, dryness-heat, the tidal fever in the afternoon, spontaneous sweating, the short voidings of reddish urine, polydipsia, the vigorous heat in muscles, and headache. It is good to relieve the headache of yangming meridians, which is forbidden to take without other symptoms.

Xin [《用药心法》, *Gist for the Use of Medicinal Herbs*] says: Shigao [石膏, gypsum, Gypsum Fibrosum] is sweet in taste and cold in nature, among which the one with the fine texture and the white lustrous color is better. It is a medicinal with cold property that goes through the stomach meridians, and it is used to moisten the lung and eliminate heat, disperse the yin pathogen, and moderate the spleen and replenish qi.

Zhen [《珍珠囊》, *Pouch of Pearls*] says: It is pungent and sweet in taste, and it pertains to yang within yin. It can be used to treat the headache in yangming meridians. It is forbidden to take for the patient who has a weak stomach. Xiangbaizhi [香白芷, Dahurian angelica, Angelicae Dahuricae Radix] needs to be used to treat toothache.

Ben Cao says: It is mainly used to treat the alternate cold and heat caused by the wind strike, the counter-flow qi below the heart, the startled panting, the thirst and the parched tongue, the failure of breath, the hardness and pain in the abdomen, the evil pathogen, the disease after the delivery of babies and the incised wound. It is effective to remove the headache due to the seasonal epidemic pathogens, the generalized fever, the great heat in the triple energizer, the skin fever, and the diaphragm qi in the stomach and intestines. It is also useful to expel pathogenic factors from muscles, promote sweating, and treat the consumptive thirst, dysphoria, the abdominal distention, the panting caused by the fulminant irritation, and the heat in throat. It can also be added to bath water.

Taishang said: Shigao [石膏, gypsum, Gypsum Fibrosum] can promote sweating. It is pungent in taste and cold in nature. It enters the meridian of the hand-taiyin.

Li Dongyuan said: It is slightly cold in nature, so it pertains to the meridian of the foot-yangming. It is also effective to treat the severe skin heat in the triple energizer, so it enters the meridian of the hand-shaoyang. Zhang Zhongjing used Shigao [石膏, gypsum, Gypsum Fibrosum] to treat the yangming disease caused by the cold damage, the generalized fever, pain of eyes and the dryness of the nose, and the inability to lie flatly. The stomach channel is located in the front part of the body while the chest is the chamber of the stomach and lung. If the pathogen exists in yangming meridians, the lung will suffer from the pathogenic fire. Therefore, Baihu Decoction, cold and pungent in nature, is used to clear away the lung-heat. Eggs can serve as the guiding medicinal. It is averse to Mangcao [莽草, leaf of lanceleaf anisetree, Folium Illicii Lanceolati], and Mamu Dugong [马目毒公, Common Dysosma Rhizome, Rhizoma Dysosmae Versipellis].

Yao Xing Lun [《药性论》, *Treatise on Medicinal Properties*] says: Shigao [石膏, gypsum, Gypsum Fibrosum] can serve as the envoy herb. It is averse to Badou [巴豆, Croton Fruit, Fructus Crotonis]. *Tang Ben* [《唐本伤寒论》, *Treatise on Febrile Disease of Tang Version*] annotates: It is used to treat the wind disease, expel heat, and expel pathogenic factors from muscles.

滑 石

气寒,味甘。大寒。无毒。

入足太阳经。

《象》云:治前阴不利,性沉重,能泄上气令下行。故曰滑则利窍。不可与淡渗同用。白者佳。杵细、水飞用。

《本草》云:主身热泄澼,女子乳难,癃闭。利小便,荡肠胃积聚寒热,益精气。通九窍六腑津液,去留结,止渴,令人利中。入足太阳。滑能利窍,以通水道,为至燥之剂。猪苓汤,用滑石与阿胶同为滑利,以利水道。葱、豉、生姜同煎去渣,澄清以解利。淡味渗泄为阳,解表、利小便也。若小便自利,不宜以此解之。

《衍义》云:暴吐逆,不下食,以生细末二钱匕,温水调服,后以热面压之。

Huashi [滑石, talc, Talcum]

It is cold in property and sweet in taste. It is greatly cold in property and nontoxic.

It enters the meridian of the foot-taiyang.

Xiang [《药类法象》, *Rules for the Use of Medicinal Herbs*] says: It is used to treat the acatharsia in the external genitalia. Being heavy in property, it can conduct qi downward. Thus it is said that orifices can be dredged by herbs with lubricant action. It can not be taken together with herbs milder in flavor to eliminate dampnes. The white one is better in quality. Pestle it first, and then leave it for water grind.

Ben Cao says: It is mainly used to treat the generalized fever, diarrhea, the difficulty in delivering baby and anuresis. It is effective to promote urination, clear away the accumulated cold and heat in the stomach and intestines, and benefit the essential qi. Huashi [滑石, talc, Talcum] is used to regulate the body fluid in the nine orifices and six fu-organs, dissipate binds, relieve thirst, and benefit the middle energizer. It enters the meridian of the foot-taiyang. Orifices can be dredged by herbs with lubricant action, so it is used to regulate the water passage, and is a medicinal herb to dry. Zhuling Decoction uses Huashi [滑石, talc, Talcum] and Ejiao [阿胶, ass hide glue, Colla Corii Asini], both with lubricant action, to regulate the water passage. You can boil it with Congbai [葱白, scallion white, Allii Fistulosi Bulbus Recens], Xiangchi [香豉, fermented soybean, Semen Sojae Preparatum] and Shengjiang [生姜, fresh ginger, Rhizoma Zingiberis Recens], and then remove residues. The clear decoction is good to release diarrhea. The bland medicinal herbs with straining and purging function pertain to yang, which is used to release the exterior and promote urination. If patients have the uninhibited urination, the prescription mentioned above is not suitable for them.

Yan Yi [《本草衍义》, *Extension of the Materia Medica*] says: For those who suffer from the violent vomiting and the retention of food, 2 Qian of Huashi [滑石, talc, Talcum] pestled into powder should be taken with warm water, and hot noodles should be taken to avoid vomiting.

朴 硝

气寒,味辛、苦。

《象》云:除寒热邪气,逐六腑积聚,结瘕血癖,胃中食饮热结。去血闭,停痰痞满。消毒。揉细,生用。

Puxiao [朴硝, crystallized sodium sulfate, Natrii Sulfas]

It is cold in property, and pungent and bitter in taste.

Xiang [《药类法象》, *Rules for the Use of Medicinal Herbs*] says: It is used to expel the pathogenic factors due to cold and heat, the accumulations in the six fu-organs, the chronic binds, the blood aggregation, and the heat binding in the stomach. It is effective to treat the blood stasis, the retention of phlegm and fullness. Detoxify it first. Then rub it into fine granules and use it raw.

盆 硝(即芒硝)

气寒,味咸。

《心》云:去实热。《经》云:热淫于内,治以咸寒,此之谓也。

《珍》云:纯阴,热淫于内,治以咸寒。

《本草》云:主五脏积聚,久热胃闭。除邪气,破留血,腹中痰实结,转通经脉及月水。破五淋。消肿毒,疗天行热病。

《药性论》云:使。味咸。有小毒。通月闭症瘕,下瘰疬,黄疸,主漆疮,散恶血。

《圣惠方》云:治代指用芒硝煎汤,淋渍之,愈。

Penxiao [盆硝, crystallized sodium sulfate, Natrii Sulfas] (also named Mangxiao)

It is cold in property and salty in flavor.

Xin [《用药心法》, *Gist for the Use of Medicinal Herbs*] says: It is used to remove the excessive heat. *Jing* says: The pathogenic heat that arises from the inner body should be treated by medicine that is salty in flavor and cold in nature, thereby Penxiao [盆硝, crystallized sodium sulfate, Natrii Sulfas] is suitable.

Zhen [《珍珠囊》, *Pounch of Pearls*] says: It pertains to pure yin. The pathogenic heat that arises from the inner body should be treated by medicine salty in flavor and cold in nature.

Ben Cao says: It is mainly used to treat the accumulations in the five zang-organs, and the stomach block caused by enduring heat. It is effective to remove the evil qi, break the retention of blood, the diaphragm phlegm in abdomen, regulate channels and promote menstruation. It is also used to break five types of stranguria, disperse swelling and toxin, and treat acute contagious febrile diseases.

Yao Xing Lun [《药性论》, *Treatise on Medicinal Properties*] says: Penxiao [盆硝, crystallized sodium sulfate, Natrii Sulfas] serves as the assistance in compatibility. It is salty in taste and slightly toxic. It is used to treat the menstrual block, concretions and conglomerations, the cervical scrofula, jaundice, lacquer sore, and the malignant blood.

Shen Hui Fang [《太平圣惠方》, *The Great Peace Sagacious Benevolence Formulary*] says: It is very effective to treat the acute pyogenic infection of finger tip with the decoction of Mangxiao [芒硝, crystallized sodium sulfate, Natrii Sulfas].

硝 石

气寒，味甘、辛。一作苦、辛，大寒。无毒。又云：咸。又云：甜，甜微缓于咸。

《液》云：硝石者硝之总名也，但不经火者谓之生硝、朴硝，经火者谓之盆硝、芒硝。古人用辛，今人用咸。辛能润燥，咸能软坚，其意皆是，老弱虚人可下者宜用。若用此者，以玄明粉代之尤佳。《本经》谓利小便而堕胎，伤寒妊娠，可下者用此，兼以大黄引之，直入大肠，润燥、软坚、泻热，子母俱安。《经》云：有故无殒，殒亦无殒也。此之谓欤。以在下言之，则便溺俱阴；以前后言之，则前气后血；以肾言之，总主大小便难，溺涩秘结，俱为水少。《经》云：热淫于内，治以咸寒，佐以苦，故以芒硝、大黄，相须为使也。

Xiaoshi [硝石, niter, Sal Nitri]

It is cold in property, and sweet and pungent in taste. It is also said to be bitter and pungent in taste, and greatly cold in nature. It is nontoxic. It is also said to be salty in taste. It is also said to be more salty than sweet.

Ye [《汤液本草》, *Materia Medica for Decoctions*] says: Xiaoshi [硝石, niter, Sal Nitri] is the common name for all kinds of niters, among which Puxiao [朴硝, crystallized sodium sulfate, Natrii Sulfas] (also named as Shengxiao [生

硝, crystallized sodium sulfate, Natrii Sulfas]) refers to those that have not undergone fire, while Penxiao [盆硝, crystallized sodium sulfate, Natrii Sulfas] (also named as Mangxiao [芒硝, crystallized sodium sulfate, Natrii Sulfas]) refers to those that have undergone fire. The ancient people used it for its pungency, but nowadays people use it for its saltiness. As pungency is effective to moisten dryness and saltiness is good for softening hardness, it is suitable to be used for the old and weak who have difficulty in discharging. When it is compared with Xuanmingfen [玄明粉, sodium sulfate powder, Natrii Sulfas Exsiccatus], the latter may be a better choice. *Ben Jing* [《神农本草经》, *Agriculture God's Cannon of Materia Medica*] says: It is used for promoting urination, inducing abortion and treating the cold damage during pregnancy. For the patients who need purging it is recommended to be used. With Dahuang [大黄, rhubarb root and rhizome, Radix et Rhizoma Rhei] as the medicinal guide, it can go down to the large intestines, moisten dryness, soften hardness, and purge heat to guarantee the safety of both mother and child. *Jing* says: As long as the medicine is suitable to treat the disease, it will not cause abortion even it is a bit toxic. So it is. In terms of the disease location, the lower pertains to yin and the stool and urine belong to the lower. In terms of the front and hind position, the front is in charge of qi while the hind is in charge of blood. In terms of the kidney, the difficulty in stool and urine and constipation are all caused by shortage of water in the body. *Jing* says: The pathogenic heat in the interior part of the body should be treated by the medicine salty in flavor and cold in nature, and assisted by bitterness. Thus Mangxiao [芒硝, crystallized sodium sulfate, Natrii Sulfas] and Dahuang [大黄, rhubarb root and rhizome, Radix et Rhizoma Rhei] should be its assistance.

玄 明 粉

气冷,味辛、甘。无毒。

《液》云:治心热烦躁,五脏宿滞,症瘕。明目,逐膈上虚热,消肿毒。注中有治阴毒一句,非伏阳不可用。若止用此除阴毒,杀人甚速。牙硝条下,太清炼灵砂补注,谓阴极之精,能化火石之毒。

《仙经》云:阴中有阳之物。

Xuanmingfen [玄明粉, sodium sulfate powder, Natrii Sulfas Exsiccatus]

It is cold in property, and pungent and sweet in taste. It is nontoxic.

Ye [《汤液本草》, *Materia Medica for Decoctions*] says: It is used to treat the heart heat and dysphoria, the food stagnation in the five zang-organs, concretions and conglomerations. Xuanmingfen [玄明粉, sodium sulfate powder, Natrii Sulfas Exsiccatus] is effective to brighten eyes, expel the heat of deficiency-type above the diaphragm, and disperse swelling and toxin. It is annotated as being effective to treat the yin toxin only when there is latent yang in the body. If Xuanmingfen [玄明粉, sodium sulfate powder, Natrii Sulfas Exsiccatus] is used alone to treat yin pathogen, it may cause death soon. Under the category of Yaxiao [牙硝, horse-tooth niter, Nitrum Equidens], Taiqing added that Xuanmingfen [玄明粉, sodium sulfate powder, Natrii Sulfas Exsiccatus] pertains to extreme yin, so it is effective to remove the toxin of flint.

Xian Jing [《仙经》, *Immortal Canon*] says: Xuanmingfen [玄明粉, sodium sulfate powder, Natrii Sulfas Exsiccatus] pertains to yang within yin.

硫　黄

气温,大热,味酸。有毒。

《本草》云:主妇人阴蚀,疽痔,恶血。坚筋骨,除头秃。疗心腹积聚邪气,冷癖在胁,咳逆上气,脚冷疼弱无力,及鼻衄,恶疮,下部䘌疮。止血,杀疥虫。

《液》云:如太白丹佐以硝石,来复丹用硝石之类,至阳佐以至阴,与仲景白通汤佐以人溺、猪胆汁,大意相同,所以去格拒之寒。兼有伏阳,不得不尔;如无伏阳,只是阴证,更不必以阴药佐之也。硫黄亦号将军,功能破邪归正,返滞还清,挺出阳精消阴,化魄生魂。

Liuhuang [硫黄, sulfur, Sulphur]

It is warm in property, sour in flavor and severely hot. It is toxic.

Ben Cao says: It is mainly used to treat the erosion of vulva, hemorrhoids, and the malignant blood. It is effective to strengthen the tendons and bones, and treat baldness. It is also used to treat the accumulation of the evil qi in the heart and abdomen, the coldness in the rib-side, the cough with dyspnea and the counter-flow of qi, and cold, pain, or weak in the foot, epistaxis, obstinate sore, and the invisible-worm sores of the lower body. It is used to cease bleeding and kill scabies.

Ye [《汤液本草》, *Materia Medica for Decoctions*] says: Taibai Pill is assisted with Xiaoshi [硝石, niter, Sal Nitri] and so is Laifu Pill. They follow the rule that the consummate yang is assisted with the consummate yin, which is similar to the way Zhang Zhongjing put the human urine and the pig's bile into his Baitong Decoction. Therefore, it is effective to treat the coldness caused by the cold and heat repulsion. If the syndrome is accompanied by the latent yang, the yin medicinal herb should be used; if there is no latent yang, it is not necessary to assist the yin syndrome with yin medicinal herbs. Liuhuang [硫黄, sulfur, Sulphur] is also named as the general medicinal herb, because it can remove the pathagethic factors and restore the healthy qi, expel retention and clear stagnation, make the essence of yang stand out, dispel the hyperactive yin, and invigorate the spirit and soul.

雄 黄

气温,寒,味苦、甘。有毒。

《本草》云:主寒热鼠瘘恶疮,疽痔死肌。疗疥虫䘌疮,目痛,鼻中息肉,及绝筋破骨,百节中大风,积聚癖气,中恶,腹痛,鬼疰。

Xionghuang [雄黄, realgar, Realgar]

It is warm in property, cold in nature, and bitter and sweet in taste. It is toxic.

Ben Cao says: It is mainly used to treat the cold and heat, the mouse fistula and the obstinate sore, as well as hemorrhoids and muscle necrosis. It is effective to expel scabies, eyepain, the nasal polyp, the muscular exhaustion and bone damage, the wind-stroke of joints, the accumulation of pathogenic factors, malignity stroke, the abdominal pain, and the demonic infixation.

赤石脂

气大温,味甘、酸、辛。无毒。

《本草》云:主养心气,明目益精。疗腹痛泄澼,下利赤白,小便利,及痈疽疮痔,女子崩中漏下,产难,胞衣不出。久服,补髓、好颜色、益志不饥、轻身延年。五色石脂,各入五脏补益。

东垣云:赤石脂、白石脂并温无毒。畏黄芩、芫花,恶大黄。

《本经》云:涩可去脱,石脂为收敛之剂。胞衣不出,涩剂可以下之。赤入丙、白入庚。

《珍》云:赤、白石脂俱甘酸,阳中之阴,固脱。

《心》云:甘温,筛末用。去脱,涩以固肠胃。

《局方本草》云:青石脂,养肝胆气,明目;黑石脂,养肾气,强阴,主阴蚀疮;黄石脂,养脾气,除黄疸。余与赤、白同功。

Chishizhi [赤石脂, red halloysite, Halloysitum Rubrum]

It is greatly warm in property, and sweet, sour and pungent in taste. It is nontoxic.

Ben Cao says: It is mainly used to nourish the heart qi, brighten eyes and boost the essence. It is used to treat the abdominal pain and aggregation, the leukorrhagia and bloody dysentery, the difficult urination, welling-abscesses and flat-abscesses, sore and hemorrhoid, metrostaxis, the difficult delivery, and the retention of the placenta. The long-term taking of it can tonify the marrow, luster the skin, boost the mind and make one feel no hunger, relax the body, and prolong the life span. The five colors of Shizhi [石脂, halloysite, Halloysitum] can tonify the five zang-organs respectively.

Li Dongyuan said: Both Chishizhi [赤石脂, red halloysite, Halloysitum Rubrum] and Baishizhi [白石脂, white halloysite, halloysitum album] are warm and nontoxic. It is restrained by Huangling [黄芩, baical skullcap root, Radix Scutellariae] and Yuanhua [芫花, immature flower of lilac daphne, Flos Genkwa], and it is averse to Dahuang [大黄, rhubarb root and rhizome, Radix et Rhizoma Rhei].

Ben Jing [《神农本草经》, *Agriculture God's Canon of Materia Medica*] says: As an astringent medicinal herb, Shizhi [石脂, halloysite, Halloysitum] is effective to treat depletion and collapse syndrome. If there is the retention of the placenta, the astringent medicinal herb is helpful. Red corresponds to Bing, which governs the small intestines and is ranked the third in the heaven stems, and white corresponds to Geng, which governs the large intestines and is ranked the seventh in the heaven stems.

Zhen [《珍珠囊》, *Pounch of Pearls*] says: Both Chishizhi [赤石脂, red halloysite, Halloysitum Rubrum] and Baishizhi [白石脂, white halloysite, halloysitum album] are sweet and sour in taste, pertaining to yin within yang, and they are effective to prevent prolapse with its astringent action.

Xin [《用药心法》, *Gist for the Use of Medicinal Herbs*] says: It is sweet in taste and warm in nature, often sieved to use the powder. It is effective to prevent prolapse, as the astringent medicinal herb is befenicial to reinforce the stomach and intestines.

Ju Fang Ben Cao [《局方本草》, *Materia Medica of Bureau Prescription*] says: The green-blue Shizhi [石脂, halloysite, Halloysitum] is good for nourishing the liver and gallbladder qi and brightening eyes. The black Shizhi [石脂, halloysite, Halloysitum] is mainly used to preserve the kidney qi, and invigorate yin and treat the erosion of vulva. The yellow Shizhi [石脂, halloysite, Halloysitum] is effective to tonify the spleen qi and remove the jaundice. They are similar to red and white ones in other functions.

禹 余 粮

气寒,味甘。无毒。

《本草》云:主咳逆寒热烦满,下痢赤白,血闭,症瘕大热。

《本经》云:重可去怯。禹余粮之重,为镇固之剂。

《本草》注云:仲景治伤寒下病不止,心下痞硬,利在下焦者,赤石脂禹余粮汤主之。赤石脂、禹余粮各一斤,并碎之,以水六升,煎取二升,去渣,分二服。

雷公云:看如石,轻敲便碎,可如粉也。兼重重如叶子雌黄,此能益脾,安五脏。

Yuyuliang [禹余粮, limonite, Limonitum]

It is cold in property and sweet in taste. It is nontoxic.

Ben Cao says: It is mainly used to treat choking cough, alternate cold and heat, vexation and fullness, bloody dysentery, blood stasis, and the severe heat due to concretions and conglomerations.

Ben Jing [《神农本草经》, *Agriculture God's Cannon of Materia Medica*] says: Heavy medicinal herbs can eliminate timidity. Yuyuliang [禹余粮, limonite, Limonitum], being heavy in property, is a herb with tranquilizing and reinforcing function.

Ben Cao is annotated: When Zhang Zhongjing treated the patients who suffer from the cold damage, the persistent leukorrheal disease, the glomus and hardness below the heart, and the diarrhea in the lower energizer, Chishizhi Yuyuliang Decoction was mainly adopted. The decoction is composed of 1 Jin of Chishizhi [赤石脂, red halloysite, Halloysitum Rubrum] and 1 Jin of Yuyuliang [禹余粮, limonite, Limonitum] respectively. Smash them and boil them in 6 Sheng of water, decoct them until 2 Sheng was left, remove residues, and take 1 Sheng of it at a time, twice a day.

Lei Gong (Lei Xiao) said: It looks like a stone, and it is easily broken into powder when it is dabbed. It looks like the leaves of Cihuang [雌黄, orpiment, Auripigmentum], which is effective to benefit the spleen and tranquilize the five zang-organs.

代 赭 石

气寒，味甘、苦。无毒。一名须丸。出姑幕者，名须丸；出代郡者，名代赭。入手少阴经、足厥阴经。

《本草》云：主鬼疰，贼风蛊毒。杀精物恶鬼，腹中毒邪气，女子赤沃漏下，带下百病，产难，胞衣不出，堕胎。养血，除五脏血脉中热，血痹、血瘀，大人、小儿惊气入腹，及阴痿不起。

《圣济经》云：怯则气浮，重则所以镇之。怯者亦惊也。

Daizheshi [代赭石, hematite, Haematitum]

It is cold in property and sweet and sour in taste. It is nontoxic. It is also named Xuwan [须丸, hematite, Haematitum]. If the hematite is produced in Gumu County, it is called Xuwan [须丸, hematite, Haematitum]. If the hematite is found in Dai County, it is named Daizheshi [代赭石, hematite, Haematitum].

It enters the meridian of the hand-shaoyin and the meridian of the foot-jueyin.

Ben Cao says: It is mainly used to treat the demonic infixation, the wind pathogen and the parastic toxin. It is effective to kill the strange pathogenic factors like monster and ghost, and treat the diseases caused by the toxin and evil qi in the abdomen, the constant vaginal bleeding, various diseases caused by the vaginal discharge, the difficult delivery, the retention of the placenta, and abortion. It is also used to nourish the blood, eliminate the heat in the blood and vessels of the five zang-organs, and treat the blood impediment, the stagnation of blood, the fright entering the abdomen of adults and children, and impotence.

Sheng Ji Jing [《圣济经》, *Sages' Salvation Classic*] says: Timidity causes the floating of qi, so the heavy medicinal herbs can eliminate timidity. The timid one is also easy to be frightened.

铅 丹

气微寒,味辛。黄丹也。

《本草》云:主吐逆反胃,惊痫癫疾,除热下气。止小便利,除毒热筋挛,金疮溢血。又云:镇心安神,止吐血。

《本经》云:涩可去脱而固气。

成无己云:铅丹收敛神气,以镇惊也。

《药性论》云:君。治消渴。煎膏,止痛、生肌。

Qiandan [铅丹, minium, Minium]

It is slightly cold in property and pungent in taste. It is also named Huangdan.

Ben Cao says: It is mainly used to treat vomiting, stomach reflux, fright epilepsy and madness, eliminate heat and descend qi. It stanches the uninhibited copious urine, expels the toxic heat and convulsions, and cures the blood spillage caused by incised wounds. It is also said to be effective in setting the heart, calming the mind, and stopping haematemesis.

Ben Jing [《神农本草经》, *Agriculture God's Canon of Materia Medica*] says: It is the astringent medicinal herb that prevents prolapse and reinforces qi.

Cheng Wuji said: By restraining vitality, Qiandan [铅丹, minium, Minium] can relieve convulsion.

Yao Xing Lun [《药性论》, *Treatise on Medicinal Properties*] says: It is a monarch medicinal herb. It is used to treat consumptive thirst. Brewing it into paste can help patients relieve pain and promote granulation.

白 粉

《本草》云：一名胡粉，一名定粉，一名瓦粉。仲景猪肤汤用白粉，非此白粉，即白米粉也。黄延非治胸中寒，是治胸中塞，误写作寒字。

《药性论》云：胡粉，使。又名定粉，味甘、辛，无毒。能治积聚不消，焦炒，止小儿疳痢。

陈藏器云：主久痢成疳。粉和水及鸡子白服，以粪黑为度。为其杀虫而止痢也。

Baifen [白粉, processed galenite, Galenitum Praeparatum]

Ben Cao says: It is also called Hufen [胡粉, processed galenite, Galenitum Praeparatum], Dingfen [定粉, processed galenite, Galenitum Praeparatum], or Wafen [瓦粉, processed galenite, Galenitum Praeparatum]. It is the rice flour rather than Baifen [白粉, processed galenite, Galenitum Praeparatum] that is in Zhang Zhongjing's Zhufu Decoction. Huang Yan actually cures the blockage in the chest rather than the cold in the chest. The misunderstanding was resulted from the recorder who mistook Se (塞, blockage) for Han (寒, cold).

Yao Xing Lun [《药性论》, *Treatise on Medicinal Properties*] says: Hufen [胡粉, processed galenite, Galenitum Praeparatum] can be used as the assistance. It is also named Dingfen [定粉, processed galenite, Galenitum Praeparatum], sweet and pungent in taste, and nontoxic. It is used to treat the prolonged accumulation, and stop the infantile dysentery after it is fried.

Chen Cangqi said: It is mainly used to treat the dysentery caused by the chronic diarrhea. Mix Baifen [白粉, processed galenite, Galenitum Praeparatum] with water and egg-albumen, and then take them several times until the defecation turns black. That is out of its function of killing worms and stopping diarrhea.

紫石英

气温,味甘、辛。无毒。

入手少阴经、足厥阴经。

《本草》云:主心腹咳逆邪气,补不足,女子风寒在子宫,绝孕十年无子。疗上气,心腹痛,寒热邪气,结气。补心气不足,定惊悸,安魂魄,填下焦,止消渴。除胃中久寒,散痈肿。令人悦泽。久服温中,轻身延年。得茯苓、人参、芍药,共疗心中结气;得天雄、菖蒲,共疗霍乱。长石为之使。畏扁青、附子,不欲鮀甲、黄连、麦句姜。

《衍义》云:仲景治风热瘛疭,风引汤。紫石英、白石英、寒水石、石膏、干姜、大黄、龙齿、牡蛎、甘草、滑石等分。上㕮咀,以水一升,煎去三分。食后,量多少温呷之。不用渣,立效。

Zishiying [紫石英, fluorite, Fluoritum]

It is warm in property and sweet and pungent in taste. It is nontoxic.

It enters the meridian of hand-shaoyin and the meridian of the foot-jueyin.

Ben Cao says: It is mainly used to treat the cough and counter-flow in the heart and abdomen caused by the evil qi, and tonify insufficiency. It treats the wind-cold syndrome in the womb, and the long-term infertility. It is used to treat the qi ascent, the pain in the heart and abdomen, the cold and heat due to evil qi, and the qi stagnation. It tonifies the insufficiency of the heart qi, removes the palpitation with fright, pacifies the ethereal soul and corporeal soul, fills up the lower energizer, and stops consumptive-thirst. It can eliminate the enduring cold in the stomach, disperse the swollen welling-abscess, and luster the complexion. The long-term taking of it may warm the middle internal organs, relax the body and prolong the life span. When it is used together with Fuling [茯苓, Indian bread,

Poria], Renshen [人参, ginseng, Radix Ginseng] and Shaoyao [芍药, Chinese herbaceous peony, Paeonia lactiflora Pall.], the qi stagnation in the heart could be treated. When used together with Tianxiong [天雄, aconite, Aconiti Radix Lateralis] and Changpu [菖蒲, acorus, Acorus Calamus], cholera could be treated. Changshi [长石, anhydrite, Anhydritum] is its assistance. It is restrained by Bianqing [扁青, azurite, Azuritum] and Fuzi [附子, aconite, Radix Aconiti Praeparata], and is inhibited by Tuojia [鼍甲, Kyphosus Shell, Kyphosidae], Huanglian [黄连, golden thread, Rhizoma Coptidis] and gingers.

Yan Yi [《本草衍义》, *Extension of the Materia Medica*] says: Zhang Zhongjing treated the convulsions due to the wind-heat with Fengyin Decoction, which is composed of Zishiying [紫石英, fluorite, Fluoritum], Baishiying [白石英, white quartz, Quartz Album], Hanshuishi [寒水石, glauberite, Gypsum seu Calcitum], Shigao [石膏, gypsum, Gypsum Fibrosum], Ganjiang [干姜, dried ginger, Rhizoma Zingiberis], Dahuang [大黄, rhubarb root and rhizome, Radix et Rhizoma Rhei], Longchi [龙齿, dragon tooth, Mastodi Dentis Fossilia], Muli [牡蛎, oyster shell, Concha Ostreae], Gancao [甘草, liquorice root, Glycyrrhiza uralensis Fisch.] and Huashi [滑石, talc, Talcum] with equal amount. Chew them and boil them in 1 Sheng of water until 3 Fen is reduced. After dinner, it may be sipped warm. It takes effect without using the residue.

伏 龙 肝

气温,味辛。

《时习》云:主妇人崩中吐血。止咳逆,止血,消痈肿。

《衍义》云:妇人恶露不止,蚕砂一两(炒),伏龙肝半两,阿胶一两。同为末,温酒调,空心服三二钱。以止为度。

《药性论》云:单用亦可。咸,无毒。

《日华子》云:热,微毒。治鼻洪、肠风、带下、血崩、泄精、尿血,催生下胞衣,及小儿夜啼。一云:治心痛及中风心烦。陶隐居云:此灶中对釜月下黄土也。

Fulonggan [伏龙肝, oven earth, Terra Flava Usta]

It is warm in property and pungent in taste.

Shi Xi [《时习》, *Constant Practice*] says: It is mainly used to treat the profuse vaginal bleeding and haematemesis, stop cough and counterflow, cease bleeding, and dispel abscess.

Yan Yi [《本草衍义》, *Extension of the Materia Medica*] says: 1 Liang of Cansha [蚕砂, silkworm droppings, Bombycis Faeces] (fry), half a Liang of Fulonggan [伏龙肝, oven earth, Terra Flava Usta] and 1 Liang of Ejiao [阿胶, ass hide glue, Colla Corii Asini] can be used to stop the persistent flow of lochia. Grind them into powder, mix them with warm liquor, and take 2 or 3 Qian on an empty stomach. Once the persistent flow of lochia is stopped, patients should stop taking that medicinal formula.

Yao Xing Lun [《药性论》, *Treatise on Medicinal Properties*] says: Fulonggan [伏龙肝, oven earth, Terra Flava Usta] can also be used alone. It is salty in taste and nontoxic.

Ri Hua Zi [《日华子》, *Materia Medica of Ri Hua-Zi*] says: It is hot in property and slightly toxic. It is used to treat nosebleed, intestinal wind, vaginal discharge, flooding, seminal discharge, hematuria, hasten the child delivery and discharge placenta, and stop the infantile night cry. It is also said to be effective to treat heart pain, stroke and vexation. Tao Yinju says: It is like Zaozhong Huangtu [灶中黄土, oven earth, Terra Flava Usta] in some way.

白 矾

气寒,味酸。无毒。

《本草》云:主寒热泄泻,下痢白沃,阴蚀恶疮。消痰止渴,除痼热。治咽喉闭,目痛。坚骨齿。

《药性论》云:使,有小毒。生含咽津,治急喉痹。

Baifan [白矾, alum, Alumen]

It is cold in property and sour in taste. It is nontoxic.

Ben Cao says: It is mainly used to treat the diarrhea caused by cold and heat, the dysentery and morbid leucorrhea, the genital erosion, and the malign sore. It can clear away phlegm, relieve thirst, and expel the enduring heat. It is used to cure the swelling of the throat and eye pain, and strengthen bones and teeth.

Yao Xing Lun [《药性论》, *Treatise on Medicinal Properties*] says: It is slightly toxic when served as the assistant medicinal herb. When raw Baifan [白矾, alum, Alumen] is held in the mouth, it can help swallow the salica, and treat the acute throat impediment.

朱 砂

味甘。

《珍》云：心热者，非此不能除。

《局方本草》云：丹朱味甘，微寒。无毒。养精神，安魂魄，益气明目，通血脉，止烦渴。

《药性论》云：君。有大毒。镇心，抽风。

《日华子》云：凉，微毒，润心肺。恶磁石，畏咸水。

Zhusha [朱砂, cinnabar, Cinnabaris]

It is sweet in taste.

Zhen [《珍珠囊》, *Pounch of Pearls*] says: It is very effective to treat the heart heat.

Ju Fang Ben Cao [《局方本草》, *Materia Medica of Bureau Prescription*] says: It is sweet in taste and slightly cold in nature. It is nontoxic. It cultivates spirit, pacifies the ethereal soul and corporeal soul, replenishes qi and brightens eyes, disinhibits vessels, and stops vexation and thirst.

Yao Xing Lun [《药性论》, *Treatise on Medicinal Properties*] says: It is the monarch medicinal herb. It is very toxic. It can calm the mind and stop convulsion vulsion.

Ri Hua Zi [《日华子》, *Materia Medica of Ri Hua-Zi*] says: It is cold in property and slightly toxic, and it nourishes the heart and lung. It is averse to Cishi [磁石, loadstone Magnetitum] and restrained by the salt water.

硇 砂

味咸。

《本草》云：破坚癖，独不用，入群队用之。味咸、苦、辛，温。有毒，不宜多服。主积聚，破结血，烂胎止痛，下气，疗咳嗽宿冷。去恶肉，生好肌。柔金银，可为焊药。

《药性论》云：有大毒。畏浆水，忌羊血。味酸咸，能腐坏人肠胃，生食之化人心为血。能除冷病，大益阳事。

《日华子》云：北庭砂，味辛、酸，暖。无毒，畏一切酸。补水脏，暖子宫，消冷癖瘀血，宿食，气块痃癖，及妇人血气心痛，血崩带下。凡修制，用黄丹、石灰作匮，煅赤使用。无毒。柔金银，驴马药亦用。

Naosha [砀砂, sal ammoniac, Sal Ammoniacum]

It is salty in taste.

Ben Cao says: It can break the hard aggregation, but it can not be used alone. It is salty, bitter and pungent in taste, and warm in property. It is toxic, so it can not be taken too much. It is mainly used to treat accumulation, break the stagnation of blood, eliminate the retention of dead fetus, relieve pain, descend qi, and cure the cough with abiding cold. It can remove slough and promote granulation. It can melt gold and silver as a kind of fluxing agent.

Yao Xing Lun [《药性论》, *Treatise on Medicinal Properties*] says: Naosha [硇砂, sal ammoniac, Sal Ammoniacum] is very toxic. It is restrained by Jiangshui [浆水, sour millet water, Setariae Praeparatum Liquidum] and the goat blood. It is sour and salty in taste, eroding the stomach and intestines of human beings. If it is eaten raw, it can help produce more blood from the heart. It is effective to remove cold pathogen and benefit the male sexuality.

Ri Hua Zi [《日华子》, *Materia Medica of Ri Hua-Zi*] says: Beitingsha [北庭砂, sal ammoniac, Sal Ammoniacum] is pungent and sour in taste, and warm in nature. It is nontoxic, restrained by all kinds of sour substances. It replenishes the water viscus, warms the womb, eliminates coldness and the blood stasis, removes the abiding food, expels the strings and aggregations of qi, treats the female heart pain due to the poor circulation of blood and qi, flooding and the vaginal discharge. When processing Naosha [硇砂, sal ammoniac, Sal Ammoniacum], one should use Huangdan [黄丹, minium, Minium] and Shihui [石灰, quicklime, Calx Viva] to help decay and forge. It is nontoxic. It can melt gold and silver, and it can also be used in the medicine for donkeys and horses.

东 流 水

味平,无毒。

《时习》云:千里水及东流水,主病后虚弱。扬之万过,煮药,收禁神效。二者皆堪荡涤邪秽。此水洁净,诚与诸水不同。为云母所畏,炼云母粉用之。

Dongliushui [东流水, water running toward the east, Materia Medica Dongliushui]

It is mild in taste and nontoxic.

Shi Xi [《时习》, *Constant Practice*] says: It is also called Qianlishui, and mainly used to treat the weakness after illness. As this kind of water has been winnowed thousands of times, it is very effective to astringe and restrain. Both of them can clean up the evil foulness. It is quite clean, and different from other water. It is restrained by Yunmu [云母, muscovite, Muscovitum] and can be used to refine the mica powder.

甘 澜 水

《时习》云:扬之水上成珠者是也。治霍乱,及入膀胱。治奔豚药用之,殊胜。

Ganlanshui [甘澜水, worked water, Aqua Manipulata]

Shi Xi [《时习》, *Constant Practice*] says: It refers to the beads of water after being poured and splashed thousands of times. It treats cholera and enters the bladder channel. It is also used as the medicinal herb to treat Bentun.

禽 部
Fowl Herbs

鸡子黄

气温,味甘。

《本草》云:阴不足,补之以血。若咽有疮,鸡子一枚,去黄,苦酒倾壳中,以半夏入苦酒中,取壳,置刀环上,熬微沸。去渣,旋旋呷之。又主除热,火疮痫痓。可作琥珀神物。黄,和恒山末,为丸,竹叶汤服,治久疟不瘥;黄,合须发,煎消为水,疗小儿惊热、下痢。

Jizihuang [鸡子黄, egg yolk, Galli Vitellus]

It is warm in property and sweet in taste.

Ben Cao says: If there is the deficiency of yin, nourish it with blood. If there is sore in the throat, use an egg with the yolk removed, put Kujiu [苦酒, vinegar, Acetum] into the egg shell, add Banxia [半夏, pinellia tuber, Rhizoma Pinelliae] into Kujiu [苦酒, vinegar, Acetum], and then put the shell on the ring of knife and boil it. Remove the residue and sip it. It is also effective to eliminate heat, and treat the scalded sore, epilepsy and convulsion. It can be made into the magic product like amber. The yolk, made into pills with Hengshan [恒山, dichroa, Dichroae Radix] powder, is used to treat the stubborn malaria if taken with Zhuye Decoction. The yolk, mixed with beard and hair and decocted in water, is effective to treat the infantile fever due to fright and dysentery.

兽 部
Beast Herbs

龙 骨

气平微寒,味甘。阳也。无毒。

《本草》云：主心腹鬼疰，精物老魅，咳逆，泄利脓血，女子漏下，症瘕坚结，小儿热气惊痫。疗心腹烦满，四肢萎枯，汗出，夜卧自惊。恚怒伏气在心下，不得喘息。肠痈内疽，阴蚀。止汗，缩小便，溺血。养精神，定魂魄，安五脏。

《本经》云：涩可去脱而固气。

成无己云：龙骨、牡蛎、铅丹，皆收敛神气以镇惊。凡用，烧通赤为粉。畏石膏。

《珍》云：固大肠脱。

Longgu [龙骨, dragon bone, Mastodi Ossis Fossilia]

It is mild in property, slightly cold in nature, and sweet in taste. It pertains to yang. It is nontoxic.

Ben Cao says: It is mainly used to treat the demonic infixation in the heart and abdomen, expel the severe pathogenic factors like monsters and ghosts, the cough with dyspnea, diarrhea, the blood with purulent blood, vaginal bleeding, the abdominal mass with hard lump, and the infantile epilepsy due to heat. It is used to treat the vexation and fullness in the heart and abdomen, convulsions in limbs, sweating, and awakening with fright during the night. It also treats resentment, anger, the latent qi below the heart, and inability to breathe. It is used to treat the intestinal welling-abscess and genital erosion, stop sweating, reduce urination, treat the bloody urine, cultivate the mind, calm the soul and spirit, and tranquilize the five zang-organs.

Ben Jing [《神农本草经》, *Agriculture God's Canon of Materia Medica*) says: It is an astringent medicinal herb that prevents prolapse and strengthens qi.

Cheng Wuji said: Longgu [龙骨, dragon bone, Mastodi Ossis Fossilia], Muli [牡蛎, oyster shell, Concha Ostreae] and Qiandan [铅丹, minium, Minium] are all effective for astringing vitality and relieving convulsion. Burn it into powder for use. It is restrained by Shigao [石膏, gypsum, Gypsum Fibrosum].

Zhen [《珍珠囊》, *Pouch of Pearls*] says: It can strengthen the large intestines by preventing prolapse.

麝 香

气温,味辛。无毒。

《本草》云:主辟恶气,杀鬼精物,疗温疟,蛊毒痫痉,去三尸虫。疗诸凶邪鬼气,中恶心腹暴痛,胀急痞满,风毒。妇人产难,堕胎。

Shexiang [麝香, musk, Moschus]

It is warm in property and pungent in taste. It is nontoxic.

Ben Cao says: It is mainly used to expel the malign qi, kill the severe pathogenic factors like monster and ghost, treat warm malaria, parastic toxin, epilepsy and convulsion, and eliminate three kinds of parasitosis. It also treats various evil pathogenic factors like ghost, the sudden pain in the heart and abdomen due to the malignity stroke, the abdominal distension and fullness, and the wind toxin. It can be used to treat the difficult delivery and abortion.

牛 黄

气平,味苦。有小毒。

《本草》云:主惊痫寒热,热盛狂痉。逐鬼除邪。疗小儿百病,诸痫热,口噤不开,大人癫狂。又堕胎。久服,令人不忘。又云:磨指甲上黄者,为真。又云:定魂魄。人参为使。得牡丹、菖蒲,利耳目。恶龙骨、龙胆、地黄,畏生漆。

Niuhuang [牛黄, bovine bezoar, Bovis Calculus]

It is mild in property, bitter in taste and slightly toxic.

Ben Cao says: It is mainly used to treat the fright epilepsy caused by cold and heat and the convulsions due to excessive heat. It expels the ghostlike pathogens and removes the evil things. It treats most of the infantile diseases, the epilepsy caused by heat, the clenched jaw, and the adult mania. It can induce abortion. The long-term taking of it may help prevent amnesia. It is also said that authentic Niuhuang [牛黄, bovine bezoar, Bovis Calculus] can dye nail yellow. Niuhuang [牛黄, bovine bezoar, Bovis Calculus] is also said to be effective in pacifying the ethereal soul and corporeal soul. Renshen [人参, ginseng, Radix Ginseng] is its assistance. When it is used together with Mudan [牡丹, moutan, Cortex Moutan Radicis] and Changpu [菖蒲, acorus, Acorus Calamus], it can improve hearing and vision. It is averse to Longgu [龙骨, dragon bone, Mastodi Ossis Fossilia], Longdan [龙胆, root of rough gentian, Radix Gentianae], Dihuang [地黄, unprocessed rehmannia root, Rehmannia glutinosa Libosch. ex Fisch. et Mey.] and restrained by Shengqi [生漆, fresh lacquer, Toxicodendri Resina Recens].

犀 角

气寒,味苦。酸、咸,微寒。无毒。

《象》云:治伤寒温疫头痛,安心神,止烦乱,明目镇惊。治中风失音,小儿麸豆,风热惊痫。镑用。

《本草》云:主百毒蛊疰,邪鬼瘴气。杀钩吻、鸩羽、蛇毒,除邪不迷惑,魇寐。疗伤寒温疫头痛、寒热,诸毒气。能治一切疮肿,破血。

《液》云:升麻代犀角说,并见升麻条下。易老疗畜血分三部:上焦畜血,犀角地黄汤;中焦畜血,桃仁承气汤;下焦畜血,抵当汤、丸,丸但缓于汤耳。三法的当,后之用者,无以复加。

Xijiao [犀角, rhinoceros horn, Rhinoceros Unicornis L.]

It is cold in property and bitter in taste. It is sour and salty, and slightly cold in nature. It is nontoxic.

Xiang [《药类法象》, *Rules for the Use of Medicinal Herbs*] says: It is used to treat the headache caused by the cold damage and the warm epidemic, calm the mind, resolve vexation, brighten eyes and relieve convulsion. It treats the aphonia due to stroke, the infantile rash, and the fright epilepsy caused by wind-heat. It is processed into flakes.

Ben Cao says: It is mainly used to treat the diseases caused by various worm toxins, eliminate the pathogenic factors like evil and ghost, and expel miasma. It can eliminate the toxin in Gouwen [钩吻, graceful jessamine herb, Herba Gelsemii Elegantis], Zhenyu (a legendary bird with toxinous feathers) and snakes. It can remove obnubilation and nightmare. It treats the headache caused by the cold damage and the warm epidemic, and removes various toxins. It is also effective to treat all kinds of obstinate sore and abscessus, and break the blood stasis.

Ye [《汤液本草》, *Materia Medica for Decoctions*] says: Shengma [升麻, large trifoliolious bugbane rhizome, Rhizoma Cimicifugae] may replace Xijiao [犀角, rhinoceros horn, Rhinoceros Unicornis L.], and the detailed information can be seen in the clause of Shengma [升麻, largetrifoliolious bugbane rhizome, Rhizoma Cimicifugae]. Yi Lao (Zhang Yuansu) treated the blood stasis by three parts: If there is blood stasis in the upper energizer, Xijiao Dihuang Decoction is recommended. If there is blood stasis in the middle energizer, Taoren Chengqi Decoction is a good choice. If there is blood stasis in the lower energizer, both Didang Decoction and Didang Pill are suggested, but the latter functions more slowly than the former. If the three methods are used properly, there is no need for modifications in later times.

阿　胶

气微温，味甘、辛。无毒。甘、辛，平。味薄，气厚，升也，阳也。

入手太阴经、足少阴经、厥阴经。

《象》云：主心腹痛内崩。补虚安胎，坚筋骨，和血脉，益气止病。炮用。

《心》云：补肺金气不足。除不足，其温补血。出东阿，得火良。

《本草》云：主心腹内崩，劳极洒洒如疟状，腰腹痛，四肢酸痛，女子下血，安胎，丈夫小腹痛，虚劳羸瘦。阴气不足，脚酸，不能久立。养肝气，益肺气。肺虚极损，咳嗽，唾脓血，非阿胶不补。仲景猪苓汤，用阿胶，滑以利水道。《活人书》四物汤加减例，妊娠下血者，加阿胶。

Ejiao [阿胶, ass hide glue, Colla Corii Asini]

It is slightly mild in property, and sweet and pungent in taste. It is nontoxic. It is sweet and pungent in taste and mild in property. It is thin in flavor and thick in property, and it pertains to yang with ascending function.

It enters the meridians of the hand-taiyin, the foot-shaoyin and jueyin.

Xiang [《药类法象》, *Rules for the Use of Medicinal Herbs*] says: It is mainly used to treat the pain in the heart and abdomen, and the uterine bleeding. It can tonify deficiency, prevent miscarriage, strengthen tendons and bones, coordinate the blood and vessels, replenish qi and precent diseases. It should be processed before use.

Xin [《用药心法》, *Gist for the Use of Medicinal Herbs*] says: It is effective to replenish the lung qi. It eliminates the deficiency and tonifies the blood. It is originated from Dong'e County, and the function of it can be better if heated.

Ben Cao says: It is mainly used to treat the pain in the heart and abdomen, the uterine bleeding, the disease due to overexertion like malaria, the pain of the waist and abdomen, the pain of the limbs, the vaginal bleeding during menstruation, prevent miscarriage, treat the abdominal pain of male, the emaciation due to vacuity taxation, the deficiency of yin qi, the pain of feet, and the inability to stand for a long time. It nourishes the liver qi and replenishes the lung qi. Ejiao [阿胶, ass hide glue, Colla Corii Asini] is a necessity to treat the deficiency and detriment of the lung, coughing, and the spitting of blood. Zhang Zhongjing put Ejiao [阿胶, ass hide glue, Colla Corii Asini] in his Zhuling Decoction in order to regulate the water passage. *Huo Ren Shu* [《活人书》, *Book to Safeguard Life*] says: If there is metrorrhagia during pregnancy, Ejiao [阿胶, ass hide glue, Colla Corii Asini] can be added into Siwu Decoction to treat that symptom.

猪 肤

气寒，味甘。

入足少阴经。

《液》云：猪皮，味甘，寒。猪，水畜也，其气先入肾。解少阴客热，是以猪肤解之，加白蜜，以润燥除烦；白粉，以益气断痢。

Zhufu [猪肤, pig skin, Suis Corium]

It is cold in property and sweet in taste.

It enters the meridian of the foot-shaoyin.

Ye [《汤液本草》, *Materia Medica for Decoctions*] says: Zhupi [猪皮, pig skin, Suis Corium] is sweet in taste and cold in nature. Being an animal that pertains to water, the qi of pig enters the kidney first. It relieves the external heat in the meridian of the foot-shaoyin. A mixture of Baimi [白蜜, honey, Mel] and Zhufu [猪肤, pig skin, Suis Corium] can moisten dryness and eliminate vexation. If Baifen [白粉, processed galenite, Galenitum Praeparatum] is added, it is good for replenishing qi and stopping diarrhea.

猪 胆 汁

气寒,味苦、咸。苦,寒。

《液》云:仲景白通汤,加此汁,与人尿咸寒,同与热剂合,去格拒之寒。又,与醋相合,内谷道中,酸苦益阴,以润燥泻便。

《本经》云:治伤寒热渴。又白猪蹄,可用;杂青色者,不可食,疗疾亦不可。

《心》云:与人尿同体,补肝而和阴引置阳,不被格拒,能入心而通脉。

Zhudanzhi [猪胆汁, pig's bile, Suis Bilis]

It is cold in property, and bitter and salty in taste.

Ye [《汤液本草》, *Materia Medica for Decoctions*] says: The Baitong Decoction of Zhang Zhongjing is added with Zhudanzhi [猪胆汁, pig's bile, Suis Bilis] and Renniao [人尿, human urine, Hominis Urina]. As both of them are salty and cold, a mixture of them with heat formula is effective to eliminate the cold and heat repulsion. When it is combined with vinegar, it is also good for promoting urination and defecation because sourness and bitterness replenish yin, which can help moisten dryness and move the bowels.

Ben Jing [《神农本草经》, *Agriculture God's Canon of Materia Medica*] says: It is used to treat the thirst caused by the cold damage. It can also be used with Baizhuti [白猪蹄, white pig's trotter, Suis Pes]. However, if the bile is variegated blue, it can neither be taken nor be used as medicinal.

Xin [《用药心法》, *Gist for the Use of Medicinal Herbs*] says: It is the same as Renniao [人尿, human urine, Hominis Urina] in nature, tonifying the liver and harmonizing yin, freeing the yin-yang repulsion, entering the heart and regulating vessels.

獭 肝

味甘,有毒。

《本草》云:主鬼疰蛊毒,却鱼鲠,止久嗽。烧灰服之。

Tagan [獭肝, otter's liver, Lutrae Iecur]

It is sweet in taste and toxic.

Ben Cao says: It is mainly used to treat the chronic infectious disease and the disease due to the noxious agents produced by various parasites, eliminate fish bones, and stop long-time cough. Burn it into ash and then take it.

豭鼠粪

治伤寒劳复。《经》言:牡鼠粪两头尖者,是。或在人家,诸物中遗者。

Jiashufen [豭鼠粪, cornus, Corni Fructus]

It treats the taxation relapse attacked by the cold damage. Jing says: It is also named Mushufen [牡鼠粪, cornus, Corni Fructus] or Liangtoujian [两头尖, cornus, Corni Fructus]. It may be found in houses or in various things deserted.

人 尿

《时习》云:疗寒热头疼,温气。童男子者,尤良。

《衍义》云:人尿,须用童男者,产后温一杯,压下败血恶物。久服,令人反虚。气血无热,尤不可多服。此亦性寒,故治热劳方中亦用也。

《日华子》云:小便,凉。止劳渴嗽,润心肺,疗血闷热狂,扑损瘀血,晕绝,及蛇犬等咬,以热尿淋患处。难产胞衣不下,即取一升,用姜、葱煎,乘热饮,即下。

Renniao [人尿, human urine, Hominis Urina]

Shi Xi [《时习》, Constant Practice] says: It is used to treat the headache caused by cold and heat, and remove the warm pathogen. The urine of virgin boy is better in quality.

Yan Yi [《本草衍义》, *Extension of the Materia Medica*] says: Renniao [人尿, human urine, Hominis Urina] should be collected from virgin boys. The vanquished blood can be purged for women by taking a cup of warm Renniao [人尿, human urine, Hominis Urina] after delivery. However, the long-term taking of it will make people weak. The people who suffer from the absence of heat in qi and blood can not take too much of it. Renniao [人尿, human urine, Hominis Urina] is cold in nature, so it is also used in the formula to treat overstrain due to heat.

Ri Hua Zi [《日华子》, *Materia Medica of Ri Hua-Zi*] says: The urine is cold in property. It stops taxation relapse and cough, nourishes the heart and lung, treats the blood stuffiness and the heat mania, regulates the static blood, and relieves dizziness. It is also effective to cure the bite by snakes or dogs through pouring the fresh urine on the affected wound. When it comes to the difficult delivery and the retention of the placenta, the patient can take 1 Sheng of urine, decoct it with ginger and scallion, and take the decoction when it is hot.

虫 部
Insect Herbs

牡 蛎

气微寒，味咸，平。无毒。

入足少阴经。

《象》云：治伤寒寒热温疟，女子带下赤白，止汗，止心痛气结，涩大小肠，治心胁痞。烧白杵细用。

《珍》云：能软积气之痞。《经》曰：咸能软坚。

《心》云：咸，平。熬，泄水气。

《本草》云：主伤寒寒热，温疟洒洒，惊恚怒气。除拘缓，鼠瘘，女子带下赤白。除留热在关节，荣卫虚热，往来不定，烦满。止汗，心痛气结。止渴，除老血。涩大小肠，止大小便。疗泄精，喉痹咳嗽，心胁下痞热。能去瘰疬，一切疮肿。入足少阴。咸为软坚之剂，以柴胡引之，故能去胁下之硬；以茶引之，能消结核；以大黄引之，能除股间肿；地黄为之使，能益精收涩，止小便，本肾经之药也。久服，强骨节，杀邪鬼延年。贝母为之使。得甘草、牛膝、远志、蛇床子，良。恶麻黄、吴茱萸、辛夷。

《药性论》云：君主之剂。治女子崩中，止血及盗汗，除风热，定痛。治温疟。又和杜仲服，止盗汗。为末蜜丸，服三十丸，令人面光白，永不值时气。又治鬼交精出，病人虚而多热，加用之，地黄、小草。

陈士良云：牡蛎捣粉，粉身，治大人小儿盗汗。和麻黄根、蛇床子、干姜为粉，粉身，去阴汗。《衍义》意同。

Muli [牡蛎, oyster shell, Concha Ostreae]

It is slightly cold in nature, salty in taste, and mild in property. It is nontoxic.

It enters the meridian of the foot-shaoyin.

Xiang [《药类法象》, *Rules for the Use of Medicinal Herbs*] says: It treats the warm malaria due to the cold damage and alternate cold and heat, cures the bloody dysentery and leukorrhagia, checks sweating, stops the heart pain and qi stagnation, astringes the intestines, removes the glomus between the heart and the ribs. Boil it to white first, then pestle it, and keep that for usage.

Zhen [《珍珠囊》, *Pounch of Pearls*] says: It can remove the lump in the abdomen due to pneumatosis. *Jing* says: It is salty in taste so it can soften hardness.

Xin [《用药心法》, *Gist for the Use of Medicinal Herbs*] says: It is salty in taste and mild in property. You can decoct it in order to discharge the retained fluid.

Ben Cao says: It is mainly used to treat the cold damage, alternate cold and heat, warm malaria, resentment and anger. It eliminates convulsions, the mouse fistula, the leukorrhagia and bloody dysentery. It removes the heat retained in the joints, the deficiency-heat in the nutrient qi and the defensive qi, the alternate attacks of chills and fever, vexation and fullness. It checks sweating, treats heart pain and qi stagnation. It relieves thirst, eliminates blood stasis, astringes the large and small intestines, controls defecation and urination, and cures the seminal emission, the cough caused by the throat impediment, and the glomus heat below the heart and the ribs. It can remove the cervical scrofula, obstinate sore and abscessus. It enters the meridian of the foot-shaoyin. The salty taste is for softening hardness. Therefore, it can remove the hardness below the ribs with Chaihu [柴胡, Chinese thorowax root, Radix Bupleuri] as its assistant drug. Assisted by tea, it can eliminate tuberculosis; assisted by Dahuang [大黄, rhubarb root and rhizome, Radix et Rhizoma Rhei], it can remove the femoral swelling; assisted by Dihuang [地黄, unprocessed rehmannia root, Rehmannia glutinosa Libosch. ex Fisch. et Mey.], it can replenish the essence, induce the astringency of intestines, and stop the uninhibited copious urine. It belongs to the medicinal herb of the kidney meridian. The long-term taking of it can strengthen joints, remove the evil pathogens, and prolong the life span. Beimu [贝母, fritillaria, Bulbus Fritillaria] is its assistance. It functions better with Gancao [甘草, liquorice root, Glycyrrhiza uralensis Fisch.], Niuxi [牛膝, twotoothed achyranthes root, Radix Achyranthis Bidentatae], Yuanzhi [远志, polygala root, Radix Polygalae] and Shechuangzi [蛇床子, fruit of common cnidium, Fructus Cnidii]. It is averse to Mahuang [麻黄, ephedra, Herba Ephedrae], Wuzhuyu [吴茱萸, evodia, Fructus Evodiae] and Xinyi [辛夷, immature flower of biond magnolia, Flos Magnoliae].

Yao Xing Lun [《药性论》, *Treatise on Medicinal Properties*] says: It is the monarch medicinal herb. It is used to treat the profuse vaginal bleeding, cease bleeding and night sweating, dispel wind-heat and pain, and cure the warm malaria. If it is taken together with Duzhong [杜仲, eucommia bark, Cortex Eucommiae], it can stop night sweating. Mix it with honey, make them into pills, take thirty pills, and it may luster the skin and protect one from the seasonal epidemic pathogens. It is also effective to treat the seminal emission due to the dreamed coitus, deficiency and the excessive heat with the help of Dihuang [地黄, unprocessed rehmannia root, Rehmannia glutinosa Libosch. ex Fisch. et Mey.] and Xiaocao [小草, polygala leave, Leafy Polygalae].

Chen Shiliang said: Pestle Muli [牡蛎, oyster shell, Concha Ostreae] into powder to treat the night sweating of adults or infants. Pestle it together with the root of Mahuang [麻黄, ephedra, Herba Ephedrae], Shechuangzi [蛇床子, fruit of common cnidium, Fructus Cnidii] and Ganjiang [干姜, dry ginger, Rhizoma Zingiberis] into powder, and they can remove the perineal sweating. *Yan Yi* [《本草衍义》, *Extension of the Materia Medica*] also records similar methods and efficacy.

文 蛤

气平,味咸。无毒。

《本草》云:主恶疮,蚀五痔,咳逆胸痹,腰痛胁急,鼠瘘,大孔出血,崩中漏下。能利水。治急疳蚀口鼻,数日尽欲死,烧灰,腊猪脂和涂之。坠痰软坚,止渴,收涩固济,蛤粉也。咸能走肾,可以胜水。文蛤尖而有紫斑。

Wenge [文蛤, meretrix clam shell, Concha Meretricis]

It is mild in nature and salty in taste. It is nontoxic.

Ben Cao says: It is mainly used to treat the malign sore, erode five kinds of hemorrhoids, and treat the cough with dyspnea, chest impediment, lumbago, mouse fistula, anal bleeding, profuse vaginal bleeding and metrostaxis. It can regulate the water passage. It treats the urgent malnutrition and the erosion of the mouth and nose that may lead to critical condition if not cured in several days. Burn Wenge [文蛤, meretrix clam shell, Concha Meretricis] into ash and apply it to the sore with the wax lard. The powder is effective to disperse phlegm, soften hardness, relieve thirst, and induce the astringency of intestines. As it is salty, it pertains to the kidney, which is helpful to restrict the water. Wenge [文蛤, meretrix clam shell, Concha Meretricis] is pointed in shape and purple colored.

虻 虫

气微寒,味苦,平。有毒。

《本草》云:主目中赤痛,眦伤泪出,瘀血血闭,寒热酸惭,无子。炒,去翅、足。

Mengchong [虻虫, tabanus, Tabanus]

It is slightly cold in nature, bitter in taste, and mild in property. It is toxic.

Ben Cao says: It is mainly used to treat the redness and pain of eyes, the injury of canthus with tearing, the amenorrhea due to blood stasis, the cold-heat disease, the severe pain and infertility. It is usually stir-fried with wings and feet removed.

水 蛭(一名蚂蟥)

气微寒,味咸、苦,平。有毒。

《本草》云:主逐恶血,瘀血月闭,破血瘕积聚,无子,利水道,堕胎。炒用,畏盐。苦走血,咸胜血,仲景抵当汤用虻虫、水蛭,咸苦以泄畜血。故《经》云:有故无殒也。虽可用之,亦不甚安。莫若四物汤加酒浸大黄各半,下之极妙。

Shuizhi [水蛭, Leech, Hirudo] (also named Mahuang)

It is slightly cold in nature, salty and bitter in taste, and mild in property. It is toxic.

Ben Cao says: It removes the malignant blood, treats the amenorrhea due to blood stasis, breaks the lump due to blood stasis, treats infertility, regulates the water passage, and induces abortion. It is usually stir-fried, and restrained by salt. The bitter taste promotes blood circulation and the salty taste removes blood stasis. Mengchong [虻虫, tabanus, Tabanus] and Shuizhi [水蛭, Leech, Hirudo] are used in Zhang Zhongjing's Didang Decoction, which is used to release the stagnated blood. Therefore, as *Jing* [《黄帝内经》, *Yellow Emperor's Canon of Medicine*] says: As long as the medicine is targeted to the cause of disease, it will not cause abortion even it is a bit toxic. Although Shuizhi [水蛭, Leech, Hirudo] may be used in that way, it is not always so safe. Soak it in liquor with the same amount of Dahuang [大黄, rhubarb root and rhizome, Radix et Rhizoma Rhei], put them into Siwu Decoction to achieve better purging efficacy.

䗪 虫

味咸,寒。有毒。

《本草》云:主心腹寒热洒洒,血积症瘕,破坚,下血闭,生子大良。仲景主治久瘕积结,有大黄䗪虫丸。

《衍义》云:乳汁不行,研一枚,水半合,滤清汁服。勿令服药人知之。

Zhechong [䗪虫, ground beetle, Corydiidae]

It is salty in taste and cold in nature. It is toxic.

Ben Cao says: It is mainly used to treat the cold-heat disease in the heart and abdomen with chilliness and shivering as well as the conglomeration due to blood stagnation, and break the obstinate amenorrhea. It is more effective in promoting conception. Zhang Zhongjing treated concretions, conglommerations, accumulations with Dahuang Zhechong Pill.

Yan Yi [《本草衍义》, *Extension of the Materia Medica*] says: If there is galactostasis, grind a Zhechong [䗪虫, ground beetle, Corydiidae], mix it with a half He of water, and then leach it to take the juice. The processing should be left unknown for the patients.

鼠 妇

气温,微寒,味酸。无毒。

《本草》云:主气癃不得小便,妇人月水闭,血瘕,痫痓寒热,利水道。仲景治久疟,大鳖甲丸中使之。以其主寒热也。

《衍义》云:鼠妇,湿生虫也。

Shufu [鼠妇, pillbug, Armadillidium]

It is warm in property, slightly cold in nature, and sour in taste. It is nontoxic.

Ben Cao says: It is used to treat the qi stranguria, dysuria, the amenorrhea with blood conglomeration, the epilepsy with suffocation and cold-heat disease, and promote the waterway. Zhang Zhongjing used Shufu [鼠妇, pillbug, Armadillidium] as the assistance of Dabiejia Pill to treat the enduring malaria, for it can treat alternate cold and heat.

Yan Yi [《本草衍义》, *Extension of the Materia Medica*] says: Shufu [鼠妇, pillbug, Armadillidium] can be found in damp places.

蜘　蛛

微寒。

《本草》云：主大人小儿癞疝。七月七日取其网，疗喜忘。仲景治杂病狐疝，偏有大小，时时上下者，蜘蛛一十四个（熬焦），桂半两。研细为散。八分匕，酒调服，日再。蜜丸亦通。

Zhizhu [蜘蛛, spider, Aranea]

It is slightly cold in nature.

Ben Cao says: It is mainly used to treat the scrotal hernia of adults and infants. On July 7th of the lunar calendar, collect the spider web and it is effective to treat amnesia. Zhang Zhongjing used it to treat hernia—a kind of miscellaneous disease, which is different in size and often goes up in the daytime and goes down to scrotum at night. He decocted 14 Zhizhu [蜘蛛, spider, Aranea] with half a Liang of Guizhi [桂枝, cassia twig, Ramulus Cinnamomi] until they were parched. Grind them into powder. Mix 8 Feng of it with liquor. Take it two times one day. You can also mix them with honey pills.

蛴　螬

微寒，微温，味咸。有毒。

《本草》云：主恶血血瘀，痹气破折，血在胁下，坚满痛，月闭，目中淫肤，青翳白膜。吐血，在胸中不去，及破骨踒折血结。金疮血塞。产后中寒，下乳汁。仲景治杂病方，大黄䗪虫丸中用之，以其主胁下坚满也。《续传信方》治喉痹，取虫汁点在喉中，下即喉开也。《时习》补入。

Qicao [蛴螬, June beetle grub, Holotrichiae Vermiculus]

It is slightly cold in nature, slightly mild in property, and salty in taste. It is toxic.

Ben Cao says: It is mainly used to treat the blood stasis and the impediment of qi due to blood stasis and the fullness and pain below the rib-side due to blood stasis, and treat amenorrhea, pterygium, blue nebula and albuginea. It also treats haematemesis, the blood retained in the chest, the blood bind caused by bone breaking, and the blockage of blood caused by incised wounds. It is effective in curing the cold stroke after delivery, and promoting lactation. Zhang Zhongjing used Dahuang Zhechong Pill to treat miscellaneous diseases, because it is effective to treat the hardness and fullness below the ribs. *Xu Chuan Xin Fang* [《续传信方》, *Subsequent to Letters of Prescription*] says its succus can be dripped in the throat to treat impediment with good effect, *Shi Xi* [《时习》, *Constant Practice*] adds an entry for it.

蜜

气平，微温，味甘。无毒。

《本草》云：主心腹邪气，诸惊痫痓。安五脏诸不足，益气补中，止痛解毒，除众病，和百药。养脾气，除心烦，饮食不下，止肠澼，饥中疼痛，口疮，明耳目。

《液》云：凡炼蜜，必须用火熬开，以纸覆经宿，纸上去蜡尽，再熬色变，不可过度，令熟入药。

Mi [蜜, honey, Mel]

It is mild in nature, slightly warm in property, and sweet in taste. It is nontoxic.

Ben Cao says: It is mainly used to treat the pathogenic factors in the heart and abdomen, epilepsy and convulsion. It tranquilizes the five zang-organs, replenishes qi and tonifies the middle energizer, relieves pain and removes toxin, eliminates various diseases, and regulates different medicinal herbs. It can be used to cultivate the spleen qi, expel vexation, remove the retention of food, stop the intestinal afflux, remove the pain due to hunger and the mouth sore, and improve hearing and vision.

Ye [《汤液本草》, *Materia Medica for Decoctions*] says: Whenever refining Mi [蜜, honey, Mel], one should decoct it to boiling, wrap it with paper and leave it for a night, and then decoct it again until the color changes, which can be used as medicine.

蜣 螂

气寒，味酸。有毒。

《本草》云：治小儿惊风瘈疭，腹胀寒热，大人癫疾狂易。手足端寒，支满奔豚。

《日华子》云：堕胎，治疰忤。和干姜，敷恶疮，出箭头。

《图经》云：心，主丁疮。

《衍义》云：大小二种。一种大者，为胡蜣螂，身黑光，腹翼下有小黄子，附母飞行，昼不出，夜方飞至人家户庭中，见灯光则来；一种小者，身黑暗，昼方飞出，夜不出。今当用胡蜣螂，以其小者，研三十枚，以水灌牛、马肠结，佳。

Qianglang [蜣螂, dung beetle, Catharsius]

It is cold in property and sour in taste. It is toxic.

Ben Cao says: It is mainly used to treat the infantile convulsion, the chronic convulsion and epilepsy, the abdominal distension and the cold-heat disease, and the psychosis and mania in adults. It treats the coldness in hands and feet, the fullness and Bentun.

Ri Hua Zi [《日华子》, *Materia Medica of Ri Hua-Zi*] says: It is used to induce abortion and cure infixation. If used together with Ganjiang [干姜, dry ginger, Rhizoma Zingiberis] and applied on the malign sore, it can help patients extract the sore arrow from the body.

Tu Jing [《图经》, *Illustrated Classics of Materia Medica*] says: It is used to treat furuncls.

Yan Yi [《本草衍义》, *Extension of the Materia Medica*] says: There are two kinds of Qianglang [蜣螂, dung beetle, Catharsius]. One type is big in size, which is called Huqianglang [胡蜣螂, dung beetle, Catharsius]. Its body shines black light with yellow dots under its abdominal wings. It is nocturnal and likely to gather around lights in household. The other type is small in size with dark body, belonging to the diurnal creature. Presently it is Huqianglang [胡蜣螂, dung beetle, Catharsius] that is used. Grind 30 Huqianglang [胡蜣螂, dung beetle, Catharsius] into powder, and mix them with water to be used as enema. They are effective to cure the intestinal accumulation of cattle and horses.

鳖 甲

气平,味咸。无毒。

《本草》云:主心腹症瘕坚积,寒热。去鼻间息肉,阴蚀痔,恶肉。疗温疟,血瘕,腰痛,小儿胁下坚。

《衍义》云:治劳瘦,除骨中热,极佳。

Biejia [鳖甲, turtle shell, Trionycis Carapax]

It is mild in nature and salty in taste. It is nontoxic.

Ben Cao says: It is mainly used to disperse the hard lump and the fixed accumulation in the heart and abdomen, and treat symptoms due to cold and heat. It is also used to eliminate the nasal polyp, vulval sore and rotten flesh. It treats the warm malaria, the lump due to blood stasis, the pain in the loins, and the hardness below the ribs of infants.

Yan Yi [《本草衍义》, *Extension of the Materia Medica*] says: It is also very effective to treat the emaciation due to fatigue, and remove the heat in bones.

蛇 蜕

《心》云:去翳膜用之,取其意也。

《日华子》云:止呕逆,小儿惊悸客忤,催生。瘰疬、白癜风,煎汁傅。入药炙用。

Shetui [蛇蜕, snake slough, Serpentis Periostracum]

Xin [《用药心法》, *Gist for the Use of Medicinal Herbs*] says: It is used to eliminate epiletogenic membrane.

Ri Hua Zi [《日华子》, *Materia Medica of Ri Hua-Zi*] says: It mainly treats vomiting and counter-flow, the palpitation with fright and epilepsy in infants, and expedites the child delivery. It treats the cervical scrofula and leucoderma by the external application. It can be used as medicine for moxibustion.

蝉 蜕

《心》云：治同蛇蜕。

《药性论》云：使。治小儿浑身壮热惊痫，兼能止渴。又云：其蜕壳，头上有一角如冠状，谓之蝉花，最佳。味甘，寒。无毒。主小儿天吊、惊痫瘈疭，夜啼，心悸。

Chantui［蝉蜕, cicada molting, Cicadae Periostracum］

Xin［《用药心法》, Gist for the Use of Medicinal Herbs］says：It is similar in effect to that of Shetui［蛇蜕, snake slough, Serpentis Periostracum］.

Yao Xing Lun［《药性论》, Treatise on Medicinal Properties］says：Chantui［蝉蜕, cicada molting, Cicadae Periostracum］serves as the assistance. It is used to treat the fever and the epilepsy of infants, and relieve thirst. It is also said that Chanhua［蝉花, cordyceps-infested cicada larva, Cordyceps cum Larva Cicadae］, looking like a corona on the head of cicada molting, is the best among Changtui［蝉蜕, cicada molting, Cicadae Periostracum］. It is sweet in taste, cold in nature and nontoxic. It is mainly used to treat the convulsion in infants, the epilepsy due to fright, spasm, the night cry and palpitation.

白 僵 蚕

味咸，平。无毒。

《本草》云：主小儿惊痫夜啼，去三虫。灭黑黚，令人面色好。男子阴疡病，女子崩中赤白，产后余痛。灭诸疮瘢痕。生颖川平泽，四月取自死者，勿令中湿。湿中有毒，不可用。

Baijiangcan［白僵蚕, silkworm larva, Larva Bombycis］

It is salty in taste, mild in property and nontoxic.

Ben Cao says：It is mainly used to treat the infant epilepsy and the night crying, and remove three kinds of parasites. It reduces the black spots and lusters the complexion. It is effective in treating the genital ulcer in men, the metrorrhagia and leukorrhagia in women, and the pain after delivery. It removes all sorts of sore scars. It grows in lakes and pools. In April, collect the naturally dead silkworm body and keep dry. The wet one is toxic, so it is forbidden to use.

斑 蝥

味辛,寒。有毒。

《本草》云:主寒热,鬼疰蛊毒,鼠瘘,疥癣,恶疮疽蚀,死肌。破石癃血积,伤人肌,堕胎。畏巴豆。

Banmao [斑蝥, mylabris, Mylabris]

It is pungent in taste, cold in nature and toxic.

Ben Cao says: It is mainly used to treat alternate cold and heat, tuberculosis and parasitic diseases, mouse fistula, scabies, obstinate sores, and muscle necrosis. It breaks the retention of urine and blood stasis. It may damage muscles and induce abortion. It is restrained by Badou [巴豆, Croton Fruit, Fructus Crotonis].

乌 蛇

无毒。

《本草》云:主诸风瘙瘾疹,疥癣,皮肤不仁,顽痹诸风。用之炙,入丸散,浸酒,合膏。背有三棱,色黑如漆,性善,不噬物。江东有黑梢蛇,能缠物至死,亦是其类。生商洛山。

Wushe [乌蛇, black-striped snake, Zaocys]

It is nontoxic.

Ben Cao says: It is mainly used to treat the itching dormant papules caused by various wind diseases, scabies, numbness in the skin, and the obstinate impediment. It can be used by moxibustion, mixed into pills, being soaked in liquor, or made into paste. Wushe [乌蛇, black-striped snake, Zaocys], whose body is as black as paint and covered with three burred tubers on the back, is mild and does not devour anything. Heishaoshe [黑梢蛇, black-tail snake, Zaocys], living at the east area of the Yangtze River and being the same type, can twine around creatures and cause them to die. It grows in Shangluo Mountains.

五灵脂

味甘,温。无毒。
《本草》云:主疗心腹冷气,小儿五疳,辟疫,治肠风,通利气脉,女子月闭。出北地,此是寒号虫粪也。

Wulingzhi [五灵脂, squirrel's droppings, Trogopteri Faeces]

It is sweet in taste and mild in property. It is nontoxic.

Ben Cao says: It is mainly used to treat the cold qi in the heart and abdomen, five kinds of infantile malnutrition, prevent invasion of pestilence, remove the intestinal wind, promote the circulation of blood and the flow of qi, and regulate amenorrhea. If found in the north of China, it is called Hanhaochong Fen [寒号虫粪, squirrel's droppings, Trogopteri Faeces].

绯 帛

《液》云:主恶疮丁肿,毒肿,诸疮有根者。作膏:用帛如手大,取露蜂房、弯头棘刺、烂草节二寸许、乱发。烧末,作膏。主丁疮肿。又主小儿初生脐未落时,肿痛、水出,烧,为末,细研,敷之。又,五色帛主盗汗,拭干讫,弃五道头。仲景治坠马,及一切筋骨损方中用。

Feibo [绯帛, red silk, Rubei Serica]

Ye [《汤液本草》, *Materia Medica for Decoctions*] says: It is mainly used to treat the swelling due to malign sore, the toxin swelling, and various sores with root inside the body. Make it into paste by using a piece of silk as big as a palm. Prepare some Lufengfang [露蜂房, honeycomb of paper wasps, Nidus Polistis Mandarini], Ciji [棘刺, spiny jujube, Ziziphi Spinosi Flos], about 2 Cun of rotten grass with nodes, and tousle. Burn them to ash and make them into paste. It is mainly used to treat the obstinate sore and abscessus. It is also effective in treating the infantile swelling and pain, and the abscess with pus caused by the retention of umbilical cord. Burn Feibo [绯帛, red silk, Rubei Serica], grind it, and then apply it on the sore. The colorful silk is used to treat night sweats, dry the sweat and drop it on the crossroads. Zhang Zhongjing used it to treat the diseases due to falling from the horse, and all kinds of damages of tendons and bones.